MINIMALLY INVASIVE THORACIC SURGERY

PRINCIPLES AND PRACTICE OF THORACOSCOPIC TECHNIQUE

MINIMALLY INVASIVE THORACIC SURGERY

PRINCIPLES AND PRACTICE OF THORACOSCOPIC TECHNIQUE

Edited by

MARCO SCARCI MD FRCS(Eng) FCCP
Consultant Thoracic Surgeon
University College London Hospital
London, UK

PIERGIORGIO SOLLI MD PhD
Director of Thoracic Surgery
Maggiore 'Carlo Alberto Pizzardi' Hospital
Bellaria 'Carlo Alberto Pizzardi' Hospital
Bologna, Italy

ALAN DL SIHOE MBBChir MA(Cantab) FRCSEd(CTh) FCSHK FHKAM FCCP
Clinical Associate Professor
Department of Surgery
Li Ka Shing Faculty of Medicine
The University of Hong Kong
Hong Kong
Chief of Thoracic Surgery
The University of Hong Kong Shenzhen Hospital
Shenzhen, China

JP medical publishers

London • New Delhi • Panama City

Published by JP Medical Ltd, 83 Victoria Street, London, SW1H 0HW, UK
Tel: +44 (0)20 3170 8910 Fax: +44 (0)20 3008 6180
Email: info@jpmedpub.com Web: www.jpmedpub.com

ISBN: 978-1-909836-40-2

British Library Cataloguing in Publication Data
A catalogue record for this book is available from the British Library

Library of Congress Cataloging in Publication Data
A catalog record for this book is available from the Library of Congress

Publisher: Richard Furn
Development Editor: Gavin Smith
Editorial Assistant: Katie Pattullo
Design: Designers Collective Ltd

Preface

Minimally Invasive Thoracic Surgery is intended for practicing thoracic and cardiothoracic surgeons who are new to the world of advanced video-assisted thoracic surgery. Experienced surgeons will also find a wealth of information and tips to improve their procedures.

The book is written by leaders in the field, with proven experience in minimally invasive techniques. We have aimed to deliver a concise yet comprehensive guide on how to treat a wide spectrum of conditions using the thoracoscopic approach.

Minimally Invasive Thoracic Surgery covers a wide range of minimally invasive procedural techniques with detailed explanations of how the reader can reproduce them. Chapters 1–5 outline the general principles of minimally invasive thoracic surgery: history, rationale, anesthetic techniques and, in an era of the multi-disciplinary team approach, how to set up a surgical program. Chapters 6–13 discuss all aspects of lung resections, from wedge resections to complex resections (pneumonectomies, en-bloc chest wall resections). Later chapters cover a number of benign conditions that can be successfully treated using video-assisted thoracic surgery (VATS), with two chapters on the more recent role of robotic surgery, now emerging as a standard technique performed by most thoracic surgeons. The last two chapters are dedicated to endobronchial ultrasonography (EBUS) and navigational bronchoscopy which, even if not firmly in the surgical arena, are still relevant to many thoracic surgeons.

We hope *Minimally Invasive Thoracic Surgery* will help the reader consolidate his or her understanding of clinical concepts and technical procedures, and provide an overview of the latest best practice perioperative care in minimally invasive thoracic surgery.

Marco Scarci
Piergiorgio Solli
Alan DL Sihoe
August 2017

Dedications

To my mother and father: vobis pagina nostra dedicatur. MS

To my wife Manuela and my daughters Aurora and Sabrina, who have always understood and supported the rather chaotic life I lead. PS

I would like to dedicate this work to Kok Keng and Sun Ming Sihoe – the best father and mother in the world. As the Chinese saying goes: 'A doctor has the heart of a parent'; my parents showed me what caring with a parental heart truly means. **AS**

Contents

Contributors

Thirugnanam Agasthian MD
Senior Consultant
Department of Cardiothoracic and Vascular Surgery
National University Hospital
Singapore

Vittorio April MD
Resident Thoracic Surgeon
Multidisciplinary Robotic Center
University of Pisa
Pisa
Italy

Benedetta Bedetti MD
Department of Thoracic Surgery
Malteser Hospital
Bonn
Germany

Luca Bertolaccini MD PhD FCCP
Resident Thoracic Surgeon
Department of Thoracic Surgery
AUSL Romagna Teaching Hospital
Ravenna
Italy

Nicholas R Carroll MA FRCP FRCR
Consultant Radiologist
Department of Radiology
Addenbrooke's Hospital
Cambridge
UK

Ilenia Cavaliere MD
Thoracic Surgeon
Division of Thoracic Surgery
University of Pisa
Pisa
Italy

Robert J Cerfolio MD MBA FACS FCCP
Professor of Thoracic Surgery
UAB Hospital
Pelham, AL
USA

Sumit Chatterji MA MB BChir FRCP (Lond)
Consultant in Respiratory Medicine
Department of Interventional Pulmonology
Pulmonary Institute
Chaim Sheba Medical Center
Tel Hashomer
Israel

Liu Chengwu MD PhD
Attending Surgeon of Thoracic Surgery
Department of Thoracic Surgery
West China Hospital of Sichuan University
Chengdu
China

Joyce Chew MBChB MRCP (UK)
Respiratory Specialist Registrar
Department of Respiratory Medicine
Addenbrooke's Hospital
Cambridge
UK

Simon Chow MBChB (Hons) MRCSEd
Senior Resident of Cardiothoracic Surgery
Department of Surgery
Division of Cardiothoracic Surgery
Prince of Wales Hospital
Hong Kong
China

Miguel Congregado MD PhD
Professor of Surgery
Department of Thoracic Surgery
Virgen Macarena University Hospital
University of Seville
Seville
Spain

John P Costello MD
General Surgery Resident
Department of Surgery
MedStar Georgetown University Hospital
Washington DC
USA

Donna Cummins MRCPUK MR
Specialist Registrar
Addenbrooke's Hospital
Cambridge
UK

Thomas A D'Amico MD
Gary Hock Endowed Professor of Surgery
Division of Thoracic Surgery
Duke Cancer Institute
Durham, NC
USA

Frederico Davini MD
Thoracic Surgeon
Division of Thoracic Surgery
University of Pisa
Pisa
Italy

Todd L Demmy MD FACS
Professor of Oncology and Surgery
Department of Thoracic Surgery
Roswell Park Cancer Institute
Jacobs School of Medicine and Biomedical Sciences
Buffalo, NY
USA

Joel Dunning PhD
Consultant Thoracic Surgeon
Department of Thoracic Surgery
James Cook University Hospital
Middlesbrough
UK

Tom Dymond BSc
Respiratory Research Practitioner
Cambridge University Hospitals NHS Foundation Trust
Cambridge
UK

Robert S George PhD FRCS-CTh
Consultant Thoracic Surgeon
University College London Hospitals
London
UK

Diego Gonzalez-Rivas MD FECTS
Thoracic Surgeon
Department of Thoracic Surgery
Coruña University Hospital
Coruña
Spain

Mark W Hennon MD, FACS
Assistant Professor of Oncology and Surgery
Department of Thoracic Surgery
Roswell Park Cancer Institute
Jacobs School of Medicine and Biomedical Sciences
Buffalo, NY
USA

Luis A Hernández-Arenas MD FEBTS PhD
Thoracic Surgery Consultant
Department of Thoracic Surgery
Birmingham Heartlands Hospital
Birmingham
UK

Jürgen Herre MD PhD
Consultant Interventional Pulmonologist
Department of Respiratory Medicine
Addenbrooke's Hospital
Cambridge
UK

Joanne F Irons MBChB MRCP FRCA PGDipCU
Consultant Cardiothoracic Anaesthetist
Papworth Hospital
Cambridge
UK

Nur Aziah Ismail MBChB (Leic) MRCS (Lon)
Senior Registrar Cardiothoracic Surgery
Department of Cardiothoracic Surgery
Institute Jantung Negara
Kuala Lumpur
Malaysia

Sanghoon Jheon MD PhD
President of Seoul National University Bundang Hospital
Department of Thoracic and Cardiovascular Surgery
Seoul National University Bundang Hospital
Gyeongg-doi
Korea

Sandeep Khandhar MD
Medical Director, Thoracic Surgery
Inova Fairfax Medical Center
Inova Heart and Vascular Center
Falls Church, VA
USA

Arthur Kostron MD
Resident in Orthopedic and Trauma Surgery
Department of Pediatric, Orthopedic and
Trauma Surgery
HELIOS Klinikum Emil von Behring
Berlin
Germany

Kwhanmien Kim MD PhD
Professor and Chairman of Thoracic and Cardiovascular Surgery
Department of Thoracic and Cardiovascular Surgery
Seoul National University, Bundang Hospital
Seoul National University, College of Medicine
Seoul
Korea

Eric Lim MB ChB MD MSc FRCS(C-Th)
Consultant Thoracic Surgeon
Imperial College and The Academic Division of Thoracic Surgery
The Royal Brompton Hospital
London
UK

Liu Lunxu MD PhD FRCS
Professor of Thoracic Surgery
Department of Thoracic Surgery,
West China Hospital of Sichuan University
Chengdu
China

Ravi Mahadeva MBBS MA MD FRCP
Consultant Respiratory Physician/Associate Lecturer
Addenbrooke's Hospital
Associate Lecturer
University of Cambridge
Cambridge NIHR Biomedical Research Centre
Cambridge
UK

Amit K Mahajan MD FCCP DAABIP
Medical Director
Interventional Pulmonology
Inova Fairfax Medical Center
Inova Heart and Vascular Center
Falls Church, VA
USA

M Blair Marshall MD
Chief
Division of Thoracic Surgery
Department of Surgery
MedStar Georgetown University Hospital
Washington, DC
USA

Puja R Mehta MB BChir MA MRCP(UK)
Academic Clinical Fellow
Department of Thoracic Oncology
Papworth Hospital
Cambridge
UK

Franca Melfi MD
Thoracic Surgeon
Division of Thoracic Surgery
University of Pisa
Pisa
Italy

Pankaj Kumar Mishra MS MCh MRCS FRCS (CTh)
Consultant Cardiothoracic Surgeon
Lancashire Cardiac Centre
Blackpool Victoria Hospital
Blackpool
UK

Harish Mithiran MBBS MRCSEd FRCSEd(CTh) FAMS
Consultant Thoracic Surgeon
Department of Cardiac, Thoracic and Vascular Surgery
National University Hospital
Singapore

James Moore MB ChB FANZCA FCICM
Consultant in Cardiothoracic Anaesthesia and Intensive Care Medicine
Wellington Hospital
Wellington
New Zealand

Alfredo Mussi MD
Professor of Thoracic Surgery
Division of Thoracic Surgery
University of Pisa
Pisa
Italy

Calvin SH Ng BSc(Hons) MBBS(Hons) MD(Res)(Lond) FRCSEd(CTh) FCCP
Associate Professor of Thoracic Surgery
Department of Surgery
Division of Cardiothoracic Surgery
Prince of Wales Hospital
Hong Kong
China

Alessandro Pardolesi MD
Consultant Thoracic Surgeon
Department of Thoracic Surgery
AUSL Romagna Teaching Hospital
Forli
Italy

Cecilia Pompili MD
Thoracic Surgeon
Department of Thoracic Surgery
Leeds Institute of Cancer and Pathology -University of Leeds
Leeds
UK

David N Ranney MD
General Surgery Resident
Department of Surgery
Division of Cardiovascular and Thoracic Surgery
Duke University
Durham, NC
USA

Roberta Ricciardi MD
Neurologist
Neurologic Unit
University of Pisa
Pisa
Italy

Robert C Rintoul MB ChB PhD FRCP
Consultant in Respiratory Medicine
Department of Thoracic Oncology
Papworth Hospital
Cambridge
UK

Gaetano Rocco MD FRCSEd FEBTS
Division Chief of Thoracic Surgery
Department of Thoracic and Medical Oncology
Pascale National Cancer Institute
Naples
Italy

Michele Salati MD
Staff Thoracic Surgeon
Riuniti Hospital
Ancona
Italy

Marco Scarci MD FRCS(Eng) FCCP
Consultant Thoracic Surgeon
University College London Hospital
London
UK

Alan DL Sihoe MBBChir MA(Cantab) FRCSEd(CTh) FCSHK FHKAM FCCP
Clinical Associate Professor
Department of Surgery
Li Ka Shing Faculty of Medicine
The University of Hong Kong
Hong Kong
Chief of Thoracic Surgery
The University of Hong Kong Shenzhen Hospital
Shenzhen
China

Pasupathy Sivasothy PhD FRCP
Consultant Respiratory Physician
Addenbrooke's Hospital
Cambridge
UK

Peter Smit MD
General Surgery Resident
Department of Surgery
Jacobs School of Medicine and Biomedical Sciences
Buffalo, NY
USA

Piergiorgio Solli MD PhD
Director of Thoracic Surgery
Maggiore 'Carlo Alberto Pizzardi' Hospital
Bellaria 'Carlo Alberto Pizzardi' Hospital
Bologna
Italy

John Kit Chung Tam MD MSc MEd FRCSC
Head of Thoracic Surgery and Senior Consultant
Associate Professor of Surgery
Department of Surgery
National University of Singapore
Singapore

Carlos Velasco MD
Cardiac Surgeon
Department of Cardiac Surgery,
Coruña University Hospital
Coruña
Spain

Benjamin Wei MD
Assistant Professor of Surgery
Division of Cardiothoracic Surgery
University of Alabama Birmingham, AL
USA

Hanghang Wang MD PhD
General Surgery Resident
Department of Surgery
Division of Cardiovascular and Thoracic Surgery
Duke University Medical Center
Durham, NC
USA

Yang Yang MD
Associate Professor of Thoracic Surgery
Department of Thoracic Surgery
Shanghai Pulmonary Hospital
Tongji University
Shanghai
China

Eunjue Yi MD
Clinical Assistant Professor of Thoracic and Cardiovascular Surgery
Department of Thoracic and Cardiovascular Surgery
Korea University Anam Hospital
Seoul
Korea

Carmelina C Zirafa MD
Thoracic Surgeon
Division of Thoracic Surgery
University of Pisa
Pisa
Italy

Chapter 1 The rationale for minimally invasive thoracic surgery

Arthur Kostron, Eric Lim

INTRODUCTION

Surgery as a speciality has originated from a spirit of innovation and improvement, an innate driving force within us that strives to better outcomes and lower morbidity. What we consider to be standard practice today would have started its journey from impossible, advocated by 'irresponsible rogue surgeons' to development, refinement and acceptance. Along the way, some procedures will be proven not to be of any benefit (e.g. no improved survival with extrapleural pneumonectomy for mesothelioma), others have demonstrable improvement in outcomes (e.g. pleurodesis to reduce recurrent pneumothoraces) but most will be accepted as standard practice without question (e.g. surgery for early stage lung cancer).

One of the main reasons surgeons and patients seek minimally invasive options for procedures that can otherwise be done safely using conventional open surgery is the allure that the same benefit can be achieved with less 'trauma' resulting in reduced pain, quicker recovery and better cosmetic appearance.

DEFINING MINIMALLY INVASIVE SURGERY

Minimally invasive surgery usually refers to a procedure undertaken through a smaller skin incision(s). Often this involves the use of specialised (thoracoscopic) cameras and equipment designed to facilitate operating within the body whilst taking up as little space as possible.

While most of us are caught up in the allure of 'minimal invasion', we often fail to realise if the operation is to be equally effective, the procedure performed is the same and therefore the degree of 'invasion' is comparable (apart from that saved by incision length).

There are other benefits apart from incision length alone. Rib spreading is widely thought to contribute to post-operative intercostal nerve pain and therefore no rib spreading is an accepted definition for what constitutes a 'minimally invasive' (or VATS) lobectomy. Additional distinguishing factors include looking solely at the television screen and not into the wound whilst operating. These definitions may have originated from requirements of clinical trials[1] but are often used to segregate surgeons who claim to be undertaking a minimally invasive procedure simply by shortening the length of the usual incision for 'open' surgery.

Less consideration has been given to determine if any of the strict definitions improves patient outcome by defining a procedure using a smaller access. For example, would an open operation undertaken without rib spreading (as used in countries such as Japan) though a short incision yield similar benefits in terms of better pain control and quicker recovery?

EVIDENCE FOR MINIMALLY INVASIVE THORACIC SURGERY

There are several randomized and non-randomized trials comparing video-assisted thoracic surgery (VATS) to conventional open resection of lung cancer summarized in a systematic review and meta-analysis was performed.[2] 2641 patients from 2 randomized and 19 non-randomized trials were included and postoperative outcomes such as prolonged air leak, arrhythmia, pneumonia and surgical mortality were found to be comparable between the groups. Oncological results seem to be equal for local recurrence; however, lower systemic recurrence rates and a reduced 5-year mortality were reported. The reason might be selection bias, on the other hand it has been suggested that due to a better physical performance status more patients were eligible to complete adjuvant therapy;[3] however, a recent retrospective study comparing both modalities in patients with clinical stage I lung cancer and unsuspected lymph node metastasis found no difference in the application of adjuvant chemotherapy or number of patients completing all cycles.[4]

A meta-analysis of 7 retrospective studies suggested that VATS should be the preferred technique for lung resection in patients with limited pulmonary function as VATS was associated with significantly reducing the overall pulmonary complications, mainly the incidence of pneumonia and thus leading to a shorter stay in intensive care and overall length of stay[5] with similar benefits compared to those with normal pulmonary function.[6]

Important patient related outcomes, like postoperative pain and affection on the health-related quality of life (HRQOL) unfortunately are seldom addressed in studies and therefore conclusive data on these relevant issues is missing. HRQOL has just been reported in two trials comparing the two modalities for the resection of lung cancer; these have lately been summarized by a systematic review[7] that concluded that VATS may have a better HRQOL compared to thoracotomy; however, they admitted a high risk of selection bias.

Literature is scarce for the comparison of VATS to open thoracotomy in other indications. A systematic review of pulmonary metastasectomy consisting of 7 controlled, non-randomized trials comparing VATS to open resection concluded that the current lack of high quality data makes it impossible to favour one of the two approaches.[8]

For empyema surgery, one relatively large retrospective study comparing 289 patients undergoing VATS with 94 patients after open decortication and it was suggested, that VATS had less operating time, postoperative air leak, atelectasis, need for re-intubation, ventilator dependency, transfusion, sepsis, hospitalisation, and 30-day mortality; however, the groups were not matched well and a clear selection bias was present.[9]

For the treatment of pneumothorax, open treatment still seems to have the lowest recurrence rate (1% vs 4%).[10] However, VATS is widely recommended,[11] due to better overall tolerability, reduced length of hospitalisation, fewer analgetic requirements and perhaps less peri-operative pulmonary dysfunction.[12]

For lung volume reduction surgery (LVRS) in end-stage emphysema, the National Emphysema Treatment Trial, the largest randomized controlled trial in this field, allowed both, VATS and median sternotomy, and of the 580 patients randomly assigned to surgical treatment, 30% underwent LVRS through VATS.[13] A subgroup analysis comparing VATS to median sternotomy showed comparable complication rates, equal surgical mortality and equal functional status at 12 and 24 months; however, patients undergoing VATS had a shorter time of hospitalisation, lower cost of operation, better independent living by 30 days after surgery (81% versus 71%) and less overall cost in the 6 months after surgery.[14] Therefore, VATS has been suggested to be the preferred approach for LVRS.[15]

FUTURE OF MINIMALLY INVASIVE SURGERY

Within the standard three port VATS there continues to be modifications for the procedure. Some enthusiasts argue that it is rib spreading rather than the number of ports used and so are less concerned by the number of incisions;[16] others continue to develop less incisions and undertake lung resections through a single incision.[17] In parallel, advances continue to be made in robotic surgery.[18]

Currently, we function in an environment that lacks high quality comparative data from clinical trials, and in this circumstance, the patient should be given the opportunity to decide on the benefits and risks of traditional versus minimally invasive surgery. Whilst waiting for the generation of evidence, our current practice may or may not be influenced and in return is a function of the different capabilities of individual surgeons and patient preference for the 'right' procedure.

Ultimately, the future use and technique of minimally invasive surgery will depend on generating evidence from clinical trials. Otherwise the movement will continue to be introduced in an ad hoc and patchy manner, limited to centres and surgeons with an interest in this field. Robust data needs to be generated to support claims of improvement in patient care or acceptability and balanced against potential risks and cost. Until cost-effectiveness data is available, it would be more difficult to secure fair reimbursement and national procedure tariffs.

REFERENCES

1. Swanson SJ, Herndon JE 2nd, D'Amico TA, et al. Video-assisted thoracic surgery lobectomy: report of CALGB 39802 – a prospective, multi-institution feasibility study. J Clin Oncol 2007; 25:4993–4997.
2. Yan TD, Black D, Bannon PG, McCaughan BC. Systematic review and meta-analysis of randomized and nonrandomized trials on safety and efficacy of video-assisted thoracic surgery lobectomy for early-stage non-small-cell lung cancer. J Clin Oncol 2009; 27:2553–2562.
3. Teh E, Abah U, Church D, et al. What is the extent of the advantage of video-assisted thoracoscopic surgical resection over thoracotomy in terms of delivery of adjuvant chemotherapy following non-small-cell lung cancer resection? Interac Cardiovasc Thorac Surg 2014; 19:656–660.
4. Licht P, Schytte T, Jakobsen E. Adjuvant chemotherapy compliance is not superior after thoracoscopic lobectomy. AnnThorac Surg 2014; 98:411–416.
5. Oparka J, Yan T, Dunning J. Does video-assisted thoracic surgery provide a safe alternative to conventional techniques in patients with limited pulmonary function who are otherwise suitable for lung resection? Interactive Cardiovasc Thorac Surg 201317:159–162.
6. Ceppa DP, Kosinski AS, Berry MF, et al. Thoracoscopic lobectomy has increasing benefit in patients with poor pulmonary function: a society of thoracic surgeon's database analysis. Ann Surg 2012; 256:487–493.
7. Gazala S, Pelletier JS, Storie D, et al. A systematic review and meta-analysis to assess patient-reported outcomes after lung cancer surgery. Scientific World Journal 2013; 2013:789625.
8. Greenwood A, West D. Is a thoracotomy rather than thoracoscopic resection associated with improved survival after pulmonary metastasectomy? Interac Cardiovas Thorac Surg 2013; 17:720–724.
9. Tong BC, Hanna J, Toloza EM, et al. Outcomes of video-assisted thoracoscopic decortication. Ann Thorac Surg 2010; 89:220–225.
10. Barker A, Maratos EC, Edmonds L, Lim E. Recurrence rates of video-assisted thoracoscopic versus open surgery in the prevention of recurrent pneumothoraces: a systematic review of randomised and non-randomised trials. Lancet 2007; 370:329–335.
11. MacDuff A, Arnold A, Harvey J. Management of spontaneous pneumothorax: British Thoracic Society pleural disease guideline 2010. Thorax 2010; 65:ii18–31.
12. Vohra HA, Adamson L, Weeden DF. Does video-assisted thoracoscopic pleurectomy result in better outcomes than open pleurectomy for primary spontaneous pneumothorax? Interact Cardiovasc Thorac Surg 2008; 7:673–677.
13. Fishman A, Martinz F, Naunheim K, et al. A randomized trail comparing lung volume reduction surgery with medical therapy for severe emphysema. N Engl J Med 2003; 348:2059–2073.
14. McKenna R, Benditt J, DeCamp M, et al. Safety and efficacy of median sternotomy versus video-assisted thoracic surgery for lung volume reduction surgery. J Thorac Cardiovasc Surg 2004; 127:1350–1360.
15. Huang W, Wand WR, Deng B, et al. Several clinical interests regarding lung volume reduction surgery for sever emphysema: meta-analysis and systematic review of randomized controlled trials. J Cardiothorac Surg 2011; 6:148–156.
16. McKenna RJ Jr, Houck W, Fuller CB. Video-assisted thoracic surgery lobectomy: experience with 1,100 cases. Ann Thorac Surg 2006; 81:421–425.
17. Gonzalez-Rivas D, Fieira E, Delgado M, et al. Uniportal video-assisted thoracoscopic sleeve lobectomy and other complex resections. J Thorac Dis 2014; 6:S674–681.
18. Nasir BS, Bryant AS, Minnich DJ, Wei B, Cerfolio RJ. Performing robotic lobectomy and segmentectomy: cost, profitability, and outcomes. Ann Thorac Surg 2014; 98:203–208.

FURTHER READING

Handy JR. Minimally invasive lung surgery and postoperative quality of life. Thorac Surg Clin 2012; 22:487–495.

Moisiuc FV, Colt HG. Thoracoscopy: origins revisited. Respiration 2007; 74:344–355.

Chapter 2 The history and evolution of minimally invasive thoracic surgery

Alan DL Sihoe, Robert S George

INTRODUCTION

To operate in the human chest, a surgeon must place three things into it: a right hand, left hand and a pair of eyes to look inside.[1,2] However, the human intercostal space is too narrow to allow these through, and for a major thoracic operation, one must forcibly retract the ribs for up to several hours. This causes significant tissue trauma, pain and consequent perioperative morbidity. Video-assisted thoracic surgery (VATS) has without doubt been the most significant advance in thoracic surgery over the past half century.[1-3] With VATS, surgical instruments are used to replace the right and left hands, and a video-thoracoscope is used to replace direct vision through the wound. All of this is done using three small ports without rib-spreading. VATS therefore allows the same complex operations to be performed using the same three things put into the chest, but it does so without forcible rib-spreading, resulting in improved postoperative outcomes which have been well documented in literature.[1-3]

It has become a cliché to say that minimally invasive thoracic surgery (MITS) began when – in the late 19th century – the Swedish physician Hans Christian Jacobaeus first coupled a modified cystoscope with a simple candle as a light source to examine the pleural cavity under local anesthesia.[4,5] Jacobaeus used this technique of direct thoracoscopy technique to lyse adhesions in order to collapse the lungs as this was the prevailing treatment for tuberculosis at the time. However, modern MITS was only truly born when the surgical rod lens was coupled with solid state video systems and micro-cameras in the early 1990s. This allowed a panoramic view of the hemithorax, instead of the previous tunnel-like vision with Jacobean direct thoracoscopy. At the same time, the development of new endoscopic instruments (developed initially for laparoscopic surgery) allowed the performance of a wide spectrum of diagnostic and therapeutic procedures. Amongst the most important of these was the endoscopic mechanical stapler. This combination of video technology with endoscopic instruments ushered in the era of VATS.[6,7]

The first major meeting on VATS was held in January 1992 in San Antonio, Texas in conjunction with the Society of Thoracic Surgeons meeting, representing the baptism of a newborn technique.[8] VATS has now become established and developed in many centers in North America, Asia, Europe, Australia and South America.[3,9] Its applications as a diagnostic approach and as a therapeutic modality for benign thoracic diseases have since become firmly incorporated into mainstream thoracic surgery. Throughout the 1990s, VATS gradually became the approach of choice for thoracic procedures such as diagnosis of solitary lung nodules, diffuse pulmonary infiltrates and pleural disease; and simpler therapeutic procedures, for example, pneumothorax and excisions of mediastinal lesions.[10]

THE RISE AND FALL OF EARLY VATS LOBECTOMY

The posterolateral thoracotomy is the quintessential mode of surgical access for major surgery in the chest – including lobectomy for lung cancer.[5] Unfortunately, although the thoracotomy generally provides good surgical exposure, it is also one of the most painful incisions in surgery. It has been reported that 5–80% of patients experience significant levels of pain at 2 months or more after a standard thoracotomy.[11,12] This pain can persist in up to 30% of patients at 4–5 years after surgery. It has been suggested that the pain can result from a combination of the skin incision, muscle splitting, rib fracturing, costo-chondral dislocation, pleural injury, diathermy burning, and neuroma formation at the wound. Above all, many surgeons believe that the single most important element is the forcible spreading of the ribs during thoracotomy. It is unsurprising that surgeons soon turned to the use of VATS not just for simpler procedures, but for major lung resection surgery. The rationale was that by using video technology to minimize the surgical access required, most of these pain-causing elements can be reduced, particularly rib-spreading.[1-3]

One of the first to report a large series of lobectomies for lung cancer using the VATS approach was Dr Ralph Lewis.[6,13] The technique his group described used 4 ports and explicitly called for the avoidance of rib-spreading. With this technique, the mediastinal lymph nodes are first excised, the fissures divided with endoscopic staplers, and the hilar structures skeletalized. The hilar structures (pulmonary artery, pulmonary vein and lobar bronchus) are then simultaneously stapled in their normal anatomic configuration using two firings of a stapler device. In his first 200 consecutive patients using this technique, Lewis claimed impressively short average operating times of 79.5 minutes and an average length of hospital stay of 3.07 days.[14] There was no mortality, and minor complications occurred in 13% of patients. After a mean follow-up of 34 months, recurrence-free survival was claimed in 141 out of 171 patients with primary lung cancers (even though less than half had stage I disease), and there were 7 deaths unrelated to neoplasm. However, despite such promising results, Lewis' simultaneous stapling technique met with considerable skepticism from many in the thoracic surgery community.[15] Although Lewis and colleagues made a very sound argument that simultaneous stapling was a safe and even historically-proven technique for lobectomy, their approach failed to become established into the mainstream in the face of overwhelming conservatism. Nonetheless, Lewis' simultaneous stapling technique has never been discredited on clinical evidence. It may still play a part in the surgeon's armamentarium for selected patients with benign disease, and when an expeditious lobectomy is required.

Since then, the individual isolation-ligation strategy took over as the mainstream for VATS lobectomy. The conventional sequence of conventional open thoracotomy was adopted: with dissection of the pulmonary vessels via the interlobar fissure first, then completing the fissures, and finally dividing the bronchus.[7,9,16] The advantage of this strategy was that it was immediately familiar for conventional thoracic surgeons. To closely replicate the ergonomics and instrumentation of the open approach (where the surgeon typically stands posterior to the laterally-turned patient) Dr William Walker's group in Edinburgh famously advocated the 'posterior' approach to VATS lobectomy, where the hilar structures are isolated and divided from a posterior-to-anterior direction.[17,18] However, it became evident that simply copying the open thoracotomy approach (hilum, then fissure then bronchus) was not necessarily ideal when performing VATS.[19] In particular, the rigidity of the ribs, the narrowness of the intercostals spaces, and the lack of angulation of the early staplers meant that stapler insertion around relatively fixed positions of the hilar vessels was often difficult.

It was gradually appreciated that the slightly different views and access presented during VATS may require slightly different surgical strategies compared to open thoracotomy. With VATS, where the camera is usually placed at a lower level than the working port(s), and the latter working or 'utility' port is often placed more anteriorly to take advantage of the wider intercostal space at the front of the chest.[3] Hence, working in an anterior-to-posterior direction, and inferior-to-superior direction, tackling the vein, the artery then the bronchus, seemed to work better. The pulmonary vein is usually easiest to approach first with the video-thoracoscope, with little overlying tissue obscuring it. Once divided, the pulmonary artery branches are usually easy to expose without having to dissect laboriously through often fused interlobar fissures. Dr Robert McKenna was among the first to advocate such a strategy,[20,21] and the gradual acceptance of this approach as the mainstream meant that most VATS surgeons nowadays tend to stand anterior to the patient when performing a lobectomy, instead of behind the patient as during a lobectomy via posterolateral thoracotomy.

By the mid-1990s, emerging results of early case series were very encouraging. The overall surgical mortality of 0–2% for VATS compared favorably to the conventional open thoracotomy technique.[3,22,23] Major complications and post-operative morbidity from VATS resections were relatively uncommon,[24,25] and minor complication rates were also no higher than with open thoracotomy. Tumor implantation following VATS was an early concern.[26] However, even in a series in which wound protection was not routinely carried out, port site recurrence was noted in only 0.26%.[27] This already low figure could be further minimized by routine use of a wound protector, gentle handling of tissue, and copious irrigation of the hemithorax prior to closure.[3] Early studies further showed that VATS took similar operating times as open surgery, but consistently produced similar or lower levels of blood loss.[28,29]

In return for equivalent safety as open surgery, VATS delivered the promise of less postoperative pain for patients. Early evidence confirmed that patients who undergo resections via the VATS approach experience less immediate post-operative pain than those having the thoracotomy approach. This has been documented in several large case controlled studies either by objective assessment in terms of analgesic requirements,[17,24] or subjective assessment in terms of pain scoring, usually in the form of a visual analogue scale.[24,28,30] A trend for reduced postoperative analgesic requirement was also seen in early studies comparing VATS with thoracotomy for lobectomy.[29,30] The reduced pain translated into faster recovery, resulting in significantly shorter hospital stays and earlier return to preoperative work or activities.[28,29]

By the mid to late 1990s, although relatively few surgeons were actively performing lobectomies this way, the rise of VATS was strikingly reflected in the large volumes of publications in this field.[1] By the turn of the century, the number of papers published in indexed journals on VATS or 'thoracoscopic' lobectomy was being counted in hundreds. It almost seemed inevitable that VATS lobectomy would replace open lobectomy in our specialty. However, this honeymoon period was abruptly brought to a halt.

An early, small, multi-institutional, randomized, prospective study of lobectomy performed through VATS compared to thoracotomy showed no significant benefits for using VATS in terms of pain reduction.[31] In another cross-sectional, questionnaire-based study, Landreneau and colleagues reported that the incidence of chronic postoperative pain at 1 year following VATS was also not any different from thoracotomy.[32] Soon, a number of similar papers followed suit, questioning whether VATS gave patients any real benefit at all. In a separate study comparing VATS and open lobectomy, no statistical differences could be found in the pain assessment after 1 week, nor were any differences detected between groups with respect to respiratory muscle strength or 6-minute walking distance.[33] Over the years, these studies have frequently been quoted by opponents of VATS to suggest that the benefits of VATS may not extend to the long-term or were not clinically important. Without doubt, these reports slowed the general acceptance of VATS lobectomy by surgeons in some countries for a number of years.

Unsurprisingly, a survey of the General Thoracic Surgery Club members in 1997 showed that the majority considered the use of VATS unacceptable.[34] In that survey, 60% of respondents used VATS less than 20% of the time and 38.1% expressed concern regarding overuse. In particular, several other concerns were raised. First, the safety of fine anatomical dissection of the hilum in an essentially closed chest was questioned. Second, there was skepticism over the adequacy of clearance for oncological lung resections with curative intent. Third, although the short term benefits of VATS to patients were intuitively obvious, its long term advantages over conventional surgery remained unclear. Fourth, the relatively high costs of the endoscopic equipment and VATS-related consumables cast doubt on the cost-effectiveness of this technique.

It is no accident that despite the birth of VATS lobectomy in the early 1990s, in most countries VATS lobectomy was used in only a minority of lung cancer operations well into the first and even second decades of the 21st century.

THE RENAISSANCE OF VATS LOBECTOMY

Although some reports of VATS were emerging showing poorer than expected outcomes, it soon became clear that not all those reports were describing the same operation. Careful comparison of published reports confirmed that the 'VATS lobectomy' being reported was not a unified technique, but several variations existed.[1,35,36] During the initial scramble to become the first to report results with this new surgical technique, this procedure was performed almost simultaneously at different centers, with each unit developing its own characteristics.[5] For example, how long an incision does one allow for a utility 'minithoracotomy' before it becomes a 'thoracotomy'? How often should one operate through the minithoracotomy as opposed to the video monitor? How much rib-spreading can we afford before the benefits of minimal access surgery are lost?

As a result of this lack of standardization in defining the VATS lobectomy procedure, some authors had been loosely applying the term

'VATS' to describe any thoracic surgery in which a video-thoracoscope is prepared, often for little more than illumination of the thoracic space while the operation is performed essentially via an open approach. Some authors were even tolerating a degree of rib-spreading when performing supposed 'VATS lobectomy'. The number and position of ports used also varied considerably between centers. At first, the VATS community was very tolerant of such variations.[1,3] After all, what did it matter if the surgeon was looking at the monitor throughout the operation or if they frequently chose to peek through the wounds directly? As it turned out, it mattered a great deal.

In a couple of landmark papers, Shigemura and colleagues compared three well-defined surgical approaches for lobectomy: 'complete' VATS (c-VATS) using purely endoscopic techniques with 100% monitor vision without rib-spreading minithoracotomy; 'assisted' VATS (a-VATS) performed using some degree of rib-spreading and a minithoracotomy (10 cm long) for both monitor and direct vision; and open thoracotomy (20 cm long) with direct vision only.[37,38] In these studies, the average operative time was longer for c-VATS (246 ± 47 minutes) than for a-VATS (169 ± 27 minutes) or open surgery (159 ± 28 minutes) ($p < 0.05$), but estimated blood loss was lower for c-VATS (96 ± 65 mL), and there was no significant difference in the number of dissected lymph nodes. Recovery time objectively analyzed by an accelerometer was shorter in patients undergoing c-VATS than in patients undergoing a-VATS or open surgery ($p < 0.05$). Median length of hospitalization was shorter for patients undergoing c-VATS (11.8 ± 2.7 days) than for patients undergoing a-VATS and open procedures ($p < 0.05$). It was therefore elegantly demonstrated that strict adherence to a completely endoscopic approach could give measurably better outcomes. In effect, it became no longer possible to consider any compromise in technique (as in a-VATS) as acceptable when describing a proper VATS lobectomy.

As a consequence of this realization, VATS surgeons have since applied much stricter definitions when describing VATS lobectomy. The Cancer and Leukemia Group B (CALGB) 39802 trial of the American Society of Clinical Oncology has produced perhaps the most widely accepted definition of the approach thus far.[39] In this trial of the safety and feasibility of c-VATS, VATS lobectomy has been defined by: no rib-spreading; a maximum length of 8 cm of the access incision for removal of the lobectomy specimen; individual dissection of the vein, arteries and airway for the lobe in question; and standard node sampling or dissection (identical to an open thoracotomy). All specimens were placed in an impermeable bag and removed through the access incision. This definition carries the key points emphasized by the pioneers of VATS lobectomy to reduce surgical access trauma, filtering out 'pseudo-VATS' techniques that gave compromised results.[1,3,40] However, it also allowed enough flexibility for individual surgeons to adapt the approach to their own preferences.

Once the definition of VATS lobectomy was re-established, it became once more possible to clearly demonstrate the benefits of the minimally invasive approach over thoracotomy. Since the turn of the century, we have witnessed a second burst of publications espousing the virtues of VATS, no less compelling than the first burst of the early to mid-1990s. A large systematic review of 39 papers involving over 6000 patients compared VATS with thoracotomy with the majority of those papers published since the turn of the century.[41] Acknowledging the CALGB definition of VATS lobectomy, this study reaffirmed that compared with thoracotomy, VATS lobectomy was associated with significantly shorter chest tube duration, shorter length of hospital stay, and improved survival at 4 years after resection. Furthermore, in a secondary analysis of data from the American College of Surgeons Oncology Group Z0030 randomized clinical trial comparing VATS with open lobectomy for lung cancer, it was also found that VATS was associated with fewer bronchoscopies for atelectasis (0% versus 6.3%, $p = 0.035$), lower incidence of prolonged chest tubes duration of greater than 7 days (1.5% versus 10.8%; $p = 0.029$), and shorter median length of stay (5 days versus 7 days; $p < 0.001$).[42]

It is therefore confirmed that VATS gives clinical advantages once clearly defined. However, this in turn raises the question: 'why?' What is so special about the criteria used for defining VATS that they can significantly impact on outcomes?

Looking at the four listed criteria of the CALGB definition, it is clear that the length of the main incision is not that important. Even when a large number of reports using a large range of wound lengths are considered together, the advantage of VATS over thoracotomy is well maintained.[41] Neither is the use of individual isolation-ligation of the hilar structures that important – as evidenced by the excellent results reported by surgeons using a simultaneous stapling technique.[6,13] Even the extent of lymph node dissection is not the critical issue, as similar outcomes in terms of morbidity are seen regardless of how much dissecting is done.[43,45] What is left of the CALGB criteria is perhaps the most important: avoidance of rib-spreading.

As noted earlier, pain or aching can occur in up to 80% of patients at 2 months or more after thoracotomy.[11,12] In 5% of these patients, the pain has been described as 'severe and disabling,' and over 40% of patients may still have some degree of pain at 1 year after surgery. Patients with such post-thoracotomy pain typically describe their pain as being burning, aching, electrical and/or shock-like in quality,[11,46] and responding poorly to the use of opiates.[47] These characteristics are the same as those of recognized neuropathic pain syndromes, such as post-herpetic neuralgia and diabetic peripheral neuropathy.[48,49] These all suggest that one of the key mechanisms of postthoracotomy pain may be neuropathic. Specifically, the rib-spreading during thoracotomy may be causing substantial compression and hence neuropraxic damage to the intercostals nerves. Emerging physiological studies are now gradually confirming this hypothesis.[46,50] In turn, this means that the benefits of VATS over thoracotomy may to a large degree be explained by the eschewing of rib-spreading and intercostal nerve trauma.

IMPROVING THE QUALITY OF VATS LOBECTOMY STUDIES

Although the reduction of morbidity with VATS was being reaffirmed, there remained continued skepticism over the growth of VATS. Critics complained that outcome measures being studied were too crude or subjective. Measures such as pain scores, chest drain durations and lengths of stay were inherently susceptible to confounding variables, especially since blinded and randomized trials were not feasible. In response to these valid criticisms, it was necessary to improve the quality and sophistication of the studies looking at VATS.[1]

It was quickly realized that pain assessment by patient self-reporting of levels of pain – often using a visual-analog scale or a simple 10-point numeric score – were easily subject to a wide range of confounding variables. For example, these may include patient socio-economic factors, chronic pain or analgesic use pre-operatively, other sources of post-operative satisfaction or dissatisfaction, and so on. This may have contributed to some of the more negative findings about VATS in the aforementioned studies of the mid and late 1990s.[31-33]

In response to this problem, more objective measures of morbidity were used. One of the methods is to compare pre- and postoperative Quality of Life (QoL). One detailed survey used the EORTC QLQ-C30 and EORTC QLQ-LC13 questionnaires designed to assess QoL in lung cancer patients, supplemented by a self-designed, nine-item surgery-specific questionnaire.[51] The survey was conducted on patients who received lung resections with curative intent for early stage lung cancer either by a VATS approach (median follow-up time of 33.5 months) or by an open thoracotomy approach (39.4 months). Statistically comparable levels of QoL and functional status were noted in both groups, although there was a trend for the VATS group to show better QoL scores and lower incidences of fatigue, dyspnea, coughing, and pain. Since then, an increasing number of papers have confirmed that VATS offers patients better QoL following lobectomy than thoracotomy, providing a much more reliable, quantifiable proof of its advantage.[52,53]

Another important composite measure of both post-operative pain and QoL after thoracic surgery is the impairment of shoulder function following thoracic surgery. It had been reported that the strengths of the latissimus dorsi and serratus anterior muscles may be better preserved following VATS when compared to thoracotomy.[30,32] In a prospective study, Li et al. reported that short-term shoulder strength and range of movement were significantly better in patients who received VATS pulmonary resection than those who received thoracotomy.[54]

There was also emerging evidence that VATS causes less depression of pulmonary function after lung resection surgery than thoracotomy. Kaseda reported that both the forced expiratory volume in one second (FEV1) and forced vital capacity (FVC) values measured at 3 months postoperatively were significantly preserved relative to preoperative values in patients who underwent lobectomy by a VATS approach compared to those receiving a thoracotomy approach ($p < 0.0001$).[55] In another similar study, post-operative Pao_2, SaO2, peak flow rates, FEV1 and FVC were all found to be better on postoperative days 7 and 14 in patients who had VATS rather than thoracotomy for lung resection.[56] Blood oxygenation, lung diffusion capacities, 6-minute walk test results, and recovery of vital capacity and cardiopulmonary function after surgery all tend to be better after VATS than after various forms of open thoracotomy for pulmonary resections.[57-59]

Arguably the most exciting attempt to objectively demonstrate that VATS causes less trauma may have come from looking at the impact of surgery on inflammatory and immune markers. In a landmark study, it was demonstrated that patients with clinical stage I lung cancer undergoing VATS lobectomy had significantly reduced postoperative release of both pro-inflammatory (interleukins 6 and 8) and anti-inflammatory cytokines (interleukin 10) into the plasma compared to those having conventional resection.[60] Similar findings were also reported in a smaller Japanese study which showed significantly reduced cytokine release (interleukins 6 and 8) into the pleural fluid in the VATS lobectomy group compared to the open group.[61] In a small randomized, prospective study from Edinburgh, it was also shown that VATS lobectomy was associated with a lesser effect on the postoperative fall in circulating T (CD4) cells and natural killer (NK) cells.[62] Lymphocyte oxidation was also less suppressed by VATS compared to open surgery. The same group also found that a range of acute phase responses – including C-reactive protein, interleukin 6, tumor necrosis factor, P-selectin, and oxygen free radical activity – were also significantly less amongst the VATS patients.[63] A separate Hong Kong study found that NK cell levels were suppressed to similar degrees on the first postoperative day following both VATS and thoracotomy lung resections for non-small cell lung cancer, but that T lymphocyte numbers were significantly more reduced following thoracotomy.[64] The levels of NK cells subsequently rose more quickly in the VATS group. These results suggest that the VATS approach was associated with less, and quicker recovery from, postoperative immunosuppression following lung resection surgery than the thoracotomy approach.

The clinical impact of these findings should not be underestimated. At least one study has shown that disturbances to postoperative interleukin levels may be correlated with complications.[65] More importantly, it has also been hypothesized that as immunosurveillance may play an important role in the progression of cancer, surgically induced immunosuppression may predispose to increased tumor growth or recurrence. Whether better preservation of the immune system by VATS may lead to improved long term survival is unclear but certainly deserves further investigation.[40,41]

Critics of the VATS approach for lung cancer research will say – quite rightly – that all the above benefits of VATS are meaningless if the operation cannot fulfil its primary obligation to provide effective oncologic treatment.

As a surrogate measure of the oncological 'adequacy' of the surgery, the quantity of nodal tissue dissected during lung cancer surgery is often taken as a battleground. Opponents of VATS have long suggested that even if a lobe can be removed by VATS, the approach does not allow radical nodal clearance. However, there is now growing evidence that the adequacy of VATS radical lymphadenectomy approaches that of open surgery both in terms of number and mass of nodal tissue removed. In one study, an open thoracotomy immediately after VATS nodal dissection in the same patient could yield only 3% more nodal tissue – an insignificant amount.[43] Two retrospective studies on non-contemporary cohorts of VATS and thoracotomy patients found that VATS gave similar or slightly less nodal tissue, but survival and staging were not affected.[44,45]

More important, though, is the need to demonstrate similarity between VATS and thoracotomy in terms of 'cure' rates postoperatively. A large volume of evidence has been accumulated over the past two decades in this regard. These have consistently demonstrated similar survival rates between VATS and open lobectomy patients.[53,66] However, a trend has long been noticed by VATS surgeons for a trend of longer survival amongst VATS patients. Studies from Japan have time and again reported remarkable 5-year survival rates of around 90% for stage IA lung cancer patients receiving VATS lobectomy.[44,55,66] In a 2008 systematic review of 39 studies comparing VATS with open lobectomy, patients who underwent VATS lobectomy were finally confirmed to have improved survival versus patients with open lobectomy (88.4% versus 71%; $p = 0.003$).[41] More recently, another similar systematic review reported that 5-year survival was significantly improved for patients who undergo VATS lobectomy for early-stage NSCLC (VATS relative risk, 0.72; $p = 0.04$), further suggesting that VATS lobectomy is at least oncologically equivalent to open lobectomy.[67]

It is still premature to declare with certainty that VATS gives better survival than open lobectomy. Nonetheless, many surgeons have already begun to speculate over reasons why this phenomenon should be possible. The theory gaining most recent attention is that of the effect of VATS on perioperative immunosurveillance. It has been shown that tumor cells may be shed into the circulation during lung cancer surgery.[68] In other surgical specialties, it has been demonstrated that the body's own immune system can help kill or remove such circulating tumor cells – a process often called 'immunosurveillance'.[69,70] In theory, if the body's immune function is somehow impaired this may inhibit the perioperative removal of tumor cells shed during the operation, which can then manifest as subsequent recurrence or metastasis. It has already been mentioned above that studies now show that VATS causing less immune system disruption than open surgery. Therefore, according to this theory, it should be expected that VATS is associated with better long-term survival.[41]

THE EVOLUTION OF MINIMALLY INVASIVE THORACIC SURGERY

The VATS lobectomy that has established itself as a viable – if not superior – alternative surgical approach to open lobectomy is now practiced widely around the world. In some centers, such as in Hong Kong, VATS lobectomy has been routinely performed for the majority of patients with early stage lung cancer since the mid-1990s.[3,9] As said above, other countries have taken up VATS lobectomy at a rather slower pace because of lingering doubts generated by the negative reports of the mid to late 1990s. What is most noticeable about the current resurgence of VATS lobectomy compared to the initial rise in the early 1990s is that this time most surgeons are performing the operation according to the same consensus definition of what VATS lobectomy should be.[39] The result is that operations in different centers around the world are now much more similar in the basic characteristics: no rib-spreading; a single access incision for specimen retrieval; individual isolation-ligation of the vessels; and systematic nodal dissection.

Multi-port VATS

In the classic approach to VATS lobectomy, a three-port strategy is used, with two 10 mm incisions for the camera and instruments respectively, and a third 3–5 cm utility port in the 4th or 5th intercostal space (with no rib-spreading) for specimen retrieval.[2,3] Both the surgeon and assistant stand anterior to the patient, and both watch the same video-monitor throughout the operation, facilitating camera handling by the assistant (instructions from the surgeon are easier to follow without the hinderance of paradoxical movement or resorting to awkward camera orientations). Dissection is from an anterior-to-posterior direction, typically taking the pulmonary vein first, then pulmonary artery, then bronchus. The fissures are taken last of all, and staplers are used in a 'fissureless' technique to minimize postoperative air leak.[71] A systematic dissection at all the ipsilateral mediastinal lymph node stations in routinely carried out in all patients.

This totally endoscopic c-VATS lobectomy performed in Hong Kong is essentially the same operation found throughout the world nowadays.[21,72] However, certain detail variations exist of course.

As noted earlier, the Edinburgh group has long championed the 'posterior approach'.[17,18] The sequence of hilar dissection is reversed, so that for a right upper lobectomy, e.g. the lobar bronchus may be divided first, followed by the pulmonary artery and then the pulmonary vein. This technique more closely resembles traditional open surgery, and remains an attractive alternative when classic VATS lobectomy from an anterior approach is not feasible for any reason.

Instead of always standing at the anterior side of the patient, surgeons at several centers in Asia (particularly Korea) prefer always standing on the right side of the operating table for a VATS lobectomy, regardless of whether the operation is on the right or left lung.[72] In other words, the surgeon would stand anterior to the patient for a left lung operation, but posterior to the patient for a right lung operation. The rationale for this is because for a right-handed surgeon, it is usually ergonomically more comfortable to reach around the patient with the dominant right arm and face the video-monitor placed in a more cephalad direction. Proponents of this positioning claim that for the surgeon to stand on the left side of the table, the right arm can be tucked too close to the surgeon's own body for comfortable operating. They claim that by always standing on the right side of the patient, back problems may also be possibly avoided.

Dr Tadasu Kohno of Tokyo, Japan is another leading VATS surgeon in Asia who has developed a rather distinctive strategy for surgeon and assistant positioning.[73] In this strategy, for a right-sided resection, the surgeon stands posterior to the patient and the camera-holding assistant anterior to the patient. The camera is inserted in the port most anterior on the patient, with the other working ports closer to the surgeon. To ensure the correct orientation of the image on the video-monitor for the surgeon, the camera on the video-thoracoscope is turned so that 'upwards' on the camera and image is toward the anterior of the patient. Because the video-thoracoscope enters the chest via the most anterior camera port, this usually means the camera itself is held almost upside-down by the assistant. The advantage of this strategy is that it best approximates the surgeon's position and views during a traditional open lobectomy via a posterolateral thoracotomy. This facilitates the transition from open to VATS lobectomy for some surgeons. However, handling the camera in a virtually upside-down position on the opposite side of the operating table from the surgeon requires a very skilled and experienced assistant.

Regardless of the exact details of the operation used, patients today can expect rapid recovery after a classic VATS lobectomy.[41,42,53,67] Data collected around the world suggest that mortality is no higher than after open lobectomy, and morbidity rates (typically around 15–20%) are usually lower. Chest drain durations average around 4–5 days, and patients are generally discharged around 4–7 days after surgery. For an ultra-major operation that a mere 30 years ago had a mortality rate approaching 10% and a complication rate of almost 60%,[74,75] these modern figures achieved with VATS are commendable.

ROBOT-ASSISTED THORACIC SURGERY

The emergence of the da Vinci robotic surgical system (Surgical Intuitive, Mountain View, CA) captured considerable attention amongst surgeons and the lay public around the dawn of the 21st century. Such 'robot-assisted thoracic surgery' (RATS) allowed the surgeon at a console to 'remote control' robot limbs inserted into the patient to perform the operation. The purported advantages of using robot assistance include precise tremor-free manipulations, 3D binocular visualization, excellent ergonomics for the surgeon, and the ability of the robotic arms to minimize torquing of the instruments at each working port.[76] Early published series have demonstrated the safety and feasibility of robot assisted surgery within the thorax, even for major lung resection.[77] However, good results have so far mainly been reported by a small number of specialist centers with particular experience using robots, and a couple of recognized drawbacks still remain. The first issue is the complete absence of tactile feedback throughout the operation.[78] For many operations, the 3D visual information can partly compensate for this, but many continue to harbor doubts. The other disadvantage of RATS is the costs – both of the initial outlay for the advanced hardware and of the bespoke instruments and consumables that must be purchased for each operation. Furthermore, there is 'cost' in terms of time. Especially early on in the adoption of RATS, the surgical team will expend considerable operating room time setting up and docking the robot system. The extra surgical times may result in fewer operations being performed per day.

Because of the very low morbidity rates and excellent outcomes with conventional VATS, it may prove difficult – if not impossible – to ever demonstrate any significant superiority of the robot system over VATS. Conceptually, it is see how a robot-assisted lobectomy using four ports can ever be convincingly proven to cause less trauma than a typical c-VATS lobectomy using three ports. Consequently, for the foreseeable future at least, making a compelling case for robot-assisted surgery in terms of cost-effectiveness will almost certainly prove futile.

In the inevitably upcoming debates over the relative merits of robot-assisted surgery and VATS, it is worth making one telling observation. Many centers using RATS acknowledge that their standard approach to lung lobectomy was through thoracotomy, not VATS.[77] Conversely, few of the established VATS lobectomy centers have switched to using the robot at all. This peculiar phenomenon suggests that for surgeons used to open surgery, the very intuitive and user-friendly robot systems interface may be easier to master than the different set of hand-eye skills demanded by VATS lobectomy. This provides non-VATS surgeons an excellent route into the world of MITS. However, for those who have mastered VATS lobectomy, the robot systems do not seem to offer any advantage or incentive to switch.[79] It has now been well over 15 years since robot systems first appeared, and some may wonder whether RATS has already peaked and is becoming obsolete.

'Next generation' VATS

Instead of improving VATS by using technology (RATS), another direction has been to improve VATS by using more advanced techniques. These new approaches are often termed the 'next generation' of VATS.[2] **Figure 2.1** shows our view of the 'generations' of thoracic surgery approaches. **Figure 2.2** shows the progression of approaches from conventional multi-portal VATS to uniportal VATS.

With needlescopic VATS (nVATS), video-thoracoscopes and instruments of only 2–3 mm in diameter are used, requiring much smaller ports than the typical 5–15 mm ports used in conventional VATS. The wounds are typically so small that only barely detectable 'pinpoint' scars remain after surgery – leading to the term 'needlescopic'. The principle is that if VATS can improve on open thoracotomy by using smaller wounds, then nVATS should give better outcomes than conventional VATS by using even smaller wounds. Compared to robot-assisted surgery, this approach uses far smaller ports and is much cheaper. Needlescopic VATS has already been used for a variety of diagnostic and simple therapeutic procedures, such as sympathectomy for palmar hyperidrosis.[80-82] The nVATS approach has been used for pleurodesis surgery in the management of pneumothorax, achieving equivalent efficacy as conventional VATS but with less pain and faster recovery.[83,84] The natural evolution of this has now seen nVATS being applied to lobectomy for lung cancer.[2] This is described more fully in a later chapter of this book. Briefly, while a 2–4 cm utility incision is still needed for retrieval of the resected lobe, the 10 mm camera and instrument ports of classic three-port VATS can be replaced with 3 mm ports instead. This retains that same basic ports strategy and ergonomics of conventional three-port VATS, but allows the potential benefits of the smaller wounds.

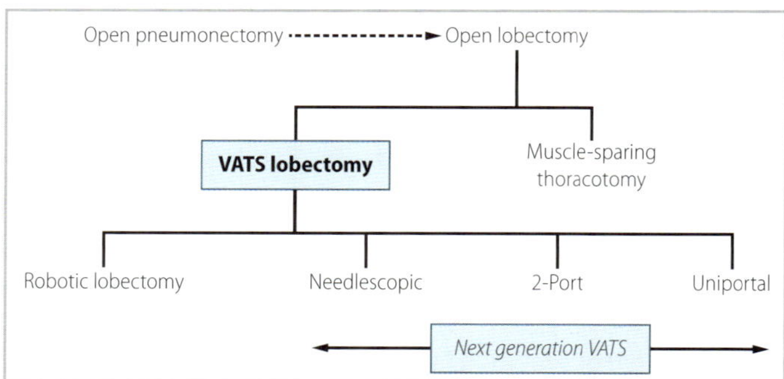

Figure 2.1 The 'family tree' of thoracic surgery approaches for lung cancer surgery. In the early days of lung cancer surgery, all tumors were treated surgically by a pneumonectomy in the belief that radical surgery represented the best chance of a 'cure'. By the 1970s, it became established that a lobectomy was sufficient for cure in most cases, and resulted in much less mortality and morbidity than pneumonectomy. As described in the text, lobectomy via the 'classic' multi-portal VATS approach began in the early 1990s. VATS thrived and outlived attempts to perpetuate open surgery through 'muscle sparing' thoracotomy. Robot-assisted thoracic surgery emerged as a possible successor for VATS in the 2000s, but has become the preferred approach in only a minority of centers thus far. 'Next generation' VATS represented another branch of evolution from classic VATS. These 'next generation' approaches include needlescopic, two-port and uniportal approaches, which in turn can be seen as different steps along an evolutionary path.

The next step was the transition to two-port VATS.[2] In Hong Kong, it was noted that the posterior 3 mm instrument port for nVATS lobectomy was often of very limited usefulness. It was therefore omitted altogether, and all instrumentations with both hands were performed together via the 2–4 cm utility port. Again, the technical details of this approach are presented in a later chapter in this book. This was a relatively painless transition for the surgical team: the surgeon needed to get used to working with both hands' instruments through one small wound, but the visualization was from the same angle as with three-port VATS and nVATS – making it easy for the camera assistant to adapt. For the patient, the reduction in number of wounds promised further potential benefits. In Hong Kong, the two-port VATS approach was arrived at from an evolution through nVATS, and hence the camera wound was a minute 3 mm skin incision. However, other centers arrived at a two-port strategy directly from conventional three-port VATS, and the camera port remained a 10–15 mm one with use of a plastic or metal trocar.[85,86]

Perhaps the most exciting development since the birth of conventional VATS has been the rise of uniportal (or single post) VATS. The concept of using only a single incision to perform simpler thoracic procedures was first proposed by Dr Gaetano Rocco.[87] Using curved endoscopic instruments co-axially with the video-thoracoscope through the same incision, a variety of diagnostic procedures, simple wedge resections, and even pneumothorax surgery could be achieved. Early results suggested some potential benefit even compared to conventional VATS.[88] It was further suggested that the visualization achieved through this coaxial approach better approximated the natural human hand-eye approach, perhaps offering superior optics for MITS.[89]

Starting in 2011/12, Dr Diego Gonzalez Rivas took the uniportal concept to the next level by using it for lobectomy for lung cancer.[90] Again, using instruments coaxially with the video-thoracoscope, a complete lobectomy with full nodal dissection could be performed safely via only a single 3–5 cm incision. Dr Gonzalez Rivas has since gone on to describe the uniportal technique for increasingly complex resections, including segmentectomy, bronchoplasty and even vascular sleeve resections.[91-93] The technique has since gradually gained popularity around the world, particularly in Asia. In Hong Kong, the first author of this chapter was the first to perform uniportal lobectomy, arriving at the approach from a natural evolution from two-port VATS.[2] Once experience was gained performing both hands' instruments through one small wound, it was only a relatively simple matter of bringing the camera up to the main utility port for a truly single portal operation.

The uniportal approach itself has gone on to inspire other 'next generation' variants. In Asia, some surgeons have started using a single-port placed at the sub-xiphoid location to perform a variety of procedures – ranging from thymic surgery to complete lobectomy.[94] The theoretical advantage here is the potential complete avoidance of any intercostal neuralgia. On the negative side, technical challenges such as the impacting of the beating heart against the thoracoscope,

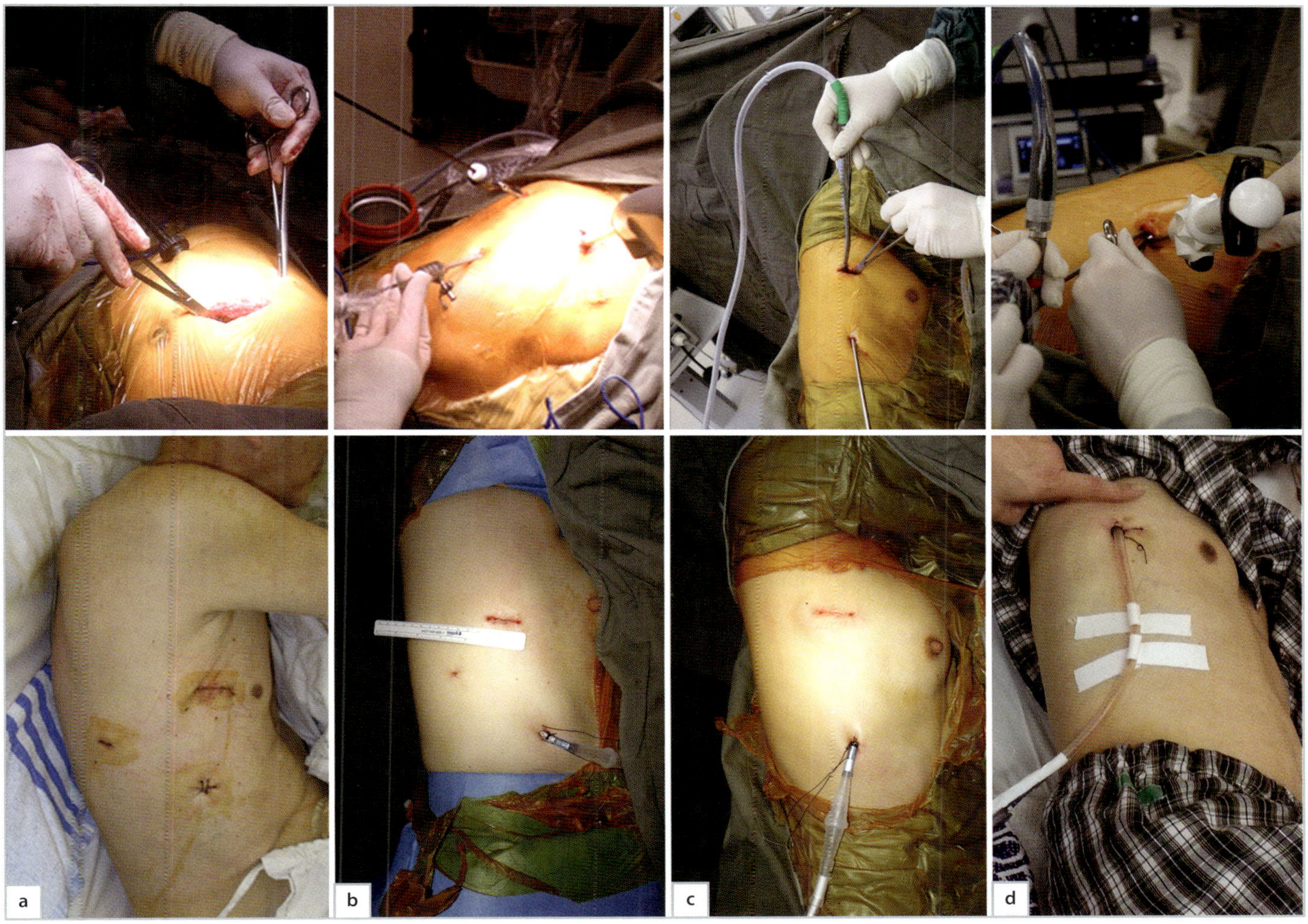

Figure 2.2 The evolution of VATS approaches. Progressing from one step to the next means that only incremental changes are necessary, making learning of each approach relatively easy. (a) The 'classic' 3-port VATS approach: one 3–5 cm utility port, one lower 10 mm camera port, one 10 mm posterior instrument port. (b) Needlescopic VATS: a 2–5 cm utility port remains, but the camera and posterior instrument ports have been reduced to 3 mm ports (alternatively, a 5-mm video-thoracoscope can be used with no trocar, giving similar incision size as a 3-mm video-thoracoscope with a trocar used). The ports layout and operative ergonomics are essentially the same as with 'classic' VATS, with visualization and instrumentation angles largely unchanged. (c) two-port VATS: a 2–5 cm utility port remains, a 3-mm (or 5 mm without trocar) camera port remains, but the posterior instrument port is abandoned. Visualization angles are the same as classic or needlescopic VATS, and only instrumentation is changed with the surgeon's left and right hand instruments sharing the same access via the utility port. (d) Uniportal VATS: a 2–4 cm utility port remains, but the camera port is abandoned. Instrumentation is the same as two-port VATS, and now only the visualization angle is changed so that the video-thoracoscope becomes co-axial with the instruments.

and access to some nodal stations, still remain as issues for concern. The concept of natural orifice surgery is also being explored. Although a direct natural orifice into the chest for surgery does not seem immediately obvious, there has been at least one group reporting thoracic sympathectomy being performed using a transumbilical approach.[95]

A potential future development may be the marriage of robotic technology with the uniportal approach. It is well known that industry is already developing advanced robot systems that allow visualization and complex, multi-arm instrumentation through a robotic insert via a single surgical incision.[96] Should such systems succeed, the combination of intricate robot-enabled surgery with the minimal invasiveness of a uniportal access promises to offer unprecedented benefits for patients.

COMPLEMENTARY ADVANCES

The evolution of minimally invasive surgery in the thorax extends beyond the use of video-assisted surgical access. Further development of the surgery can also be influenced by reducing how much is resected once that access is gained, by the need to manage the footprint of surgery postoperatively, and by the assimilation of new technology.

Sublobar resection

Despite the current success and popularity of VATS lobectomy, surgery can no longer claim to be the least traumatic mode of curative therapy for lung cancer. Today, ablative therapy (using radio-frequency or microwave energy), stereotactic ('cyberknife') radiosurgery, and stereotactic body radiation therapy (SBRT) all have potential claims for that title.[97-99] Despite the fact that the effectiveness of these modalities compared to respective surgery is still under investigation, to the lay patient they represent an astonishing option that may 'treat' cancer without requiring major surgery. Unless the surgical option is made more palatable for patients, there is no doubt that increasing numbers of patients who are marginally or even completely suitable for surgery may be tempted away from the operating room.

One of the ways in which surgery is fighting back against these non-operative options is the re-emergence of sublobar resection in recent years. In 1995, the only randomized trial of sublobar resection versus lobectomy for T1N0 NSCLC suggested that survival and especially loco-regional recurrence was significantly worse in the sublobar group.[100] This result confirmed fears at the time that sublobar resection was inadequate in terms of oncologic treatment, and negatively affected the adoption of sublobar resection as a mainstream surgical option for NSCLC for many years thereafter. However, over the past decade, many modern case series have shown that in selected patients, survival rates after sublobar resection can actually approach those after lobectomy.[101-106] Review of the literature suggests that sublobar resection can be equally as effective as lobectomy for patients found to have confirmed stage IA disease with a peripherally located tumor up to 2–3 cm in diameter, and which is predominantly with a ground-glass opacity (GGO) appearance on CT imaging.[107] It is also noted that to achieve the best results, the evidence suggests that segmentectomies rather than wedge resections be performed.

Traditionally, the concern about segmentectomy is that this is often technically more difficult than an anatomic lobectomy. If a segmentectomy is seen as 'difficult' enough that conversion to thoracotomy is considered, one has to ponder whether it is less traumatic to the patient to persevere with VATS but perform a lobectomy, or to convert to a thoracotomy to complete the segmentectomy. However, the evolution of VATS approaches as described above have demonstrated that segmentectomies can be safely and reliably achieved via two-port or even uniportal VATS.[108] The chance of requiring conversion seems to be low in experienced hands. Furthermore, the use of the 'next generation' VATS approaches perfectly complements the goal of sublobar resection, which is to minimize the impact of surgery for patients. In this way, the current trends for both sublobar resection and for 'next generation' approaches are driving each other forward. Against the uncertain alternative of the above non-surgical therapies, the rise of minimally invasive sublobar resection promises to be a very important development promising hope for patients with a small, peripheral GGOs in the coming years.

Perioperative care

To make VATS lobectomy even better, it is first necessary to appreciate that it is not perfect. Despite the smaller wounds and avoidance of rib-spreading, 52.9% of patients receiving VATS pleurodesis for pneumothorax (in which no rib-spreading is used) experience paresthetic chest wall discomforts which are distinct from classical localized wound pain.[81,109] VATS reduced pain compared to thoracotomy, but was itself still associated with a certain level of neuropathic injury – most likely caused by the torquing of the video-thoracoscope and instruments at the ports during surgery, and by the placement of a chest tube that is kept for a few days postoperative. Pharmacotherapy aimed specifically at treating neuropathic pain (specifically the use of gabapentin) has been suggested to be effective in alleviating postoperative pain after thoracic surgery.[110] Another strategy has been to make use of 'pre-emptive' analgesia. A randomized trial in patients undergoing nVATS has now demonstrated that giving local anesthesia at the ports sites prior to making the surgical incisions can significantly reduce postoperative pain for up to a week after surgery.[82]

Aside from the above, postoperative care following VATS requires a detailed co-ordination of multiple practices into a clinical pathway.[3,111] In a typical pathway, the analgesic regime is revised to reduce the use of opiates – which are both unnecessary given the reduced pain with VATS, and detrimental because the sedation and dizziness caused could delay patient mobilization. All patients are mobilized fully within 24 hours of surgery. Physiotherapy is implemented earlier and more aggressively. Chest drain removal is also expedited. Even postoperative investigations, when a patient opens his/her bowels, and schedules for meeting the patient's relatives are included in the overall clinical pathway package. Using such a clinical pathway in Hong Kong, the literally dozens of items of changes have significantly improved the recovery process of VATS lobectomy patients.[112] Since its implementation, chest drain durations, lengths of hospital stay, rates of complications, and rates of re-admission can all be reduced. The lesson learned is that improving operative surgical performance alone must be complemented by appropriate improvements in the ancillary services to bring out the full potential of VATS. An awareness of the importance of perioperative care to the evolution of VATS is crucial. VATS surgeons must realize that advances in operative technique do not automatically result in faster patient recovery. It is necessary to tailor the clinical pathway to take advantage of the supposedly better recovery, by appropriately speeding up the rehabilitation process.

The development of a sound clinical pathway is the key to fast-track programs in surgery. Another emerging development that promises to promote fast-tracking lies in the realm of anesthesiology. Non-intubated VATS has been shown in some centers to be an exciting new prospect.[113,114] By allowing patients to breathe spontaneously without endotracheal intubation, it has been postulated that the after-effects of general anesthesia and the risk of airways injury is reduced. Experience is only gradually accumulating, and it may be some time before any advantages or disadvantages become confirmed with this approach. However, case series have already demonstrated that it can be done in combination with multi-port and even uniportal VATS with reasonable levels of safety.[113,114] Anecdotal reports of very rapid recovery after such surgery have emerged. Reports of VATS on completely awake (non-sedated, non-intubated) also exist.[115-117] Regardless of the merits (or lack thereof) of these strategies, they provide a timely reminder that the evolution of minimally invasive approaches and enhanced recovery programs is not a uni-dimensional phenomenon led solely by surgeons, but must always be a multi-disciplinary collaboration that involves anesthesiologists, nursing staff, and other healthcare professionals and specialties.

New technology

Arguably the most common complication seen after VATS lobectomy today is air leakage. Air leaks are the single most common reason for an extended length of hospitalization.[118] Air leaks occur in up to 58% of patients after a lobectomy, and can persist for 5 days or more in 15–18% of patients.[119-121] Air leak rates after VATS lobectomy are generally no different than after open lobectomy. However, once an air leak occurs, chest drain durations and lengths of stay are determined by the leak itself and not by the wonderful minimally invasive surgical approach used. It is therefore especially important for VATS surgeons to find an effective solution to this problem. Traditional methods such suturing, pleural tent creation, and so on are possible with VATS, but not necessarily easy to perform given the small ports. Instead, studies have shown that sealants may be a simple yet effective way to reduce air leaks.[122,123] Modern surgical sealants can now be readily aerosolized and delivered via dedicated endoscopic spray applicators, allowing an effective air leak remedy that can be used during VATS without requiring conversion to open surgery. This has allowed surgeons to proceed with evolving ever less invasive techniques with fewer worries.

Postoperatively, another emerging technological advance to combat air leakage is the emergence of portable digital chest drain.

A modern digital system such as the Medela Thopaz (Medela AG, Switzerland) has an inbuilt suction system that maintains a constant, user-set negative pleural pressure without need for any external connection. The result is a compact, portable chest drain that permits complete patient mobility after lobectomy, perfectly complementing the faster recovery expected after VATS.[111] Perhaps more importantly, it has also been shown that use of the digital air flow monitor on a digital system such as the Thopaz can reduce chest drain durations and lengths of stay after surgery. This is in part due to the increase in accuracy and objectivity in measurements of postoperative air leaks.[124] It has been suggested that the greater consistency in monitoring air leaks can be translated into more decisive, confident postoperative chest drain management resulting in shortened chest drain durations and lengths of hospital stay.[1] It has also been hypothesized that the more 'regulated' pleural pressures maintained by a digital system may be more conducive to an earlier cessation of air leakage.[125] Digital drainage is gaining popularity at the same time as VATS is evolving into 'next generation' approaches, and it seems that this technology is at least in part enabling some of the potential benefits of these approaches to be better realized.

Developments in bronchoscopic technology also appear to be complementing the evolution of VATS. The rise of Endobronchial Ultrasonography (EBUS) presented a minimally invasive option for routine mediastinal nodal screening – perhaps even in the operating room immediately prior to embarking on a VATS lobectomy.[126] More recently, Electromagnetic Navigation Bronchoscopy (ENB) seems to offer an even further leap forward.[127] By allowing accurate targeting of small lung lesions that can be very peripherally located, ENB offers some potentially important clinical advantages for the surgeon. A lung lesion that may be too peripheral to be accessible by traditional bronchoscopy or too small to be biopsied by a CT-guided percutaneous needle aspiration may now be biopsied endobronchially using ENB. This can be done in the operating room, and if malignancy is confirmed, it is possible to proceed to a VATS curative resection in the same sitting. Furthermore, a small lesion as described here may be difficult to locate by digital palpation, but use of the ENB may allow its identification in the operating room. This in turn allows the possibility of a VATS sublobar resection with confidence and accuracy. Just as importantly, this method of lung nodule localization foregoes the need for preoperative CT-guided localization with all the potential risks and technical problems that that may entail.[128] In this way, ENB complements the evolution of VATS by allowing the adoption of a 'one stop' strategy for selected patients with a small GGO or lung nodule: instead of traditional attempts at pre-operative biopsy, one could consider proceeding to the operating room where the surgeon can offer potential diagnosis, localization and resection in one sitting.[129]

The above are just a few examples of how emerging technology from the medical product industry are helping the development of VATS. Many other examples of new surgical equipment and technologies can be cited. Looking to the future, these include new single-port-access quasi-robotic endoscopic surgery platforms, magnetic anchoring and guidance systems for intrathoracic surgery, sophisticated navigation systems, and others. All of these may potentially further increase the power of VATS to enable ever more complex operations with ever greater safety and efficiency. However, it would be wrong to only look in awe upon the technological and technical breakthroughs per se. Instead, it behoves surgeons appreciate that as surgical morbidity is lowered, so are thresholds for accepting patients for surgery. As the rate of postoperative recovery is hastened, clinical pathways must be rewritten to realize the full potential of modern surgery. As the human costs of surgical biopsy are minimized, one must rethink whether traditional dogma about securing diagnosis before surgery must be so strictly upheld. The 'how' of surgery is now fundamentally changing the 'who', 'when' and 'why' of our practice.

IMPLICATIONS OF EVOLUTION

Learning the technique

The fact that the above described evolution of VATS is a gradual, stepwise progression should be good news for those hoping to learn VATS. As the approach evolves from classical three-port VATS, through needlescopic and two-port VATS, to eventually uniportal VATS, this has fundamental implications for how one should approach learning these 'next generation' techniques. If one forgets the basic lesson of evolution (that all the approaches involve placing the right hand, the left hand and a pair of eyes into the chest), and try to leapfrog from open surgery to – say – uniportal VATS in one go, then that may be a leap too far. However, if one remembers to appreciate that this is an evolution – not a revolution – then one can see each step is only incremental and hence easy to learn.

The transition from open thoracotomy to basic three-port VATS is simply a matter of replacing the right and left hands with instruments that are introduced through separate small incisions, and the eyes with a video-thoracoscope placed through another camera port. The transition from conventional three-port VATS to nVATS simply means replacing the 10 mm camera with a 3-mm or 5-mm camera, and one conventional instrument port with a 3-mm instrument port. The transition from nVATS to a two-port VATS approach is then just a matter of abandoning the 3 mm instrument port and placing both right and left hand instruments through the same utility port. The instrumentation only is changed, but the visualization from a separate camera port is maintained as with conventional three-port and nVATS. From there, the transition from two-port to uniportal VATS just involves abandoning the camera port and placing the video-thoracoscope also through the same utility port. If the two-port technique of instrumentation with both hands via the same port is already mastered, this last transition then only requires the surgeon and assistant to become accustomed to the new visualization.

Details of the conventional three-port, needlescopic, two-port and uniportal approaches are covered in other chapters of this book, and hence will not be elaborated on here.

Instead, we would like to stress a few key points about the implications of evolution on learning 'next generation' VATS approaches:

- Uniportal VATS is not an 'all-or-nothing' proposition. There are many steps between open thoracotomy and Uniportal VATS. These are not only steps along the path of training, but legitimate alternative approaches in their own right. Each of the VATS approaches have already greatly reduced surgical morbidity for patients when compared to thoracotomy, and no evidence exists to say that any one approach has significant advantages over another. It is by no means necessary to 'end up' practicing uniportal VATS: a surgeon may find him/herself to be more comfortable with conventional three-port, needlescopic, or two-port, and that is fine.
- As one transitions through the different VATS approaches, there is no need to be intimidated. Going from conventional three-port, to the needlescopic, two-port and uniportal approaches, each transition is 'just' another step in the evolutionary process: the same basic principles and techniques of conventional VATS apply – including instruments, methods for trouble-shooting, and so on. The surgeon should retain all the skills and wisdom acquired if he/she moves to the next step, and should not abandon everything and start afresh

with each transition. This not only shortens the learning curve, but also gives reassurance and confidence as a new approach is learned. The main caveat in the interest of safety is that the surgeon should ideally dwell at each step long enough to master it before moving onto the next.

- The surgeon is not the only one evolving. An experienced thoracic surgeon may well find that the evolution is easy to learn. However, it is not sufficient for the surgeon him/herself to acquire the technical skills. It is necessary to train the assistant because without good camera control, the compromised visualization can ruin the surgery no matter how good the surgeon's instrumentation is. It is necessary to train and communicate with all members of the multi-disciplinary team – including anesthetists and nurses – to jointly develop a clinical pathway each time a new approach is introduced. This is necessary to realize the benefits of the surgery. It is necessary to keep abreast of the newest developments in the specialty and in related technology because the evolution of these is always ongoing, and no one step of the VATS evolution is ever the definitive 'end product'.

Clinical research

As described above, the early history of VATS was mired in trials and tribulations. These took the form of sharp criticism from conservative 'authorities' in thoracic surgery who were instinctively suspicious of any new developments in the specialty, and also of early clinical evidence that was not always favorable to the new minimally invasive approach.[1] The emergence of VATS triumphant from this difficult era brought with it some painfully learned lessons. Firstly, it was appreciated that the only way to overcome criticism (which is often fair and reasonable) is to remain objective and provide sound clinical data that will prove one's point. It took years of patiently collected data that consistently demonstrated the safety and advantages of VATS before even the critics were won over. Secondly, the data must be generated using solid study designs and meticulous analysis. As already seen above, errant studies – even randomized trials conducted by respected institutions – can be let down by inadequate stringency in patient selection, definition of key terms (including what is and is not 'VATS'), heterogeneity within study arms, and other problems. It takes only a handful of negative results from seemingly thorough (but actually flawed) studies to jeopardize the progress of a surgical technique or trend. The early years of VATS were beset with problems in this regard, and it took many years of improving the quality of clinical research before the evidence became convincing enough for everyone.

As thoracic surgery moves forward with newer techniques and newer technologies, these will inevitably face similar resistance from conservative elements within the specialty. Those already established in the use of conventional VATS may scoff at the advent of uniportal surgery, and those used to conventional anesthesia may scorn the use of non-intubated surgery, for example. At the time of writing, it is still unclear whether such newfangled strategies really possess any advantages. However, it is clear that as practitioners of medicine, we need to apply the scientific method and seek real evidence to confirm or refute our viewpoints. That is the lesson that the evolution of VATS has taught us: time and evidence speak far louder than outspoken opinions.

Drawing from the 20-plus year experience of the evolution of VATS, it becomes clear what the gauntlet that 'next generation' VATS must run looks like. It will take an accumulation of evidence in five phases that each prove a point about each of the 'next generation' approaches and their associated technologies.

Infancy

The first step for any new surgical technique is to demonstrate its safety and feasibility. This can often be demonstrated by case reports and then by case series. Taking VATS lobectomy as the example the earliest published papers on this emerged in the early 1990s and consisted of case reports and case series reporting that the technique could be safely performed in humans. In recent years, as uniportal VATS is gaining interest, case reports and case series can again be seen announcing that the approach is feasible and safe. Case reports have gone on to demonstrate the feasibility of the uniportal approach for ever more complex procedures, such as segmentectomy, bronchoplasty, double sleeve resection and so on. Case series demonstrate the safety initially for straightforward lobectomy, and later for more challenging scenarios such as advanced cancer.[130,131]

Childhood

The next step after showing a technique 'can' be done, is to provide data suggesting that perhaps it 'should' be done. To demonstrate clinical advantages of a technique, case reports and series are of no use, and comparative studies are required. In the history of VATS, these began in the early/mid 1990s with crude comparisons between a VATS cohort and historical control cohorts of patients who had received thoracotomy.[30] Gradually, the comparisons became more sophisticated, with case-matched comparisons and later by simple prospective trials, including a handful of randomized trials.[28,31] In these early comparative studies, investigators tended to rely on simple outcome measures such as pain scores, chest drain durations, lengths of stay, and crude morbidity rates. It was such early comparative studies in the 1990s that first raised awareness of the possible benefits of performing MITS. In recent years with uniportal VATS, only a few crude comparisons between uniportal and multi-port VATS have so far been published,[132,133] and more are warranted to demonstrate whether any potential advantage exists for the newer approach.

Adolescence

The problem with studies in the above 'childhood' phase is that the above outcome measures are quite crude and subject to considerable bias or influence by confounding variables. For example, pain scores are very subjective, while chest drain durations and lengths of stay can be influenced by investigator bias and other non-clinical factors. With VATS, as time went on, more objective, quantifiable, and reproducible outcome measures were called for to clearly prove any advantage. Simple pain scores were supplanted by surrogate measures of pain, including use of QoL questionnaires that had been previously validated in clinical trials, or by the quantified assessment of shoulder function after surgery.[51,54] More convincingly, the amount of trauma caused to the body by surgery was assessed by looking at perioperative changes in humoral and cellular immune function.[60-64] By measuring items such as inflammatory cytokine levels and lymphocyte numbers and activity, an objective quantification of perioperative trauma was able to prove that VATS caused less potential harm to patients. Clinical research with 'next generation' VATS techniques has not yet reached this phase.

Adulthood

It is no use showing benefit of a new technique if the resulting surgery fails to treat the disease as effectively as the older one. The greatest concern regarding VATS lobectomy in its early years was whether it offered the same survival rates for lung cancer patients as lobectomy via thoracotomy. This is a fundamental question, but because it required the accumulation of many patient-years of experience to prove, it was not until the late 1990s that 'adulthood' papers on long-term survival after VATS lobectomy began to emerge. Most were case series only. Comparisons with historical cohorts of patients receiving thoracotomy suggested similar survival rates, but of course such crude comparisons could not be reliable. It required the accumulation of many such studies involving series of both VATS and open lobectomies before well-designed systematic reviews and meta-analyses emerged.[41,67] In turn, it is because of this waiting for enough studies that this crucial phase did not really reach its apogee until the early 2000s. It is also why this critical phase of demonstrating similar survival only occurred after the demonstration of VATS advantages in the 'childhood' and 'adolescence' phases. And of course this phase was crucial to silencing the critics. Once equivalent or better survival was shown for VATS, this was coupled with the previously demonstrated advantages to reach the final inevitable conclusion: the VATS is the better approach. The culmination of this evolution of evidence resulted in official guidelines now concluding that VATS lobectomy is no longer merely an 'alternative' approach for treating lung cancer, but indeed a 'preferred' approach for patients with early stage disease.[134] For newer approaches such as uniportal VATS, there is an important lesson here: it takes many years to have enough data to convincingly show equivalency/superiority in survival, so such data collection must begin as soon as possible.

Maturity

Although many papers on conventional VATS have been published over the years, there are still papers being published on this topic today. These papers tend to address the cost-effectiveness of the technique, and how it can be taught to others.[135,136] We feel, however, that the discussion should be centred around the fundamental issues of safety, benefit and efficacy of the technique (once proven), before issues such as cost-effectiveness and 'teachability' are addressed.

CONCLUSION

To a large extent, the word 'evolution' has been overused in the medical literature. Nonetheless, it is still an entirely appropriate term to describe the story of VATS. This is a surgical technical that has shown gradual changes over successive identifiable generations, and these changes have come about as a response to forces of 'natural selection' in healthcare. The demands to make surgery less traumatic, more effective, and more applicable to more patients have led to the creation of different interpretations of VATS, and then to selection of the 'fittest' of these innovations to survive and perpetuate. Since its birth in the 1990s, VATS has undergone a progression of modifications and reinterpretations as a result. This process is slow and incremental, and hence it is truly an evolution rather than a revolution.

Understanding the evolutionary nature of VATS has important ramifications. As seen above, it means that learning a given VATS approach can also follow the step-wise sequence, enabling a logical, easy-to-grasp attainment of the skills. It means that the lessons of the past – in terms of developing clinical evidence on which to base clinical practice – can be applied to innovations of the future. It also means that, as in nature, the evolution is a never-ending process. The only certainty is that the VATS of 5 years from now will be as different from the VATS of today as the VATS of today is different from the VATS of 5 years ago. Thoracic surgeons should embrace that, and follow the clear trajectory of improvements to produce even finer surgery for the patients of the future.

REFERENCES

1. Sihoe ADL. The Evolution of VATS Lobectomy. In: Topics in Thoracic Surgery. Cardoso P (Ed). Intech, Rijeka, Croatia, 2011:181–210.
2. Sihoe ADL. The evolution of minimally invasive thoracic surgery: implications for the practice of uniportal thoracoscopic surgery. J Thorac Dis 2014; 6:S604–617.
3. Sihoe ADL, Yim APC. Video-Assisted Pulmonary Resections. In: Patterson GA, Cooper JD, Deslauriers J, et al. (Eds), Thoracic Surgery (3rd edn). Elsevier, Philadelphia, USA, 2008:970–988.
4. Jacobaeus HC. Ueber die Möglichkeit die Zystoskopie bei Untersuchung seröser Höhlungen anzuwenden. München Med Wchenschr 1910; 57:2090–2092.
5. Brainbridge MV. Thoracoscopy – a historical perspective. In: Yim APC, Hazelrigg SR, Izzat MB, et al (Eds): Minimal Access Cardiothoracic Surgery. WB Saunders, Philadelphia, USA, 2000:1–10.
6. Lewis RJ, Caccavale RJ, Sisler GE, et al. One hundred consecutive patients undergoing video-assisted thoracic operations. Ann Thorac Surg 1992; 54:421–426.
7. Roviaro CG, Varoli F, Rebuffat C, et al. Video-thoracoscopic major pulmonary resections: pneumonectomies and lobectomies. Ann Thorac Surg 1993; 56:779–783.
8. Mack MJ, Hazelrigg SR, Landreneau RJ, Naunheim KS. The First International Symposium on Thoracoscopic Surgery. Ann Thorac Surg 1993; 56:605–806.
9. Yim APC, Ko KM, Chau WS, et al. Video-assisted thoracoscopic anatomic lung resections: the initial Hong Kong experience. Chest 1996; 109:13–17.
10. Sihoe ADL, Yim APC. VATS as a diagnostic tool. In: General Thoracic Surgery (7th Edn). Shields TW, Locicero J, Ponn RB, Rusch VW (Eds). Lippincott Williams & Wilkins, Philadelphia, USA, 2009: 313–332.
11. Rogers ML, Duffy JP. Surgical aspects of chronic post-thoracotomy pain. Eur J Cardiothorac Surg 2000; 18:711–716.
12. Karmakar MK, Ho AMH. Post-thoracotomy pain syndrome. Thorac Surg Clin 2004; 14:345–352.
13. Lewis RJ. Simultaneously stapled lobectomy: a safe technique for video-assisted thoracic surgery. J Thorac Cardiovasc Surg 1995; 109:619–625.
14. Lewis RJ, Caccavale RJ. Video-assisted thoracic surgical non-rib-spreading simultaneously stapled lobectomy. In: Yim APC, Hazelrigg SR, Izzat MB, et al (Eds): Minimal access cardiothoracic surgery. WB Saunders, Philadelphia, USA, 2000:135–149.
15. Pearson FG. Commentary. In: Yim APC, Hazelrigg SR, Izzat MB, et al (Eds): Minimal access cardiothoracic surgery. WB Saunders, Philadelphia, USA, 2000:151.
16. Kirby TJ, Mack MJ, Landreneau RJ, et al. Initial experience with video-assisted thoracoscopic lobectomy. Ann Thorac Surg 1993; 56:1248–1253.
17. Walker WS, Pugh GC, Craig SR, Carnochan FM. Continued experience with thoracoscopic major pulmonary resection. Int Surg 1996; 81:255–258.
18. Richards JMJ, Dunning J, Oparka J, Carnochan FM, Walker WS. Video-assisted thoracoscopic lobectomy: The Edinburgh posterior approach. Ann Cardiothorac Surg 2012; 1:61–69.
19. Roviaro CG, Varoli F, Vergani C, Maciocco M. Anatomic lung resection. In: Yim APC, Hazelrigg SR, Izzat MB, et al (Eds): Minimal Access Cardiothoracic Surgery. Philadelphia: WB Saunders, 2000:107–114.
20. McKenna RJ. Lobectomy by video-assisted thoracic surgery with mediastinal node sampling for lung cancer. J Thorac Cardiovasc Surg 1994 107:879–882.
21. McKenna Jr RJ, Houck W, Fuller CB. Video-assisted thoracic surgery lobectomy: experience with 1100 cases. Ann Thorac Surg 2006; 81:421–425.
22. Yim APC, Liu H, Izzat MB, et al. Thoracoscopic major lung resection: an Asian perspective. Semin Thorac Cardiovasc 1998; 10:326–331.
23. McKenna RJ, Jr, Wolf RK, Brenner M, et al. Is VATS lobectomy an adequate cancer operation? Ann Thorac Surg 1998; 66:1903–1908.

24. Yim APC, Liu HP. Complications and failures from video-assisted thoracic surgery: experience from two centers in Asia. Ann Thorac Surg 1996; 61:538–541.
25. Walker WS. Complications and pitfalls in video assisted thoracic surgery. In: Yim APC, Hazelrigg SR, Izzat MB, et al (Eds): Minimal access cardiothoracic surgery. WB Saunders, Philadelphia, USA, 2000:341–348.
26. Downey RJ, McCormick P, LoCicero J, et al. Dissemination of malignant tumors after video-assisted thoracic surgery: A report of twenty-one cases. J Thorac Cardiovasc Surg 1996; 111:954–960.
27. Parekh K, Rusch V, Bains M, et al. VATS port site recurrence: a technique dependent problem. Ann Surg Oncol 2001; 8:175–178.
28. Demmy TL, Curtis JJ. Minimally invasion lobectomy directed toward frail and high-risk patients: a case control study. Ann Thorac Surg 1999; 68:194–200.
29. Sugiura H, Morikawa T, Kaji M, et al. Long-term benefits for the quality of life after video-assisted thoracoscopic lobectomy in patients with lung cancer. Surg Laparosc Endosc 1999; 9:403–408.
30. Giudicelli R, Thomas P, Lonjon T, et al. Video-assisted mini-thoracotomy versus muscle sparing thoracotomy for performing lobectomy. Ann Thorac Surg 1994; 58:712–718.
31. Kirby TJ, Mack MJ, Landreneau RJ, Rice TW. Lobectomy video-assisted thoracic surgery versus muscle-sparing thoracotomy: a randomized trial. J Thorac Cardiovasc Surg 1995; 109:997–1002.
32. Landreneau RJ, Mack MJ, Hazelrigg SR, et al. Post-operative pain-related morbidity: video-assisted thoracic surgery versus thoracotomy. Ann Thorac Surg 1993; 56:1285–1289.
33. Nomori H, Horio H, Naruke T, Suemasu K. What is the advantage of a thoracoscopic lobectomy over a limited thoracotomy procedure for lung cancer surgery? Ann Thorac Surg 2001; 72:879–84.
34. Mack MJ, Scruggs GR, Kelly KM, et al. Video-assisted thoracic surgery: has technology found its place? Ann Thorac Surg 1997; 64:211–215.
35. Lewis RJ. VATS is not thoracoscopy. Ann Thorac Surg 1996; 62:631–632.
36. Yim APC, Landreneau RJ, Izzat MB, Fung ALK. Is video assisted thoracoscopic lobectomy a unified approach? Ann Thorac Surg 1998; 66:1155–1158.
37. Shigemura N, Akashi A, Nakagiri T, Ohta M, Matsuda H. Complete vs. assisted thoracoscopic approach. A prospective randomized trial comparing a variety of video-assisted thoracoscopic lobectomy techniques. Surg Endosc 2004; 18:1492–1497.
38. Shigemura N, Akashi A, Funaki S, et al. Long-term outcomes after a variety of video-assisted thoracoscopic lobectomy approaches for clinical stage IA lung cancer: a multi-institutional study. J Thorac Cardiovasc Surg 2006; 132:507–512.
39. Swanson SJ, Herndon JE 2nd, D'Amico TA, et al. Video-assisted thoracic surgery lobectomy: report of CALGB 39802—a prospective, multi-institution feasibility study. J Clin Oncol 2007; 25:4993–4997.
40. Yim APC. VATS major pulmonary resection revisited: controversies, techniques, and results. Ann Thorac Surg 2002; 74:615–623.
41. Whitson BA, Groth SS, Duval SJ, Swanson SJ, Maddaus MA. Surgery for early-stage non-small cell lung cancer: a systematic review of the video-assisted thoracoscopic surgery versus thoracotomy approaches to lobectomy. Ann Thorac Surg 2008; 86:2008–2018.
42. Scott WJ, Allen MS, Darling G, et al. Video-assisted thoracic surgery versus open lobectomy for lung cancer: a secondary analysis of data from the American College of Surgeons Oncology Group Z0030 randomized clinical trial. J Thorac Cardiovasc Surg 2010; 139:976–983.
43. Sagawa M, Sato M, Sakurada A, et al. A prospective trial of systematic nodal dissection for lung cancer by video-assisted thoracic surgery: can it be perfect? Ann Thorac Surg 2002; 73:900–904.
44. Watanabe A, Koyanagi T, Ohsawa H, et al. Systematic node dissection by VATS is not inferior to that through an open thoracotomy: a comparative clinicopathologic retrospective study. Surgery 2005; 138:510–517.
45. Denlinger CE, Fernandez, Meyers BF, et al. Lymph node evaluation in video-assisted thoracoscopic lobectomy versus lobectomy by thoracotomy. Ann Thorac Surg 2010; 89:1730–1736.
46. Benedetti F, Vighetti S, Ricco C, et al. Neuorphysiologic assessment of nerve impairment in posterolateral and muscle-sparing thoracotomy. J Thorac Cardiovasc Surg 1998; 115:841–847.
47. Benedetti F, Vighetti S, Amanzio M, et al. Dose-response relationship of opioids in nociceptive and neuropathic postoperative pain. Pain 1998; 74:205–211.
48. Nicholson B. Gabapentin use in neuropathic pain syndromes. Acta Neurol Scand 2000; 101:359–371.
49. Laird MA, Gidal BE. Use of gabapentin in the treatment of neuropathic pain. Ann Pharmacother 2000; 34:802–807.
50. Maguire MF, Latter JA, Mahajan R, David Beggs F, Duffy JP. A study exploring the role of intercostal nerve damage in chronic pain after thoracic surgery. Eur J Cardiothorac Surg 2006; 29:873–879.
51. Li WWL, Lee TW, Lam SSY, et al. Quality of life following lung cancer resection: video-assisted thoracic surgery versus thoracotomy. Chest 2002; 122:584–589.
52. Handy JR Jr, Asaph JW, Douville EC, et al. Does video-assisted thoracoscopic lobectomy for lung cancer provide improved functional outcomes compared with open lobectomy? Eur J Cardiothorac Surg 2010; 37:451–455.
53. Rueth NM, Andrade RS. Is VATS lobectomy better: perioperatively, biologically and oncologically? Ann Thorac Surg 2010; 89:S2107–2111.
54. Li WW, Lee RL, Lee TW, et al. The impact of thoracic surgical access on early shoulder function: video-assisted thoracic surgery versus posterolateral thoracotomy. Eur J Cardiothorac Surg 2003; 23:390–396.
55. Kaseda S, Aoki T. Video-assisted thoracic surgical lobectomy in conjunction with lymphadenectomy for lung cancer. J Jap Surg Soc 2002; 103:717–721.
56. Nakata M, Saeki H, Yokoyama N, et al. Pulmonary function after lobectomy: video-assisted thoracic surgery versus thoracotomy. Ann Thorac Surg 2000; 70:938–941.
57. Nagahiro I, Andou A, Aoe M, et al. Pulmonary function, postoperative pain, and serum cytokine level after lobectomy: a comparison of VATS and conventional procedure. Ann Thorac Surg 2001; 72:362–365.
58. Nomori H, Horio H, Naruke T, Suemasu K. Posterolateral thoracotomy is behind limited thoracotomy and thoracoscopic surgery in terms of postoperative pulmonary function and walking capacity. Eur J Cardiothorac Surg 2002; 21:155–156.
59. Nomori H, Ohtsuka T, Horio H, et al. Difference in the impairment of vital capacity and 6-minute walking after a lobectomy performed by thoracoscopic surgery, an anterior limited thoracotomy, an anteroaxillary thoracotomy, and a posterolateral thoracotomy. Surg Today 2003; 33:7–12.
60. Yim APC, Wan S, Lee TW, Arifi AA. VATS lobectomy reduces cytokine responses compared with conventional surgery. Ann Thorac Surg 2000; 70:243–247.
61. Sugi K, Kaneda Y, Esato K. Video-assisted thoracoscopic lobectomy reduces cytokine production more than conventional open lobectomy. Jpn J Thorac Cardiovasc Surg 2000; 48:161–165.
62. Leaver HA, Craig SR, Yap PL, Walker WS. Lymphocyte responses following open and minimally invasive thoracic surgery. Eur J Clin Invest 2000; 30:230–238.
63. Craig SR, Leaver HA, Yap PL, et al. Acute phase responses following minimal access and conventional thoracic surgery. Eur J Cardiothorac Surg 2001; 20:455–463.
64. Ng CS, Lee TW, Wan S, et al. Thoracotomy is associated with significantly more profound suppression in lymphocytes and natural killer cells than video-assisted thoracic surgery following major lung resections for cancer. J Invest Surg 2005; 18:81–88.
65. Szczesny TJ, Slotwinski R, Stankiewicz A, et al. Interleukin 6 and interleukin 1 receptor antagonist as early markers of postoperative complications after lung cancer surgery. Eur J Cardiothorac Surg 2007; 1:719–724.
66. Sugi K, Kaneda Y, Esato K. Video-assisted thoracoscopic lobectomy achieves a satisfactory long-term prognosis in patients with clinical stage IA lung cancer. World J Surg 2000; 24:27–30.
67. Yan TD, Black D, Bannon PG, McCaughan BC. Systematic review and meta-analysis of randomized and nonrandomized trials on safety and efficacy of video-assisted thoracic surgery lobectomy for early-stage non-small-cell lung cancer. J Clin Oncol 2009; 27:2553–2562.
68. Yamashita JI, Kurusu Y, Fujino N. Detection of circulating tumor cells in patients with non-small cell lung cancer undergoing lobectomy by video-assisted thoracic surgery: a potential hazard for intraoperative hematogenous tumor cell dissemination. J Thorac Cardiovasc Surg 2000; 119:899–905.
69. Shariat SF, Lamb DJ, Kattan MW, et al. Association of preoperative plasma levels of insulin-like growth factor I and insulin-like growth factor binding proteins-2 and -3 with prostate cancer invasion, progression, and metastasis. J Clin Oncol 2002; 20:833–841.

70. Wu Y, Yakar S, Zhao L, Hennighausen L, LeRoith D. Circulating insulin-like growth factor-1 levels regulate colon cancer growth and metastasis. Cancer Res 2002; 62:1030–1035.
71. Nomori H, Ohtsuka T, Horio H, Naruke T, Suemasu K. Thoracoscopic lobectomy for lung cancer with a largely fused fissure. Chest 2003; 123:619–622.
72. Kim K, Kim HK, Park JS, et al. Video-assisted thoracic surgery lobectomy: single institutional experience with 704 cases Ann Thorac Surg 2010; 89:S2118–2122.
73. Mun M, Kohno T. Video-assisted thoracic surgery for clinical stage I lung cancer in octogenarians. Ann Thorac Surg 2008; 85:406–411.
74. Wilkins EW Jr, Scannell JG, Craver JC. Four decades of experience with resections for bronchogenic carcinoma at the Massachusetts General Hospital. J Thorac Cardiovasc Surg 1978; 76:364.
75. Keagy BA, Lores ME, Starek PJK. Elective pulmonary lobectomy: factors associated with morbidity and operative mortality. Ann Thorac Surg 1985; 40:349–352.
76. Melfi FM, Menconi GF, Mariani AM, et al. Early experience with robotic technology for thoracoscopic surgery. Eur J Cardiothorac Surg 2002; 21:864–868.
77. Veronesi G, Galetta D, Maisonneuve P, et al. Four-arm robotic lobectomy for the treatment of early-stage lung cancer. J Thorac Cardiovasc Surg 2010; 140:19–25.
78. D'Amico TA. Robotics in thoracic surgery: applications and outcomes. J Thorac Cardiovasc Surg 2006; 131:19–20.
79. Swanson, SJ. Robotic pulmonary lobectomy: the future and probably should remain so. J Thorac Cardiovasc Surg 2010; 140:954.
80. Yim APC, Sihoe ADL, Lee TW, Arifi AA. A simple maneuver to detect airleak on-table following 'needlescopic' VATS. J Thorac Cardiovasc Surg 2002; 124:1029–1030.
81. Sihoe ADL, Cheung CS, Lai HK, et al. Incidence of chest wall paresthesia after needlescopic video-assisted thoracic surgery for palmar hyperhidrosis. Eur J Cardiothorac Surg 2005; 27:313–319.
82. Sihoe AD, Manlulu AV, Lee TW, Thung KH, Yim AP. Pre-emptive local anesthesia for needlescopic video-assisted thoracic surgery: a randomised controlled trial. Eur J Cardiothorac Surg 2007; 31:103–108.
83. Sihoe ADL, Yu PA, Wong JCC, Lee KM, Heung TCY, Ho TSY. Needlescopic Video-assisted thoracic surgery for primary spontaneous pneumothorax. Respirology 2012; 17:17–24.
84. Sihoe ADL, Hsin MKY, Yu PSY. Needlescopic video-assisted thoracic surgery for primary pneumothorax. Multimed Man Cardiothorac Surg 2014; 2014. pii: mmu012.
85. D'Amico TA. Thoracoscopic segmentectomy: technical considerations and outcomes. Ann Thorac Surg 2008; 85:S716–718.
86. Kim HK, Sung HK, Lee HJ, Choi YH. The feasibility of a two-incision video-assisted thoracoscopic lobectomy. J Cardiothorac Surg 2013; 8:88.
87. Rocco G, Khalil M, Jutley R. Uniportal video-assisted thoracoscopic surgery wedge lung biopsy in the diagnosis of interstitial lung diseases. J Thorac Cardiovasc Surg 2005; 129:947–948.
88. Jutley RS, Khalil MW, Rocco G. Uniportal vs. standard three-port VATS technique for spontaneous pneumothorax: comparison of post-operative pain and residual paraesthesia. Eur J Cardiothorac Surg 2005; 28:43–46.
89. Bertolaccini L, Rocco G, Viti A, et al. Geometrical characteristics of uniportal VATS. J Thorac Dis 2013; 5:S214–216.
90. Gonzalez D, Paradela M, Garcia J, de la Torre M. Single-port video-assisted thoracoscopic lobectomy. Interact Cardiovasc Thorac Surg 2011; 12:514–515.
91. Gonzalez-Rivas D, Fieira E, Mendez L, Garcia J. Single-port video-assisted thoracoscopic anatomic segmentectomy and right upper lobectomy. Eur J Cardiothorac Surg 2012; 42:e169–171.
92. Gonzalez-Rivas D, Fernandez R, Fieira E, Rellan L. Uniportal video-assisted thoracoscopic bronchial sleeve lobectomy: first report. J Thorac Cardiovasc Surg 2013; 145:1676–1677.
93. Gonzalez-Rivas D, Delgado M, Fieira E, Mendez L. Single-port video-assisted thoracoscopic lobectomy with pulmonary artery reconstruction. Interact Cardiovasc Thorac Surg 2013; 17:889–891.
94. Liu CY, Lin CS, Liu CC. Subxiphoid single-incision thoracoscopic surgery for bilateral primary spontaneous pneumothorax. Wideochir Inne Tech Maloinwazyjne 2015; 10:125–128.
95. Zhu LH, Wang W, Yang S, et al. Transumbilical thoracic sympathectomy with an ultrathin flexible endoscope in a series of 38 patients. Surg Endosc 2013; 27:2149–2155.
96. Simaan N, Bajo A, Reiter A, et al. Lessons learned using the insertable robotic effector platform (IREP) for single port access surgery. J Robot Surg 2013; 7:235–240.
97. Fernando HC, De Hoyos A, Landreneau RJ, et al. Radiofrequency ablation for the treatment of non-small cell lung cancer in marginal surgical candidates. J Thorac Cardiovasc Surg 2005; 129:639–644.
98. Pennathur A, Luketich JD, Heron DE, et al. Stereotactic radiosurgery for the treatment of stage I non-small cell lung cancer in high-risk patients J Thorac Cardiovasc Surg 2009; 137:597–604.
99. Crabtree TD, Denlinger CE, Meyers BF, et al. Stereotactic body radiation therapy versus surgical resection for stage I non–small cell lung cancer. J Thorac Cardiovasc Surg 2010; 140:377–386.
100. Ginsberg RJ, Rubinstein LV. Randomized trial of lobectomy versus limited resection for T1 N0 non-small cell lung cancer. Ann Thorac Surg 1995; 60:615–623.
101. Fernando HC, Santos RS, Benfield JR. Lobar and sublobar resection with and without brachytherapy for small stage IA non-small cell lung cancer. J Thorac Cardiovasc Surg 2005; 129:261–267.
102. Okada M, Nishio W, Sakamoto T. Effect of tumor size on prognosis in patients with non-small cell lung cancer: the role of segmentectomy as a type of lesser resection. J Thorac Cardiovasc Surg 2005; 129:87–93.
103. Schuchert MJ, Kilic A, Pennathur A. Oncologic outcomes after surgical resection of subcentimeter non-small cell lung cancer. Ann Thorac Surg 2011; 91:1681–1688.
104. Schuchert MJ, Abbas G, Awais O. Anatomic segmentectomy for the solitary pulmonary nodule and early-stage lung cancer. Ann Thorac Surg 2012; 93:1780–1787.
105. Kates M, Swanson S, Wisnivesky JP. Survival following lobectomy and limited resection for the treatment of stage I non-small cell lung cancer ≤1 cm in size: a review of SEER data. Chest 2011; 139:491–496.
106. Altorki NK, Yip R, Hanaoka T. Sublobar resection is equivalent to lobectomyfor clinical stage 1A lung cancer in solid nodules. J Thorac Cardiovasc Surg 2014; 147:754–764.
107. Sihoe AD, Van Schil P. Non-small cell lung cancer: when to offer sublobar resection. Lung Cancer 2014; 86:115–120. .
108. Yang CF, D'Amico TA. Thoracoscopic segmentectomy for lung cancer. Ann Thorac Surg 2012; 94:668–681.
109. Sihoe ADL, Au SS, Cheung ML, et al. Incidence of chest wall paresthesia after video-assisted thoracic surgery for primary spontaneous pneumothorax. Eur J Cardiothorac Surg 2004; 25:1054–1058.
110. Sihoe AD, Lee TW, Wan IY, Thung KH, Yim AP. The use of gabapentin for post-operative and post-traumatic pain in thoracic surgery patients Eur J Cardiothorac Surg 2006; 29:795–799.
111. Pompili C, Detterbeck F, Papagiannopoulos K, et al. Multicenter international randomized comparison of objective and subjective outcomes between electronic and traditional chest drainage systems. Ann Thorac Surg 2014; 98:490–497.
112. Sihoe ADL, Cheng LC. The evolution of minimally invasive surgery for lung cancer. Hong Kong Med Assoc Bulletin 2014:11–20.
113. González-Rivas D, Fernandez R, de la Torre M, et al. Single-port thoracoscopic lobectomy in a nonintubated patient: the least invasive procedure for major lung resection? Interact Cardiovasc Thorac Surg 2014; 19:552–555.
114. Liu J, Cui F, Li S, et al. Nonintubated video-assisted thoracoscopic surgery under epidural anesthesia compared with conventional anesthetic option: a randomized control study. Surg Innov 2015; 22:123–130.
115. Pompeo E, Mineo TC. Awake operative videothoracoscopic pulmonary resections. Thorac Surg Clin 2008; 18:311–320.
116. Al-Abdullatief M, Wahood A, Al-Shirawi N, et al. Awake anaesthesia for major thoracic surgical procedures: an observational study. Eur J Cardiothorac Surg 2007; 32:346–350.
117. Rocco G, Romano V, Accardo R, et al. Awake single-access (uniportal) video-assisted thoracoscopic surgery for peripheral pulmonary nodules in a complete ambulatory setting. Ann Thorac Surg 2010; 89:1625–1627.
118. Abolhoda A, Liu D, Brooks A, Burt M. Prolonged air leak following radical upper lobectomy. An analysis of incidence and possible risk factors. Chest 1998; 113:1507–1510.
119. Brunelli A, Fianchini A. Prolonged air leak following upper lobectomy: in search of the key. Chest 1999; 116:848.
120. Isowa N, Hasegawa S, Bando T, Wada H. Preoperative risk factors for prolonged air leak following lobectomy or segmentectomy for primary lung cancer. Eur J Cardiothorac Surg 2002; 21:951.

121. Okereke I, Murthy SC, Alster JM, Blackstone EH, Rice TW. Characterization and importance of air leak after lobectomy. Ann Thorac Surg 2005; 79:1167–1173.
122. Tansley P, Al-Mulhim F, Lim E, Ladas G, Goldstraw P. A prospective, randomized, controlled trial of the effectiveness of BioGlue in treating alveolar air leaks. J Thorac Cardiovasc Surg 2006; 132:105–112.
123. D'Andrilli A, Andreetti C, Ibrahim M, et al. A prospective randomized study to assess the efficacy of a surgical sealant to treat air leaks in lung surgery. Eur J Cardiothorac Surg 2009; 35:817–821.
124. Varela G, Jiménez MF, Novoa NM, Aranda JL. Postoperative chest tube management: measuring air leak using an electronic device decreases variability in the clinical practice. Eur J Cardiothorac Surg 2009; 35:28–31.
125. Brunelli A, Salati M, Pompili C, Refai M, Sabbatini A. Regulated tailored suction vs. regulated seal: a prospective randomized trial on air leak duration. Eur J Cardiothorac Surg 2013; 43:899–904.
126. Kurimoto N, Miyazawa T. Endobronchial ultrasonography. Semin Respir Crit Care Med 2004; 25:425–431.
127. Leong S, Ju H, Marshall H, et al. Electromagnetic navigation bronchoscopy: A descriptive analysis. J Thorac Dis 2012; 4:173–185.
128. Wiener RS, Schwartz LM, Woloshin S, Welch HG. Population-based risk for complications after transthoracic needle lung biopsy of a pulmonary nodule: an analysis of discharge records. Ann Intern Med 2011; 155:137–144.
129. Sihoe ADL, Hiranandani R, Wong H, Yeung ESL. Operating on a suspicious lung mass without a pre-operative tissue diagnosis: pros and cons. Eur J Cardiothorac Surg 2013; 44:231–237.
130. Gonzalez-Rivas D, Paradela M, Fernandez R, et al. Uniportal video-assisted thoracoscopic lobectomy: two years of experience. Ann Thorac Surg 2013; 95:426–432.
131. Gonzalez-Rivas D, Fieira E, Delgado M, et al. Is uniportal thoracoscopic surgery a feasible approach for advanced stages of non-small cell lung cancer? J Thorac Dis 2014; 6:641–648.
132. McElnay PJ, Molyneux M, Krishnadas R, et al. Pain and recovery are comparable after either uniportal and multiport video assisted thoracoscopic lobectomy: an observation study. Eur J Cardiothorac Surg 2015; 47:912–915.
133. Chung JH, Choi YS, Cho JH, et al. Uniportal video-assisted thoracoscopic lobectomy: an alternative to conventional thoracoscopic lobectomy in lung cancer surgery? Interact Cardiovasc Thorac Surg 2015; 20:813–819.
134. Howington JA, Blum MG, Chang AC, Balekian AA, Murthy SC. Treatment of stage I and II non-small cell lung cancer: Diagnosis and management of lung cancer, 3rd edn: American College of Chest Physicians evidence-based clinical practice guidelines. Chest 2013; 143:e278S–313S.
135. Nakajima J, Takamoto S, Kohno T, Ohtsuka T. Costs of videothoracoscopic surgery versus open resection for patients with of lung carcinoma. Cancer 2000; 89:2497–2501.
136. Ferguson J, Walker W. Developing a VATS lobectomy programme – can VATS lobectomy be taught? Eur J Cardiothorac Surg 2006; 29:806–809.

Chapter 3 Establishing a minimally invasive thoracic surgery program

John P Costello, M Blair Marshall

INTRODUCTION

The birth of minimally invasive thoracic surgery (MITS) has revolutionized the surgical management of all aspects of lung and esophageal disease. Although individual surgeons may utilize less invasive or truly minimally invasive approaches in various forms of chest surgery in their practices, establishing an official minimally invasive program is a more substantial undertaking. Guidelines for creating a MITS program are not well-established; however, they can be extrapolated from those that have been utilized for building new surgical programs in other specialties.

Video-assisted thoracoscopic surgery (VATS) has been in use for a few decades, and although it is common and not necessarily a 'new technology', its use has not been uniformly embraced by thoracic surgeons in the United States.[1,2] Unlike other disciplines, general thoracic surgery encompasses a variety of smaller disciplines that are each associated with different new techniques and technologies. As an initiative, it would be easier for all involved to start with a focused effort in one area, and then build on each success with the introduction of additional procedures. For instance, a new program may start by transitioning to VATS lobectomy, or to minimally invasive esophagectomy, or to a minimally invasive diagnostic suite that encompasses the ability to perform EBUS, navigation bronchoscopy, and computed tomography-guided biopsies.[3] Each of these has specific strategic differences, including instrumentation, resources, and capital development, that pose their own challenges. For example, because the approach to VATS lobectomy, minimally invasive esophagectomy, and VATS resection of mediastinal masses is diverse, it will be more challenging to train a team to attempt introduction of these all at once as opposed to focusing on one new procedure at a time.

The following review will provide a framework for identifying the critical elements necessary to establish a MITS program and how these elements can be applied at one's own institution.

KEY PRINCIPLES

The National Health Service in the UK has seven pillars of governance which must be applied to all clinical practice.[4] While medical practitioners outside the UK are not bound by these seven pillars, they do address key principles that can be applied to surgical practice in any location and provide a good framework of the components with which a new surgical program can be built. These original seven pillars are:[4]

- Clinical effectiveness
- Risk management effectiveness
- Patient experience
- Communication effectiveness
- Resource effectiveness
- Strategic effectiveness
- Learning effectiveness

A key question, however, is why should one use this particular framework when building a MITS program? The decision of whether or not to support a minimally invasive program at the institutional level will be at the discretion of the hospital or health system administration. However, these seven pillars can be used to facilitate the professional discussion between practitioner and administrator when formally seeking institutional support to start a new program.[4]

When looking to establish any new program in the hospital setting, it is imperative that the clinical effectiveness of a given new approach to surgery or treatment is proven.[4] From the perspective of MITS, a robust body of data exists to prove its clinical efficacy in modern practice. This is true in both the thoracic and cardiac specialties. Although not universally utilized by all surgeons, the VATS approach to many different procedures is not only feasible but can often be superior to open techniques.[5,6,7] Minimally invasive approaches to thoracic surgery are not only effective, but represent the future for the clinical field. As the surgeon and entire team become more comfortable with these minimally invasive techniques, there is a natural progression to push the limit on what can be performed with these innovative approaches.

The concept of risk management is crucial to adapting new techniques to any practice, particularly in the operating room.[4] Surgeons must acknowledge that, regardless of their level of experience or expertise, a learning curve does exist for any procedure.[8,9] This learning curve applies not only to the operating surgeon but is equally applicable to the whole team taking care of the patient in the operating room, from the anesthesiologist to the circulating nurse. Prior to negotiating for a new program, surgeons must have a clear view of their current outcomes with which to compare the results and effectiveness of a new program. Even if being recruited to a new institution, one should know where that institution lies in regard to volume, morbidity, mortality, and length of stay. One must also have a clear vision of where the current program is situated, the future goals of the program, as well as the achievements of similar successful programs with which to compare one's program. Thoracic surgery is a fairly small community. For the inexperienced surgeon, there are often opportunities through societal funding to train with an expert in new techniques and take the opportunity not only to increase their familiarity with the technical aspects of a procedure but also to identify the key elements of a successful program.

Although intuitive to the experienced surgeon, effective communication is a mandatory component in establishing any new clinical program.[4] This includes ensuring that steps and expectations are communicated with and understood by staff members involved in all phases of the patient's care: preoperatively, in the operating room, postoperatively in the inpatient setting, and in outpatient follow-up.

Having a standardized team, particularly in the operating room, for approximately the first 20 procedures during which a new minimally invasive approach is utilized is an essential component to this communication effectiveness principle.[4,10] However, having the same team present for every case is often a challenging feat from a personnel perspective. As such, it is not enough to just have a team. The surgeon must be a leader and be able to share his vision of the program. He must inspire other members of the team to join in the program's overall endeavors. It will take extra effort by others to achieve success, and having team members who share the same vision and are inspired by the same end-goals will help the surgeon's efforts.

An evaluation of the effectiveness of new minimally invasive approaches from a resource perspective must not be underestimated by the thoracic surgeon.[4] Even if one's own clinical judgment on what surgery or treatment is best for a patient is uniformly accepted at a given institution, it must be acknowledged that the cost of the treatments being provided will be analyzed, especially when new or novel techniques are utilized.[11] If a particular hospital or practice does not have a full complement of scopes and equipment required to perform minimally invasive thoracic surgical procedures, the initial capital costs and ongoing disposable costs can be substantial and must be appreciated by any surgeon or administrator looking to establish a new minimally invasive program. Although these upfront costs can be high, they may be offset by savings in other aspects of the patient's care, including the shortened length of hospital stay for which these new procedures may allow. When it comes to resource utilization, hospital budgets are typically siloed where costs are concerned with costs incurred in the operating room being separate from inpatient costs. Thus, the surgeon must be aware and informed of all of the costs and potential savings of a new technique or procedure in order to justify the expenditures and demonstrate the opportunity for savings.

Two additional guiding principles that should be applied when establishing a new minimally invasive program are strategic and learning effectiveness.[4] The strategic effectiveness element should not be limited in its application to a new program or technique; it is good practice for any clinical surgeon and allows for monitoring results and improving outcomes. Various elements, such as procedure time, inpatient length of hospitalization, satisfaction scores, and morbidities, among others, should be tracked and analyzed on a regular basis.[4] Programs should also look ahead and envision where a clinical practice is hoping to develop in order to plan for the tracking and monitoring of future outcomes. In addition, once the program is established, the opportunity for marketing and increasing patient volume should not be missed.

Learning effectiveness should incorporate both elements of education and training, and it should apply to the entire team, not just those performing the surgery.[4] This becomes all the more important when one acknowledges that in order for a team to be effective, all team members must be valued and their opinions and suggestions welcomed.[12] This will ensure that the team grows together and that ownership of the new technique or process is shared by all members. We find that this is particularly true when developing a new program for the operating room. The additional operating room team members, comprised of nursing, scrub technicians, and anesthesia, are exposed to the patient only on the day of the operation and have minimal opportunities to appreciate the benefits of a minimally invasive approach in comparison with traditional approaches. They do not see the patients when they return nor the healed incisions. Also, at times it may be difficult for us as the operating surgeons to anticipate the specific challenges related to their respective individual roles in a new program if this open dialogue among all team members does not occur.

Once the program has been approved and one is in the planning phase, several meetings with all members of the team should take place to review the objectives of the program, the changes to the current program, and how the new technology and or instrumentation will contribute to the goals of the program. It is important that the benefits to the patient are communicated. We have found that the constant use of the camera and monitors has additional benefits for the team as it is the only time that all team members can see and understand the challenges faced by the surgeon during the entire operation. We find that it is easier for scrub technicians to play a more active role in assisting the surgeon as they are watching exactly what is taking place. In addition, everyone in the room plays a more active role in problem solving when visualization of the task at hand is appreciated by the entire team. For example, in VATS chest wall resection, given the location of the chest wall that is planned for resection and the ergonomics of the chest wall, our team is able to find me instruments that I do not know exist to aid in the division of the chest wall. These instruments are often obtained from neurosurgery, orthopedic, and craniofacial operative sets.

Performing a new procedure is not the time to be concerned about teaching a trainee – this can only add an additional level of complexity. It is important to first perform several procedures to establish the fluidity of the operation. Once the surgeon is comfortable with the procedure, the team, and the outcomes, teaching the new procedure can be introduced. This is approached in a similar methodical manner while maximizing attention to safety. For example, when teaching VATS lobectomy, we start residents in a step-by-step fashion. If they struggle on a particular step, the attending will take over the dissection from that point on. This allows for focused feedback for the resident and safe progression of the operation. In addition, routine recording of minimally invasive procedures allows one to review the technical aspects of the procedure in a de-stressed environment that is focused on resident education rather than on the objectives of the operation.

Before a surgeon starts to adopt new minimally invasive thoracic surgical techniques at an institution that is not familiar with these procedures, a stepwise progression of approval and training is suggested. A surgeon should not proceed with clinical implementation of a new approach without institutional support.[10] Additional steps that can be helpful for the thoracic surgeon developing a new minimally invasive program include establishing standardized periprocedural checklists and protocols. These tools will guide the entire team in the consistent management of each individual patient. This standardization of care will also facilitate the tracking of outcomes of each new minimally invasive approach.

As with the introduction of anything new, the benefits of simulation are significant. When possible, taking the team through a dry run of any procedure has several downstream benefits:

1. Identifying ergonomic interference in the operating room
2. Strategizing on particular challenges that could be encountered during the procedure, and
3. Team building

The latter is very important. Inadequate preoperative discussion of cases among the team has been associated with an increased risk of minor intraoperative adverse events.[13] Taking the team through a simulated procedure allows the team to work together in a less stressful environment. Minds are open to consider potential problems and solutions together. It is an opportunity to show the team how much you, as the leader, value their input and contributions

For any medical practitioner, the duty to the patient is the ultimate focus of all medical care. The concept of the patient experience remains a key component of clinical practice,[4] and recognizing its full importance is imperative in the process of establishing a new minimally invasive program. Although less invasive approaches to thoracic surgery have numerous advantages from the patient's perspective (e.g. shorter hospitalization, quicker recovery, improved cosmetic result), the patient must still understand the full benefits and risks of the procedure. Included in this disclosure should be a discussion of how the risks of any new surgical approaches are being evaluated and minimized.[4]

CONCLUSION

When contemplating the introduction of a new service line, such as a MITS program, it should be approached in a stepwise fashion. By applying minimally invasive techniques to one surgical procedure at a time, the surgeon will be able to focus on building a strong foundation with a specific patient, a specific team, and one operative technique while avoiding the pitfalls of attempting to implement multiple new techniques all at once. By following this standardized approach, the introducing surgeon will ensure strong team building, communication, understanding, and institutional support, all paramount to safe and effective patient care. Consistency and success in one operation will lay the foundation for both a clinical and institutional rationale to proceed with applying minimally invasive approaches to additional operations. This, in turn, will generate data on outcomes that will attract patients and support a strong, lasting precedent for the continued application of minimally invasive approaches to thoracic surgical care.

REFERENCES

1. Boffa DJ, Kosinski AS, Paul S, Mitchell JD, Onaitis M. Lymphnode evaluation by open or video-assisted approaches in 11,500 anatomic lung cancer resections. Ann Thorac Surg 2012; 94:347–353.
2. Ceppa DP, Kosinski AS, Berry MF, et al. Thoracoscopic lobectomy has increasing benefit in patients with poor pulmonary function: a Society of Thoracic Surgeons Database analysis. Ann Surg 2012; 256:487–493.
3. Silvestri GA, Feller-Kopman D, Chen A, et al. Latest advances in advanced diagnostic and therapeutic pulmonary procedures. Chest 2012; 142:1636–1644.
4. Hunter S. How to start a minimal access mitral valve program. Ann Cardiothorac Surg 2013; 2:774–778.
5. Falcoz PE, Puyraveau M, Thomas PA, et al. Video-assisted thoracoscopic surgery versus open lobectomy for primary non-small-cell lung cancer: a propensity-matched analysis of outcome from the European Society of Thoracic Surgeon database. Eur J Cardiothorac Surg 2016; 49:602–609.
6. Klapper J, D'Amico TA. VATS versus open surgery for lung cancer resection: moving toward a minimally invasive approach. J Natl Compr Canc Netw 2015 13:162–164.
7. Sgourakis G, Gockel I, Radtke A, et al. Minimally invasive versus open esophagectomy: meta-analysis of outcomes. Dig Dis Sci 2010; 55:3031–3040.
8. Maruthappu M, El-Harasis MA, Nagendran M, et al. Systematic review of methodological quality of individual performance measurement in surgery. Br J Surg 2014; 101:1491–1498.
9. Maruthappu M, Gilbert BJ, El-Harasis MA, et al. The influence of volume and experience on individual surgical performance: a systematic review. Ann Surg 2015; 261:642–647.
10. Kumta NA, Mehta S, Kedia P, et al. Peroral endoscopic myotomy: establishing a new program. Clin Endosc 2014; 47:389–397.
11. Tan JM, Macario A. How to evaluate whether a new technology in the operating room is cost-effective from society's viewpoint. Anesthesiol Clin 2008; 26:745–764.
12. Sax HC. Building high-performance teams in the operating room. Surg Clin North Am 2012; 92:15–19.
13. Phadnis J, Templeton-Ward O. Inadequate preoperative team briefings lead to more intraoperative adverse events. J Patient Saf 2015.

Chapter 4 Anesthetic considerations

Joanne Irons, James Moore

INTRODUCTION

The widespread adoption of video-assisted thoracoscopic surgical techniques in thoracic surgery has driven improved patient outcomes including survival, reduced complications and a shorter recovery. As a result, increasingly complex surgical procedures are now being performed on older and sicker patients. This has led to an evolution in anesthetic techniques and philosophy and reinforces the need for a close partnership between the thoracic surgeon and anesthetist.

Effective communication and teamwork are essential to protect patient safety and further improve outcomes. It is essential that thoracic surgeons have a good understanding of the anesthetic techniques that can be offered to support video-assisted thoracoscopic surgery (VATS).

Thoracic surgery provides challenges to the anesthetists which are unique from all other surgeries. These include positioning in the lateral position, managing the effects of manipulation of thoracic organs, the potential for major bleeding and the provision of surgical exposure by lung isolation techniques and one-lung ventilation.

LUNG ISOLATION

The successful conduct of minimally invasive thoracic surgery (MITS) demands optimal surgical visualization. In order to achieve maximal surgical exposure, the anesthetist must deliver rapid and complete lung collapse. Unlike open surgery, with the ability for lung retraction and periods of alternate ventilation and apnea, this is not always possible in VATS and there is limited tolerance for incomplete collapse.

Double-lumen tube

The left-sided double-lumen tube (**Figures 4.1** and **4.2**) remains the most popular choice for lung isolation. It provides reliable lung collapse with a higher margin of safety than the right-sided tube. It is relatively easy to position due to the increased length of the left main bronchus.

The correct sizing and insertion depth of the double-lumen tube is important to ensure good lung isolation. This is based on the sex and height of the patient. The availability of fiberoptic bronchoscopy makes positioning of the tube safer and more reliable (**Figure 4.3**).

The right-sided double-lumen tube (**Figures 4.1** and **4.2**) is indicated in specific circumstances such as obstruction to the left main bronchus, a short left main bronchus or surgery to the left main bronchus. Although many anesthetists choose to place a right-sided tube for a left pneumonectomy, this procedure can still be performed with a left-sided tube, providing there is good communication between the anesthetist and surgeon at the time of the bronchial division and anastomosis to allow retraction of the tube out of the left main bronchus.

The right-sided tube is more difficult to position due to the short right main bronchus, the proximal position of the right upper lobe bronchus and the multiple anatomical variations in its location. Fiberoptic bronchoscopy to guide correct positioning is mandatory. Right-sided tubes are also more likely to displace during positioning or surgical manipulation and are slightly more expensive.

Bronchial blockers

Lung isolation can also be achieved by blockade of a main-stem or selective bronchus with a bronchial blocker device (**Figure 4.4**). Successful use of these devices relies on familiarity with the device, knowledge of tracheobronchial anatomy, good fiberoptic bronchoscopy skills and awareness of their limitations and potential complications.

The bronchial blocker devices currently in use all are in the form of a catheter with one or two distal balloons at the tip that may be inflated in the bronchus. They are inserted through, or adjacent to a single-lumen endotracheal tube.

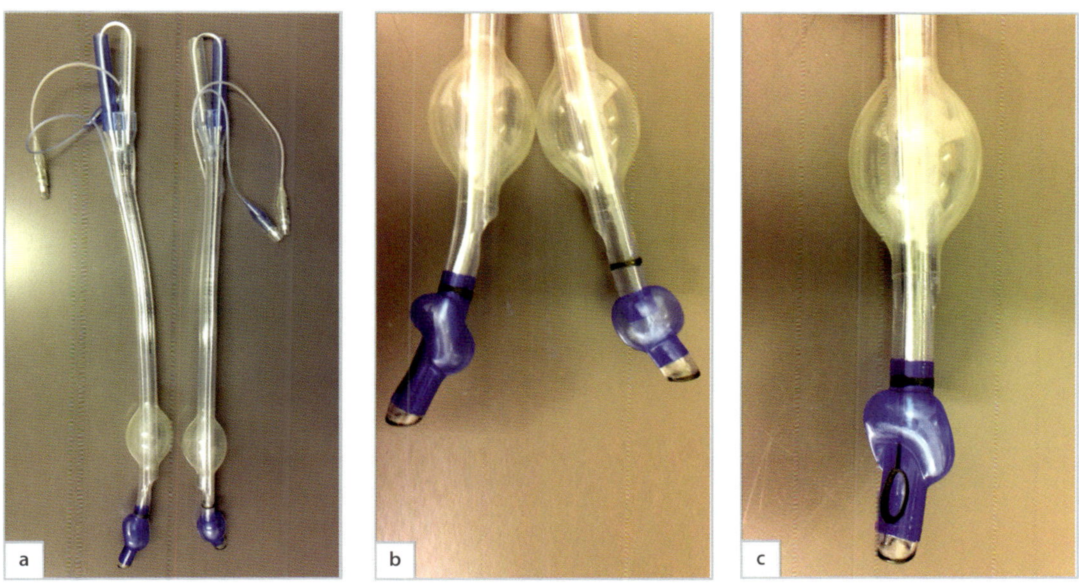

Figure 4.1 Right and left double lumen tubes (a and b). Note the difference in the right bronchial blue cuff shape and the 'murphy eye' for positioning over the right upper lobe bronchus (c).

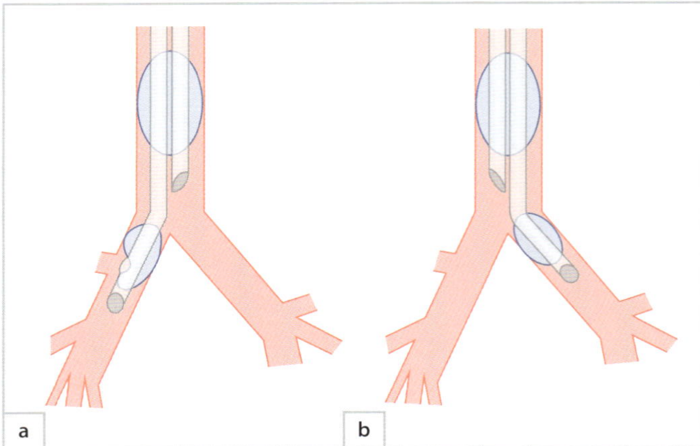

Figure 4.2 Positioning of (a) right and (b) left double lumen tube in the trachea and bronchus.

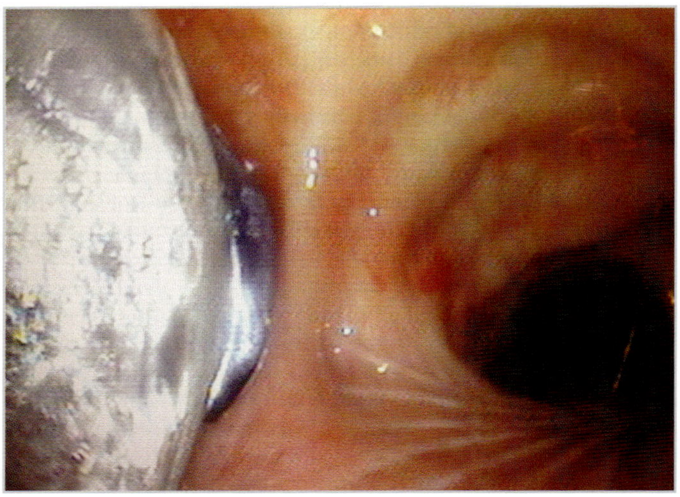

Figure 4.3 Fiberoptic bronchoscope view of a left double-lumen tube position from the tracheal lumen. Note the carina, the bronchial lumen in the left main bronchus with the edge of the blue cuff just visible and an unobstructed right main bronchus.

Bronchial blockers are preferred in patients with difficult airways (as double-lumen tube placement may be particularly difficult in this group), patients with a tracheostomy in situ, those with abnormal tracheobronchial anatomy, those with an endotracheal tube already in situ or in those where lung isolation was not expected to be required and patients requiring selective lobar collapse.

The bronchial blocker is a high maintenance device and special care and attention must be taken to avoid malposition and catastrophic complications such as occlusion of the trachea and complete airway obstruction. There is a higher risk of dislodgement and the position should be reassessed regularly using a fiberoptic scope, especially following a change in patient posture. A further limitation is the small caliber of catheter meaning that lung collapse is slower. Although lung collapse may be aided by suctioning air through the catheter, the small diameter of the suction lumen means that it is not possible to effectively suction secretions or blood (**Table 4.1**).

Spontaneous ventilation and pneumothorax

Recently there has been increased interest in performing MITS on patients who are spontaneously ventilating either under general anesthesia with a laryngeal mask airway or under sedation, with the aid of local or regional anesthesia. This allows the creation of a spontaneous pneumothorax as the surgeon enters the chest and can provide excellent lung isolation as long as there is a patent airway to allow complete lung collapse. This has the added benefit of no positive pressure ventilation on the dependant lung causing less mediastinal shifts and potentially less ventilator induced lung injury. This is discussed in more detail in Chapter 27.

Protective lung ventilation

One-lung ventilation during thoracic surgery increases the risk of ventilator induced lung injury when compared to conventional two-lung ventilation (**Table 4.2**). Larger tidal volumes and higher peak airway pressures are associated with the development of acute lung injury and pulmonary edema. Traditional management of these patients had consisted of high tidal volumes (typically 8–12 mL/kg) to prevent atelectasis and low or zero levels of positive end-expiratory pressure (PEEP) to avoid shunt. This practice is not supported by good evidence

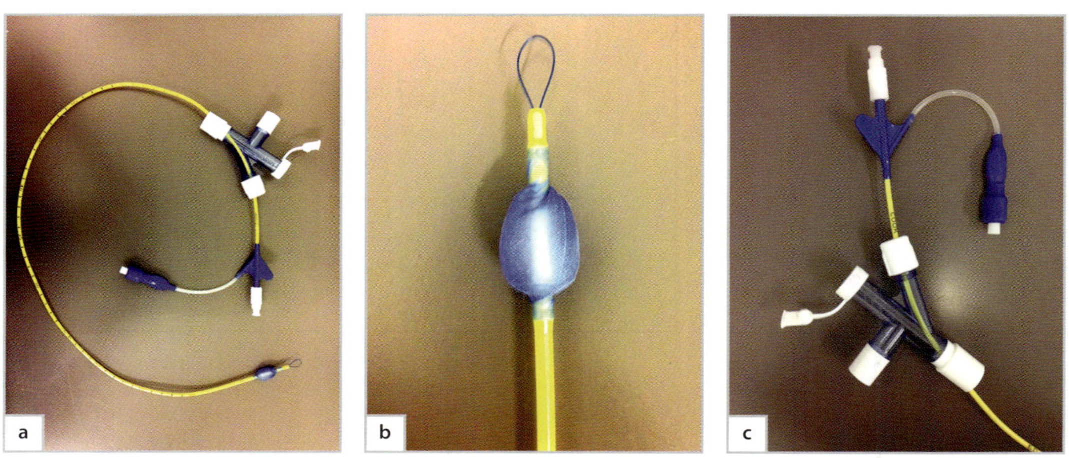

Figure 4.4 (a) Bronchial blocker. (b) Note the snare for attachment to the bronchoscope for placement, and the balloon for inflation in the bronchus. (c) Note the three-port attachment for the tube with ports for fresh gas flow, fiberoptic bronchoscope and bronchial blocker.

Table 4.1 Double-lumen tube versus bronchial blocker

Technique	Advantages versus disadvantages
Double-lumen tube	**Advantages:** Relatively easy to insert and position Reliable lung isolation Ability to inflate and deflate both lungs sequentially Ability to suction and inspect collapsed lung with bronchoscope **Disadvantages:** Need to change tube at start and end of procedure if single tube in situ or required postoperative Not suitable for infants/children More difficult to insert in difficult airways Larger tube – may produce more trauma
Bronchial blocker	**Advantages:** Easy to use if ETT in situ Can use in difficult airway Can use in infants/children Can use for selective lobar blockade **Disadvantages:** Technician dependant – requires skilled operator Requires bronchoscope for placement High maintenance device – easily displaced Cannot suction secretions Difficult to inflate and deflate both lungs sequentially

Table 4.2 Troubleshooting one lung ventilation

Complication	Management
Non-dependant lung is still ventilated	Check the correct side of the tube is clamped and disconnected Check the inflation of the bronchial cuff Re-check placement of tube in the correct bronchial lumen
Non-dependant lung is not ventilated but fails to collapse	Obstruction to airways of the non-dependant lung **Mechanical factors:** Tube clamped but not disconnected Herniation of bronchial cuff into carina Blockage of tube with secretions/gel from scope/kinked **Patient factors:** Asthma/emphysema – gas trapping/delayed collapse Obstructing lesion, e.g. tumor Inflammation/infection/adhesions adhering lung to chest wall Check for mechanical factors Suction tube Allow time for collapse
Hypoxia	Increase FiO_2 Check anesthetic machine and ventilator Check spirometry – volume/pressure loops Check tubing and connections Suction ETT Check tube position with FOB Assess and optimize cardiac output and blood pressure Insufflate oxygen to non-ventilated lung Increase/decrease PEEP to the ventilated lung Add CPAP to the non-ventilated lung Intermittently ventilate the non-ventilated lung Consider clamping the pulmonary artery Consider bypass/ECMO

and in fact appears to cause harm. Recent studies indicate that lower tidal volumes (5–6 mL/kg), the addition of a moderate amount of PEEP (5–10 cmH_2O) and the use of recruitment manoeuvers can help to reduce atelectasis, acute lung injury, intensive care unit admission and hospital length of stay. Protective lung strategies should therefore be considered in patients undergoing VATS surgery with one-lung mechanical ventilation.

FLUID MANAGEMENT

Debate remains over the optimal management of fluid administration in thoracic surgery. Pulmonary complications remain a major cause of mortality and morbidity following thoracic surgery. The incidence and severity of acute respiratory distress syndrome (ARDS) are related to the extent of pulmonary resection with a pneumonectomy posing a risk of development of 3–10% while a lesser resection poses only 2–5%. Mortality in those who develop ARDS is as high as 25–60%.

Multiple factors have been associated with the development of ARDS following thoracic surgery, one of which is fluid administration. Traditional evidence and teaching linked the excessive administration of intravenous fluids during surgery with increased lung injury. This led to the widespread practice of a restrictive fluid regimen.

Newer evidence however, raises doubts regarding the relationship with fluid administration and lung injury and there is increased concern regarding the practice of restrictive fluid administration, especially in wedge resections and lobectomies. This approach risks the development of a hypovolemic state leading to poor tissue perfusion and end organ dysfunction particularly acute kidney injury.

Protective lung ventilation strategies during one and two lung ventilation have now been shown to have the strongest link with the reduction in acute lung injury following thoracic surgery. These strategies along with a more liberal fluid regime, targeting normovolemia, may be more appropriate especially for smaller resections. One such approach suggests the use of lung protection strategies with the administration of 1.5 mL/kg/hr maintenance fluids in addition to replacement of deficit and blood loss continued into the postoperative period until oral intake is resumed. This protocol aims for normovolemia and has been found to maintain normal kidney function in thoracic patients with no increase in extravascular lung water. Goal directed therapy using less invasive hemodynamic monitors are currently being explored and may have a role in the future.

MONITORING

Minimum standards of monitoring in clinical anesthesia are set out in guidelines issued by professional bodies. Additional non-invasive and invasive monitoring devices may be included depending on the patient's condition, surgical experience, expected surgical operation time and possible intraoperative risks.

Most thoracic anesthetists will routinely place an arterial cannula for VATS lung resections. This provides accurate continuous monitoring of blood pressure and monitoring of arterial blood gases. Some anesthetists, however, no longer feel this is necessary for more minor VATS procedures depending on the patient comorbidities, surgical experience and the ability to measure accurate non-invasive blood pressure in the lateral position.

Central venous catheter insertion is not routinely indicated for VATS surgery. Indications for use are no different to other operations in that it may be useful in the high-risk cardiac patient, renal patient or to aid fluid management intra- and postoperatively during pneumothorax. Commonly central access is gained via the internal jugular vein on the same side as surgery, to prevent kinking, aid access and avoid the risk of contralateral pneumothorax. It is important to be aware that measurement of the central venous pressure may be inaccurate in a lateral position with one-lung ventilation.

Transesophageal echocardiography is not routinely utilized in VATS surgery, although it may be helpful in specific circumstances such as patients with cardiac failure or valvular dysfunction, invading tumors and to aid specific procedures such as Nuss bar insertion and placement.

ANALGESIA

Despite VATS being less invasive, patients can still experience considerable pain postoperatively, and there are still a significant proportion of patients who are left with chronic pain for months or years following their procedure. This is thought to relate to direct intercostal nerve injury, or pressure related injury from retraction or port movement during the procedure.

A major goal of anesthetic care perioperatively is control of the acute pain following the procedure to avoid postoperative respiratory complications, enable early mobilisation and reduce length of stay. There is also some evidence that control of acute pain can help to prevent progression to longer-term chronic pain states.

A 'multimodal' approach to analgesia is recommended. This involves using smaller doses of multiple agents which target pain pathways in different ways. Regional techniques are commonly used to reduce heavy opioid use, which can blunt the respiratory drive and cause further postoperative complications.

Thoracic epidural analgesia has been the mainstay of thoracic anesthetic practice for many years and provides arguably the best pain relief post-surgery. It does, however carry with it a number of rare but serious complications such as nerve injury, epidural abscess and hematoma – the burgeoning use of novel oral anticoagulant agents making the latter a significant concern to many anesthetists. Epidural placement may also be difficult, especially in the elderly or obese patient, affecting list turnover; and there is a risk of failure, or partially functioning block. Other significant disadvantages are the resulting sympathetic block and hypotension leading to fluid boluses or the need for vasopressors and the delay in patient mobility and, therefore, recovery and discharge in the postoperative period.

These factors have led to the search for alternative techniques of regional block. The most commonly used techniques in current practice are the paravertebral block, or the intercostal nerve block. Paravertebral blocks can be placed either as single shot blocks at multiple levels (e.g. with simple VATS procedures), or via placement of a catheter with an infusion of local anesthetic for longer or more complex procedures. Paravertebral catheters may be placed by the anesthetist at the beginning of the procedure, or placed directly by the surgeon at the end of the procedure. Multilevel intercostal nerve blocks are also commonly utilized and are effective at controlling acute pain following VATS.

In addition to the regional block, all patients should be prescribed paracetamol, either as an oral dose prior to coming to theatre, or loaded with an IV preparation during the case. Paracetamol should be continued regularly postoperatively. Non-steroidal anti-inflammatory agents are highly effective analgesics, but their use is limited by concerns about renal and gastrointestinal side effects. A single dose of a COX-2 inhibitor such as parecoxib intraoperatively, however, has lower rates of gastrointestinal side effects.

For second line analgesia, codeine or dihydrocodeine are effective but it should be remembered that they can impair cough, and there is significant pharmacogenetic variation in metabolism such that many patients will have little effect from codeine, and a small percentage of patients will have an exaggerated effect. Tramadol is an alternative effective second-line analgesic although it can cause nausea and occasionally hallucinations especially in elderly patients.

Opioid patient-controlled analgesia (PCA) devices are highly effective in combination with the above for postoperative analgesia in VATS patients. PCAs have multiple advantages in that patients have more control over their own analgesia rather than relying on nursing staff to attend to them. They have been shown to be safe and effective following VATS. Training for nursing staff and written institutional protocols should be in place to dictate the frequency and nature of essential vital sign observations whilst patients are on a PCA. Ideally only the patient should administer doses using the device – in this way if sedation is developing (the first sign of opioid toxicity) the patient will tend to stop activating the device. A protocol for administration of the opioid reversal agent, naloxone, should be available to nursing staff managing these patients for use in an emergency.

Other analgesic agents can be added if required. Gabapentin in particular has been shown to be effective both in acute and chronic pain management. Dosage should be adjusted to age and renal function, as it can cause sedation especially in elderly patients. Clonidine is an α-2 adrenoreceptor agonist with analgesic properties which can be useful in difficult to control postoperative pain. A single bolus or low dose ketamine infusion can also be effective.

Common side effects of opioids should ideally be prevented rather than treated once established. Routine prophylactic antiemetics should be administered during the operation, and should be available postoperatively. We also recommend routine use of laxative agents while patients are using opioid analgesia to prevent constipation which is a common reason for delayed mobility and discharge.

ENHANCED RECOVERY

Although this will be discussed in a separate chapter in this book, it is a crucial component in the anesthetic management of the VATS patient and, therefore, we discuss the key issues here briefly.

Enhanced recovery programs in a number of different surgical specialties are now heavily promoted by national bodies to produce productivity savings by driving a reduction in the length of stay. These have been successfully implemented in colorectal, gynecological, orthopedic and thoracic surgical specialties.

Enhanced recovery programs implement a number of evidence-based practices to optimise the patient before surgery, minimize the stress of the procedure and promote functional status and recovery.

Specific recommendations have been made for preoperative care including optimization of factors such as treatment of anemia, nutritional support, smoking cessation, medical therapy for chronic health conditions and pulmonary physiotherapy and 'pre-habilitation'.

All patients should attend a pre-assessment clinic for assessment of these factors and fitness for surgery. The pre-assessment clinic encounter should include a risk calculation and informed consent for anesthesia should be obtained. Patients should receive education relating to their expected perioperative journey and recovery.

A well-functioning pre-assessment service should allow for patients to be admitted to hospital on the day of surgery if possible. Premedication is no longer routinely used and ideally should be avoided if possible. If premedication is used, short-acting agents are preferred to minimize delays in postoperative recovery. Minimum fasting guidelines currently recommend no food beyond six-hours before induction of anesthesia, but clear fluids may be taken up until 2 hours before induction. Care guidelines should consider a carbohydrate drink 2 hours preoperatively and all patients should be assessed and provided with appropriate venous thromboembolism prophylaxis.

Intraoperative care should include appropriate antibiotic prophylaxis, the use of short-acting anesthetic agents and muscle relaxants to encourage early recovery, the lungs should be ventilated using a protective strategy as discussed earlier, fluid management should target euvolemia and excess fluids should be avoided and the patient should be extubated at the end of the procedure if possible. Regional analgesia should be utilized with preference for a paravertebral technique rather than thoracic epidural.

Surgery should be via a minimally invasive technique if possible with the minimal number of drains.

Postoperatively, pharmacological thromboembolic prophylaxis should be prescribed in patients with a low risk of bleeding, and there should be a low threshold for drain removal. Drain suction is not routinely required as it may delay drain removal. Patients should be mobilized as soon as possible after surgery with regular chest physiotherapy.

Because of the minimally invasive nature of the surgery, most patients can be discharged directly to a ward environment from the theatre recovery. High dependency or intensive care admission is reserved for patients with significant underlying medical conditions, or an anticipated complicated postoperative course.

Not all patients will be suitable for all the elements in the above protocol and careful patient selection and safety are paramount. Multidisciplinary input from anesthetic, surgical, nursing and physiotherapy staff is essential for a successful enhanced recovery program.

ROBOTIC THORACIC SURGERY

The development of robotic thoracic surgery over the last decade has produced another set of unique challenges to the anesthetist in addition to those already discussed.

The positioning of the patient and robot for these procedures has dramatically altered how the anesthetist plans their set up and technique. The robot is often deployed near the head end with the patient turned 90° from the anesthetist. This means that the patient's head and arms are obscured and not within easy access. It is therefore vital that the airway and vascular cannulation sites are well secured and perfectly positioned at the beginning and out of the way of the robot.

The robotic arms can cause problems with crushing injuries and nerve compression injuries especially to the brachial plexus, and therefore must be vigilantly positioned and monitored.

If carbon dioxide insufflation is to be used to create maximal surgical exposure, the anesthetist must also carefully consider the risks and complications of this. These include the risk of venous gas embolism, compromise to the venous return with resulting drop in cardiac output, bradycardia, arrhythmias from carbon dioxide absorption, arterial desaturation and hypercapnia requiring ventilator adjustments.

AWAKE VIDEO-ASSISTED THORACOSCOPIC SURGERY

General anesthesia for thoracic surgery has always been considered mandatory. However, with the introduction of minimally invasive surgical techniques, there has been increased interest in awake surgery in the last few years.

There are increasing numbers of case reports and series of thoracoscopic minor and major lung surgeries taking place under sedation and spontaneous ventilation with the use of regional techniques. Initial reports used thoracic epidural anesthesia, vagal blockade and sedation for three-port conventional VATS, however, with the development of single-port VATS, surgery is now being performed under single-shot paravertebral or intercostal nerve blocks and sedation, without the need for epidurals or vagal blockade. Initial results illustrate that these techniques appear to be feasible and safe, and may be of greater benefit to the patient with quicker recovery times, better pain scores and lower morbidity and mortality rates.

This does, however, present a greater challenge for the anesthetist. Thorough patient selection and preparation, strict planning and vigilance are essential. Complications should be anticipated and prevented if possible with preparation for conversion to general anesthesia and intubation if required.

These new techniques are innovative and exciting in a drive to reduce the invasiveness of these procedures. With further training and research, it may mean that older and sicker patients are able to undergo more major thoracic surgery, avoiding the risks of general anesthesia, tracheal intubation and mechanical ventilation. This will provide a truly minimally invasive procedure for the patient.

FURTHER READING

Assaad S, Popescu W, Perrino A. Fluid management in thoracic surgery. Curr Opin Anaesthesiol 2013; 26:31–39.

Campos J, Ueda K. Update on anesthetic complications of robotic thoracic surgery. Minerva Anestesiologica 2014; 80:83–88.

Jones N, Edmonds L, Ghosh S, Klein AA. A review of enhanced recovery for thoracic anaesthesia and surgery. Anaesthesia. 2013; 68:179–189.

Kiss G, Castillo M. Non-intubated anesthesia in thoracic surgery: general issues Ann Transl Med 2015; 3:110.

Kiss G, Castillo M. Non-intubated anesthesia in thoracic surgery: technical issues. Ann Transl Med 2015; 3:109.

Tsai J, Moon T, Vachhani S, et al. Anesthesia for Thoracic Surgical Procedures. In: Principles and Practice of Cardiothoracic Surgery. Firstenberg M (Ed.), InTech online, 2013.

Chapter 5 Clinical pathways in minimally invasive thoracic surgery

Eunjue Yi, Sanghoon Jheon

INTRODUCTION

Minimally invasive techniques have brought about a paradigm shift in thoracic surgery. Despite ongoing controversies regarding the safety and treatment effects of minimally invasive techniques, demand for these techniques is increasing from both healthcare providers and consumers. A minimally invasive approach is currently only used as the standard treatment for early stage cancers, even though numerous clinical studies have demonstrated its safety and efficacy.[1,2] However, much effort is being devoted to decreasing the invasiveness and expanding the application of minimally invasive surgery.

Numerous studies have demonstrated that minimally invasive techniques decrease surgical pain by reducing the size and number of surgical incisions, resulting in quicker functional recovery and improvement in quality of life without any negative impact on oncologic efficacy.[3] Nevertheless, minimally invasive surgery does not appear to reduce the risk of undesirable complications after major thoracic surgery. Possible serious sequelae include cardiovascular and thromboembolic complications as well as infection and pain, and these are of major concern for postoperative care. The benefits of minimally invasive surgery may be masked by the fact that this type of surgery is applied to patients with high-risk comorbidities that were previously considered inoperable.[4] As the proportion of these types of patients increases, postoperative morbidities and mortalities are of increasing concern to healthcare providers.

The concept of 'enhanced recovery after surgery' (ERAS), developed by Kehlet in the 1990s,[5] reflects the fact that conventional postoperative care cannot address this challenge.[4] Traditional postoperative care is based on the guild system, supported by traditional care plans.[6] Although this type of care is generally accepted and successful, the rapidly changing surgical environment requires more organized and active strategies for postoperative care.

THE BEGINNING OF ENHANCED RECOVERY AFTER SURGERY

Dr Kehlet first described the concept of ERAS in late 1990s.[4] This concept refers to structured multimodal approaches designed to control unnecessary surgical stress responses in postoperative patients to reduce postoperative morbidities, improve functional recovery, and decrease hospital stay.[6]

ERAS comprises controlling preoperative risk factors, reducing intraoperative surgical stress, and promoting postoperative rehabilitation by multidisciplinary collaboration among surgeons, anesthesiologists, physiotherapists, psychotherapists, nurses, and patients. The idea of ERAS can be translated into structured care strategies for individual diseases or procedures. These procedures are referred to as ERAS protocols, fast-track programs, or clinical pathways.[4-6]

A clinical pathway can therefore be defined as a structured multidisciplinary care plan. A clinical pathway is a task-oriented care plan that details essential steps in the care of patients with a specific clinical problem and describes the patients expected clinical course. Each step of a clinical pathway should be based on scientific evidence from clinical trials.[7]

In the field of colorectal surgery (where the concept of ERAS was first adopted)[2] established sets of consensus guidelines for several surgical processes have been published. Although there has been considerable interest in implementing clinical pathways and numerous studies have demonstrated the beneficial effects, no order sets for major thoracic surgeries have been published. There are, however, generally accepted goals for perioperative care.[8]

CLINICAL PATHWAYS IN MINIMALLY INVASIVE THORACIC SURGERY

A clinical pathway is usually applied to elective surgery. A carefully planned treatment strategy for an individual should be integrated into the organized multidisciplinary collaboration. Common goals for a clinical pathway for minimally invasive thoracic surgery (MITS) are as follows:

1. Preoperative risk assessment and education
2. Modulating of intraoperative factors to reduce surgical stress response
3. Rehabilitation for enhancing functional recovery
4. Assessment of impact and amendment of protocols

Preoperative factors

Evaluation of pulmonary function and smoking cessation are important check points for patients scheduled for major pulmonary resections.[9] It is still not clear whether smoking cessation benefits postoperative outcomes and when smoking should be stopped before surgery;[10,11] however, for lung cancer, smoking cessation is associated with lower risks for all types of mortality and recurrence.[12]

For patients with marginal lung function, a preoperative pulmonary rehabilitation program is a good prescription. A one-month enrollment in a preoperative rehabilitation program for 6 days one week has been shown to increase pulmonary function including Pao_2, Vo_2max, and FEV_1. Improved pulmonary function is directly related to a decrease in postoperative pulmonary complications, and therefore, a reduction in hospital stay in both major pulmonary resection and esophagectomy patients.[14]

Intraoperative factors

The use of excessive invasive monitoring systems is no longer recommended.[15] Routine adoption of central catheter or arterial blood pressure monitoring is vanishing rapidly.[16] Indwelling Foley catheter can be defended when the expected operative time is more than 4 hours. Minimizing invasive monitoring devices decreases operation time without increasing the risks for morbidities or mortalities.[16]

Minimizing invasive monitoring devices decreases operation time without increasing the risks for morbidities or mortalities.[17] It facilitates a stable surgical condition through selective lung ventilation, although adverse effects such as ventilation-related lung injury or airway impairment have been reported.[8] VATS surgery without tracheal intubation has been employed recently, and is expanding in scope from wedge resection or biopsy to lobectomies. Several studies have reported the feasibility and safety of non-intubated VATS techniques,[18] although these techniques are not yet generally used.

Protective lung ventilation, comprising an FIO_2 of 0.5, tidal volume of 6 mL/kg, positive end-expiratory pressure of 5 mm H_2O, and pressure control ventilation, as well as contraction of single lung ventilation periods have been shown to reduce postoperative pulmonary complications after a major operation.[19]

Obviously, minimizing surgical wounds and tissue manipulation are key goals in MITS,[20,21] including VATS, single VATS and robotic approaches.[22] Surgical minimalism contributes to 'stress and pain-free' surgery by reducing catastrophic neurohormonal cascades that cause organ dysfunction.[6] Although numerous clinical trials have demonstrated the superiority of single-port VATS or robotic surgeries, conventional VATS approaches are still the most widely used MITS techniques.[22]

In addition to minimizing surgical manipulation, pain control is critical. Intraoperative epidural anesthesia is well-established and has been shown to be an effective pain relief method,[23] but it can be costly in terms of time and result in urinary retention, hypotension, and nausea.[24] Paravertebral nerve blockade has been reported to have an equivalent pain control effect as intraoperative epidural anesthesia, and bupivacaine intercostal nerve blocks could have similar pain-relieving effects.[24,25]

Postoperative care

Removal of unnecessary drain systems, beyond facilitating early discharge from hospital, is associated with fast recovery of pulmonary function.[26] Drain amounts of up to 500 mL have been showed to be safe, with negligible readmission rates.[27] Suction devices have been reported to prolong air leaks, and pleurodesis should be considered when promoting early removal of chest tubes.[28] Digital air leak devices can be used to quantify air leaks, though their cost-effectiveness is still a matter of debate.[29]

Placement of nasogastric tube is no more mandatory in abdominal surgery;[30] however, digital air leak devices can be used to quantify air leaks, though their cost-effectiveness is still a matter of debate.[31] The presence of nasogastric tubes is believed to prevent the occurrence of anastomotic leaks by reducing distension of the gastric conduit; however, this is not supported by scientific evidence.[32]

Early ambulation can be encouraged by early extubation, avoidance of long-acting anesthetic agents, and early oral feeding. Traditional concepts of strict bed rest and extensive fasting are no longer accepted in rational postoperative care. In some protocols, water ingestion is permitted 2 hours before surgery, and early oral feeding 1–2 hours after surgery.[33,34]

Standards for bowel preparation and the appropriate time to restart oral feeding after esophagectomy have not yet been established; however, adoption of minimal invasive techniques can reduce the necessity for extensive bowel preparation and facilitate the beginning of oral feeding. Patients scheduled for minimally invasive esophagectomy can ingest a carbohydrate beverage 3 hours before surgery. Oral feeding can be restarted at postoperative day 4 or 5 with or without testing for anastomotic leaks.[33-35]

Postoperative pain control with oral analgesia contributes as much to early functional recovery as nerve blockade. Non-opioid analgesic drugs can be supplied at the same time with the use of epidural or paravertebral blockade or PCA.[6]

Feedback

Because not all steps in clinical pathways are supported by randomized controlled clinical trials, currently implemented protocols should be assessed and adapted as necessary. Several well-known indicators such as postoperative complication rate, pain scale, and length of hospital stay are useful. Results from the evaluation should be discussed among participating multidisciplinary groups, and the conclusions should be integrated into the revised protocols.[36,37]

Translational research activity that converts knowledge into practical methods is a defining feature of a clinical pathway.[5] Clinical pathways can be improved by the adoption of healthcare information systems and the development of efficient clinical indicators.[38]

CLINICAL INDICATORS

Clinical indicators are tools to assess the quality of specific healthcare process. Indicators can be rate- or mean-based, and provide quantitative data for evaluation of clinical outcomes, sometimes triggering further research.[39] Quality control and the amendment of a clinical pathway is impossible without monitoring clinical indicators.

Mortality, morbidity, duration of drainage, length of hospital stay, and overall costs are examples of clinical indicators for assessing postoperative outcomes. Incidence of unexpected postoperative complications could lead to further investigation, and is therefore a clinical indicator.[40] Ideal indicators are based on agreed definitions, have optimal specificity and sensitivity, provide clear comparisons, and are evidence-based.[39] They can create knowledge that can be integrated directly into practice.

MERGING WITH HEALTHCARE INFORMATION SYSTEMS

Initially, healthcare information systems were just a substitution for paper-based medical record systems. Nowadays, advanced information systems can be used for complex tasks such as healthcare delivery and medical research, and can be used to integrate new scientific evidence into clinical practice.[41]

Biomedical and health informatics, refers to any fusion of electronic information processing with medical care. For hospital-based healthcare providers, it can be used as a clinical decision support system or an integrated intelligence system based on the electronic medical records of patients. This system can be used to provide clinicians, staff, patients, and other individuals with knowledge and person-specific information, intelligently filtered and presented at appropriate times, to enhance health and healthcare.[42]

Health information technology (HIT) has outstanding data processing abilities which can translate results into knowledge, allowing healthcare providers to revise clinical pathways based on new evidence. However, the theoretical benefits of HIT do not always translate into real benefits in healthcare practice, and the cost of development and maintenance may exceed the gain.[43]

CONCLUSION

In this era of increasing cost containment and government-imposed limitations on medical administration, implementation of ERAS is no longer optional. A clinical pathway is a practical protocol which can be applied to a specific disease category, with the aim to improve cost-effectiveness of healthcare delivery. Implementation of a clinical pathway enhances the beneficial effects of MITS. Although there are still no established guidelines for thoracic disease, clinical research is expected to conclude its findings soon.

Clinical outcomes that reflect the performance of clinical pathways, often referred to as clinical indicators, can provide new knowledge and be applied to medical practice immediately. When integrated with HIT, ERAS can promote rapid and accurate delivery of healthcare services and facilitate evidence-based medical practices.

REFERENCES

1. Dziedzic D, Orlowski T. The role of VATS in lung cancer surgery: Current status and prospects for development. Minim Invasive Surg 2015; 2015:938430.
2. Anderegg MC, Gisbertz SS, van Berge Henegouwen MI. Minimally invasive surgery for oesophageal cancer. Best Pract Res Clin Gastroenterol 2014; 28:41–52.
3. Jheon S, Yang HC, Cho S. Video-assisted thoracic surgery for lung cancer. Gen Thorac Cardiovasc Surg 2012; 60:255–260.
4. Kehlet H. Multimodal approach to control postoperative pathophysiology and rehabilitation. Br J Anaesth 1997; 78:606–617.
5. Hoffmann HC, Kettelhack C. Fast-track surgery – conditions and challenges in postsurgical treatment: a review of elements of translational research in enhanced recovery after surgery. Eur Surg Res 2012. 49:24–34.
6. Kehlet H, Wilmore DW. Evidence-based surgical care and the evolution of fast-track surgery. Ann Surg 2008; 248:189–198.
7. Fearon, KC, Ljungqvist O, Von Meyenfeldt M, et al. Enhanced recovery after surgery: a consensus review of clinical care for patients undergoing colonic resection. Clin Nutr 2005; 24:466–477.
8. Jones NL, Edmonds L, Ghosh S, Klein AA. A review of enhanced recovery for thoracic anaesthesia and surgery. Anaesthesia 2013; 68:179–189.
9. Lindstrom D, Sadr Azodi O, Wladis A, et al. Effects of a perioperative smoking cessation intervention on postoperative complications: a randomized trial. Ann Surg 2008; 248:739–745.
10. Barrera R, Shi W, Amar D, et al. Smoking and timing of cessation: impact on pulmonary complications after thoracotomy. Chest 2005; 127:1977–1983.
11. Nakagawa M, Tanaka H, Tsukuma H, Kishi Y. Relationship between the duration of the preoperative smoke-free period and the incidence of postoperative pulmonary complications after pulmonary surgery. Chest 2001; 120:705–710.
12. Parsons A, Daley A, Begh R, Aveyard P. Influence of smoking cessation after diagnosis of early stage lung cancer on prognosis: systematic review of observational studies with meta-analysis. BMJ 2010; 340:b5569.
13. Divisi D, Di Francesco C, Di Leonardo G, Crisci R. Preoperative pulmonary rehabilitation in patients with lung cancer and chronic obstructive pulmonary disease. Eur J Cardiothorac Surg 2013; 43:293–296.
14. Yamana I, Takeno S, Hashimoto T, et al. Randomized Controlled Study to Evaluate the Efficacy of a Preoperative Respiratory Rehabilitation Program to Prevent Postoperative Pulmonary Complications after Esophagectomy. Dig Surg 2015; 32:331–337.
15. Brodsky JB. What intraoperative monitoring makes sense? Chest 1999 115:101S–105S.
16. King PM, Blazeby JM, Ewings P, et al. Randomized clinical trial comparing laparoscopic and open surgery for colorectal cancer within an enhanced recovery programme. Br J Surg 2006; 93:300–308.
17. Fischer GW, Cohen E. An update on anesthesia for thoracoscopic surgery. Curr Opin Anaesthesiol 2010; 23:7–11.
18. Chen KC, Cheng YJ, Hung MH, Tseng YD, Chen JS. Nonintubated thoracoscopic lung resection: a 3-year experience with 285 cases in a single institution. J Thorac Dis 2012; 4:347–351.
19. Yang M, Ahn HJ, Kim K, et al. Does a protective ventilation strategy reduce the risk of pulmonary complications after lung cancer surgery? a randomized controlled trial. Chest 2011; 139:530–537.
20. Kehlet H. Surgical stress response: does endoscopic surgery confer an advantage? World J Surg 1999; 23:801–807.
21. Sylla P, Kirman I, Whelan RL. Immunological advantages of advanced laparoscopy. Surg Clin North Am 2005; 85:1–818.
22. Flores RM, Alam N. Video-assisted thoracic surgery lobectomy (VATS), open thoracotomy, and the robot for lung cancer. Ann Thorac Surg 2008; 8:S710–S715.
23. Kehlet H, Dahl JB. Anaesthesia, surgery, and challenges in postoperative recovery. Lancet 2003; 362:1921–1928.
24. Ding X, Jin S1, Niu X, et al. A comparison of the analgesia efficacy and side effects of paravertebral compared with epidural blockade for thoracotomy: an updated meta-analysis. PLoS One, 2014; 9:e96233.
25. Rice DC, Cata JP, Mena GE, et al. Posterior Intercostal Nerve Block With Liposomal Bupivacaine: An Alternative to Thoracic Epidural Analgesia. Ann Thorac Surg 2015; 99:1953–1960.
26. Nomori H, Horio H, Suemasu K. Early removal of chest drainage tubes and oxygen support after a lobectomy for lung cancer facilitates earlier recovery of the 6-minute walking distance. Surg Today 2001; 31:395–399.
27. Bjerregaard LS, Jensen K, Petersen RH, Hansen HJ. Early chest tube removal after video-assisted thoracic surgery lobectomy with serous fluid production up to 500 ml/day. Eur J Cardiothorac Surg 2014; 45:241–246.
28. Cerfolio RJ, Tummala RP, Holman WL, et al. A prospective algorithm for the management of air leaks after pulmonary resection. Ann Thorac Surg 1998; 66:1726–1731.
29. Pompili C, Detterbeck F, Papagiannopoulos K, et al. Multicenter international randomized comparison of objective and subjective outcomes between electronic and traditional chest drainage systems. Ann Thorac Surg 2014; 98:490–496.
30. Petrowsky H, Demartines N, Rousson V, Clavien PA. Evidence-based value of prophylactic drainage in gastrointestinal surgery: a systematic review and meta-analyses. Ann Surg 2004; 240:1074–1084.
31. Shackcloth MJ, McCarron E, Kendall J, et al. Randomized clinical trial to determine the effect of nasogastric drainage on tracheal acid aspiration following oesophagectomy. Br J Surg 2006. 93:547–552.
32. Daryaei P, Vaghef Davari F, Mir M, Harirchi I. Salmasian. Omission of nasogastric tube application in postoperative care of esophagectomy. World J Surg 2009; 33:773–777.
33. Pan H, Hu X, Yu Z, et al. Use of a fast-track surgery protocol on patients undergoing minimally invasive oesophagectomy: preliminary results. Interact Cardiovasc Thorac Surg 2014; 19:441–447.
34. Das-Neves-Pereira JC, Bagan P, Coimbra-Israel AP, et al. Fast-track rehabilitation for lung cancer lobectomy: a five-year experience. Eur J Cardiothorac Surg 2009; 36:383–391.
35. Shewale JB, Correa AM, Baker CM, et al. Impact of a Fast-track Esophagectomy Protocol on Esophageal Cancer Patient Outcomes and Hospital Charges. Ann Surg 2015; 261:1114–1123.
36. Nygren J, Thacker J, Carli F, et al. Guidelines for perioperative care in elective rectal/pelvic surgery: Enhanced Recovery After Surgery (ERAS(R)) Society recommendations. Clin Nutr 2012; 31:801–816.
37. Gotlib Conn L, McKenzie M, Pearsall EA, McLeod RS.. Successful implementation of an enhanced recovery after surgery programme for elective colorectal surgery: a process evaluation of champions' experiences. Implement Sci 2015; 10:99.
38. Cohen JD, Aspry KE, Brown AS, et al. Use of health information technology (HIT) to improve statin adherence and low-density lipoprotein cholesterol

goal attainment in high-risk patients: proceedings from a workshop. J Clin Lipidol 2013; 7:573–609.
39. Mainz J. Defining and classifying clinical indicators for quality improvement. Int J Qual Health Care 2003; 15:523–530.
40. Palmer RH. Using health outcomes data to compare plans, networks and providers. Int J Qual Health Care 1998; 10:477–483.
41. Kehlet H, Mogensen T. Hospital stay of 2 days after open sigmoidectomy with a multimodal rehabilitation programme. Br J Surg 1999; 86:227–230.
42. Hunt DL, Haynes RB, Hanna SE, Smith K. Effects of computer based clinical decision support systems on physician performance and patient outcomes: a systematic review. JAMA, 1998; 280:1339–1346.
43. Garg AX, Adhikari NK, McDonald H, et al. Effects of computerized clinical decision support systems on practitioner performance and patient outcomes: a systematic review. JAMA 2005; 293:1223–1238.

Chapter 6 VATS lobectomy

Marco Scarci, Alessandro Pardolesi, Piergiorgio Solli

INTRODUCTION

Video-assisted thoracoscopic surgery (VATS) lobectomy was first described in 1993. It is used widely now, but the definition of this type of operation is variable.

We use the Cancer and Leukemia Group B (CALBG) description of VATS lobectomy as follow:

- One 5-cm maximum utility incision and two further ports
- The ribs are not resected or spread in any way. We only use a soft tissue retractor to facilitate introduction of instruments (Alexis)
- We always sample two lobe-dependent nodes and station 7. Some authors routinely use mediastinoscopy in the same session. We believe that such an approach is not necessary and lymphadenectomy can be performed safely through VATS alone
- All the anatomical structures are identified and individually divided
- All operative steps are done through the monitor and not looking through the utility incision

INDICATIONS AND CONTRAINDICATIONS

We don't believe that the size of the tumour is a contraindication to VATS. It is true, however, that the manipulation of the lobe is more difficult and potentially more hazardous with a large tumour, because of the risk of tearing small arterial branches to gain visualization.

Historically, chest wall involvement was also considered a relative contraindication to VATS surgery, but we think an extra-pleural strip, or even a chest wall resection, is achievable using a VATS approach.

While some authors will deny the potential advantages of such an approach, we feel that rib-spreading should be avoided, particularly in patients with limited pulmonary reserve.

Previous chemotherapy, in our experience, is not a contraindication to VATS. While there is the possibility of a strong periadventitial inflammatory reaction, this is unusual and, if carefully done, it is possible to dissect the vessels safely.

Similarly, we have successfully performed VATS after thoracotomies. Once the correct plane of dissection is entered, provided that there is a small space for the thoracoscope at the beginning of the dissection, it is possible to mobilize the lung. However, this procedure can be time consuming.

In our opinion, the only contraindications to VATS are large hilar tumours and bulky lymph nodes.

RIGHT UPPER VATS LOBECTOMY

Surgical technique

Patient positioning

Unlike a thoracotomy, in correct patient positioning is essential to facilitate VATS. The hip of the patient should be at the level of the table break, which allows maximum separation of the ribs. The chest is then parallel to the floor. Some authors put the upper arm on a gutter, but despite improving stability this can limit the movement of the thoracoscope. Therefore, keeping the arms together between two normal pillows is a better position for the patient.

Port position

We start with the utility incision at the level of the 4th intercostal space, usually in front of the anterior edge of the latissimus dorsi along an imaginary line between the tip of the scapula and the nipple. Even if the creation of this port may seem an easy procedure, be careful to avoid oozing from the muscle – during a lengthy procedure, the blood collecting into the chest will absorb the light and hinder the dissection of the hilar structures. Also make sure you examine the hemithorax for signs of pleural spread or any other conditions you feel will preclude resectability or a VATS procedure.

The second-port for the camera is usually two spaces below on the anterior axillary line. Be careful not to place the camera port too low. This is for two reasons:

1. The diaphragm, especially in obese patients, will interfere with the manipulation of the thoracoscope; and
2. It will be difficult to properly visualize the right upper lobe bronchus.

The third-port is usually along the same line of the camera port on the posterior axillary line. We recommend the port should be 2 cm long as this facilitates the introduction of sponge sticks for retraction and staplers. Making the port too small in an attempt to make the procedure more 'cosmetic' usually results in more nerve damage, with potential chronic pain.

Operative steps

The lung is retracted from the posterior port with a long sponge stick. This manoeuver facilitates the exposure of the superior pulmonary vein. Occasionally, if the horizontal fissure is grossly incomplete, it is possible to run a stapler along the intended fissure line. Such a manoeuver will allow independent movement of the upper and middle lobe along the horizontal axis represented by the interlobar pulmonary artery (PA). The branches to the upper lobe tend to be more vertical, while those to the middle lobe more horizontal. With a combination of blunt and diathermy dissection it is possible to isolate the branches to the upper lobe. Care must be taken to ensure that the venous anatomy is normal and an inferior pulmonary vein is present. We always incise the pulmonary ligament and send station 8 and 9, if present, during this manoeuver. We used to use a hook diathermy and while this is useful in certain cases, we think the use of an endo-dissector allows better control during the dissection and avoids poking with a very hot diathermy on the delicate vessels' surface. Once the inferior border of the vein is dissected, we create a separation between the upper and middle lobe branches until the underlying PA is visualized. Then we progress the dissection superiorly between the first branch of the PA and the superior edge of the vein. There is always a station 11 lymph node between the two vessels that needs to be removed.

Once a plane is created, we use a silicone vessel loop to retract the vessel and insert a staple from the posterior port.

This manoeuver allows exposure of the interlobar PA with its first branch. Again this is dissected and encircled with a silicone vessel loop. Although it might be tempting to push a dissector across the vessel without diving the adventia of the PA, we believe that such a manoeuver greatly facilitates further dissection.

Once the PA is divided, the next step depends on the patient's anatomy. There are two options:

1. Exposure of the recurrent apical branch of the PA. If this is visible it is advisable to dissect it before dividing the bronchus, as it makes further dissection of the airway safer.
2. Alternatively, if the recurrent apical branch is not visible we proceed directly with dissection of the upper lobe bronchus. Although classic teaching in VATS lobectomy is to move front to back, we suggest opening the pleura posteriorly and identifying the junction between the upper and intermedius bronchus. This manoeuver facilitates further dissection from the front as only very little tissue usually remains. We also recommend staying close to the bronchial wall and not forcing any instruments through. The consequences could be either laceration of lung parenchyma with lung congestion, bleeding or hemoptysis through the endo-bronchial tube and it is also possible to tear the membranous portion of the bronchus.

Once the RUL bronchus is divided it is usually easy to complete the fissure front to back. Usually, we recommend Covidien black reloads (60 mm). The first stapler goes through the utility port and is directed toward the hilum, while remaining above the middle lobe vein. The second stapler is more horizontal and must be positioned above the interlobar PA. After these two firing the remaining of the fissure is easy to complete.

The lobe is then extracted through a specimen retrieval bag.

Preference cards

1. 30°scope with HD camera. We tried several 3D systems, but we don't think they add much in VATS
2. Specifically designated VATS instruments (Scanlan)
3. LigaSure device
4. Covidien stapler with the tip at the end 30 mm for vessels
5. Alexis soft tissue retractor
6. Silicone vessel loops

Tips

1. A sponge on a stick should be mounted at all times throughout the procedure, to be used in any case of sudden bleeding.
2. There is a controversy on whether it is better to use a silk tie to retract vessels before transection instead of a vessel loop. The advocates of the silk tie believe that it does not need to be removed before staple firing. We believe that having a string attached to a vessel's stump potentially could create a point for inadvertent traction during surgery with subsequent bleeding. If removed before firing, we worry that the harsh material could saw through the back wall of delicate vessels. There are also surgeons that prefer to pass the stapler directly. While this is possible most of the time, we believe that using a vessel loop provides improved visualization and control and reduces the number of vascular injuries.
3. When performing open surgery, emphasis is not often placed on removal of N1 nodes prior to obtain vascular or bronchial control. As these nodes are often included with the specimen, they are typically not taken out separately before a planned lobectomy. In VATS lobectomy, performance of regional lymphadenectomy often facilitates dissection. Arterial branch points and lobar bronchial origins are often signaled by clusters of lymph nodes. Removal of these lymph nodes creates obvious anatomic pathways for circumferential dissection and subsequent surgical control. This is particularly true with regard to surrounding the upper lobe bronchus on the right. One or two nodes are typically present at the angle created by the inferior aspect of the upper lobe origin and the bronchus intermedius.
4. If taking the recurrent apical branch last, be careful not to exert excessive traction on the lobe to avoid tearing the small artery which is no longer supported by the bronchus.

RIGHT MIDDLE VATS LOBECTOMY

Surgical technique

Patient positioning

Unlike a thoracotomy, correct patient positioning is essential to facilitate VATS. The hip of the patient should be at the level of the table break, which allows maximum separation of the ribs. The chest is then parallel to the floor. Some authors put the upper arm on a gutter, but despite improving stability this can limit the movement of the thoracoscope. Therefore, we think keeping the arms together between two normal pillows is a better position for the patient.

Port position

We start with the utility incision at the level of the 4th intercostal space, usually in front of the anterior edge of the latissimus dorsi along an imaginary line between the tip of the scapula and the nipple. Even if the creation of this port might seem a trivial procedure, particular care must be taken to avoid oozing from the muscle as, during a lengthy procedure, the blood collecting into the chest will absorb the light and hinder the dissection of the hilar structures. At this point the hemithorax is carefully examined for signs of pleural spread or other conditions that would preclude resectability or a VATS procedure.

The second-port for the camera is usually two spaces below on the anterior axillary line. Care must be taken not to put the camera port too low because the diaphragm, especially in obese patients, will interfere with the manipulation of the thoracoscope.

The third-port is usually along the same line of the camera port on the posterior axillary line. We recommend making the port about 2 cm long as this facilitates the introduction of sponge sticks for retraction and staplers. Making the port too small in an attempt to make the procedure more 'cosmetic' usually results in more nerve damage with potential chronic pain.

Operative steps

A middle lobectomy is performed anteriorly, usually, dividing the vein, the bronchus and the artery, in this order. Each step allows exposure of the next structure.

The lung is retracted from the posterior port with a long sponge stick. This manoeuver facilitates the exposure of the superior pulmonary vein. Occasionally, if the horizontal fissure is grossly incomplete, it is possible to run a stapler along the intended fissure line. Such a manoeuver will allow independent movement of the upper and middle lobe along the horizontal axis represented by the interlobar PA. The branches to the upper lobe tend to be more vertical, while those to the middle lobe are more horizontal. With a combination of blunt and diathermy dissection it is possible to isolate the branches to the middle lobe. Care must be taken to ensure that the venous anatomy is normal and an inferior pulmonary vein is present. Occasionally, the middle lobe vein arises from the inferior pulmonary vein.

We always incise the pulmonary ligament and send station 8 and 9, if present, during this manoeuver. We used to use a hook diathermy which is useful in some cases, but we think the use of an endo-dissector allows better control during the dissection and avoids poking the delicate vessels' surface with a very hot diathermy. Once the inferior border of the vein is dissected, we create a separation between the upper and middle lobe branches until the underlying PA is seen. Similarly, the dissection is carried out to identify the inferior border of the middle lobe vein. It is quite easy to take the vein as first step.

Once a plane is created, we use a silicone vessel loop to retract the vessel and insert a staple from the posterior port.

This manoeuver allows exposure of the middle lobe bronchus. This is first felt with a cloth dissector and then dissected with diathermy to swipe the lymph nodes toward the specimen. Once the bronchus is clearly seen it is divided with a 30 or 45 mm stapler from the posterior port. Sometimes there is a certain resistance in passing the stapler through the bronchus because of soft tissue around the bronchus. Our suggestion is to keep the stapler parallel to the pericardium and to retract the lobe upward to make the bronchus more vertical.

Once the bronchus is divided, the next step depends on the patient's anatomy. There are two options:

1. Exposure of the middle lobe PA from the anterior hilum
2. Alternatively, if the fissure is relatively complete, then it is possible to find the artery in the fissure. We recommend avoiding a large fissural dissection as it is the key cause of prolonged air leak.

Once the hilar structures are divided the fissures are divided with staplers, keeping them above the underlying interlobar PA.

The lobe is then extracted through a specimen retrieval bag.

Preference cards

1. 30°scope with HD camera. We have tried several 3D systems, but feel they don't add much in VATS.
2. Specifically designated VATS instruments (Scanlan)
3. LigaSure device
4. Covidien stapler with the tip at the end 30 mm for vessels
5. Alexis soft tissue retractor
6. Silicone vessel loops

Tips

1. A sponge on a stick should be mounted at all times throughout the procedure, to be used in any case of sudden bleeding.
2. There is a controversy on whether it is better to use a silk tie to retract vessels before transection instead of a vessel loop. The advocates of the silk tie believe that it does not need to be removed before staple firing. We believe that having a string attached to a vessel's stump potentially could create a point for inadvertent traction during surgery with subsequent bleeding. If removed before firing, we worry that the harsh material could saw through the back wall of delicate vessels. There are also surgeons that prefer to pass the stapler directly. While this is possible most of the time, we believe that using a vessel loop provides improved visualization and control and reduces the number of vascular injuries.
3. When performing open surgery, emphasis is not often placed on removal of N1 nodes prior to obtaining vascular or bronchial control. As these nodes are often included with the specimen, they are typically not taken out separately before planned lobectomy. In VATS lobectomy, performance of regional lymphadenectomy often facilitates dissection. Arterial branch points and lobar bronchial origins are often signaled by clusters of lymph nodes. Removal of these lymph nodes creates obvious anatomic pathways for circumferential dissection and subsequent surgical control. This is particularly true with regard to surrounding the upper lobe bronchus on the right. One or two nodes are typically present at the angle created by the inferior aspect of the upper lobe origin and the bronchus intermedius.
4. If the middle lobectomy is performed for benign conditions such as bronchiectasis, we would recommend taking particular care in isolating the bronchial vessels and removing all the fibrous tissue around the bronchus to facilitate dissection. It is very important not to exert excessive traction behind the bronchus so as not to disrupt the membranous area.

RIGHT LOWER VATS LOBECTOMY

Surgical technique

Patient positioning

Unlike a thoracotomy, in correct patient positioning is essential to facilitate VATS. The hip of the patient should be at the level of the table break, which allows maximum separation of the ribs. The chest is then parallel to the floor. Some authors put the upper arm on a gutter, but despite improving stability this can limit the movement of the thoracoscope. Therefore, keeping the arms together between two normal pillows is a better position for the patient.

Ports position

We start with the utility incision at the level of the 4th intercostal space, usually in front of the anterior edge of the latissimus dorsi along an imaginary line between the tip of the scapula and the nipple. Even if the creation of this port might seem a trivial procedure, particular care must be taken to avoid oozing from the muscle as, during a lengthy procedure, the blood collecting into the chest will absorb the light and hinder the dissection of the hilar structures. At this point the hemithorax is carefully examined for signs of pleural spread or other conditions that would preclude resectability or a VATS procedure.

The second-port for the camera is usually two spaces below on the anterior axillary line. Care must be taken not to put the camera port too low because the diaphragm, especially in obese patients, will interfere with the manipulation of the thoracoscope.

The third-port is usually along the same line of the camera port on the posterior axillary line. We recommend making the port about 2 cm long as this facilitates the introduction of sponge sticks for retraction and staplers. Making the port too small in an attempt to make the procedure more 'cosmetic' usually results in more nerve damage with potential chronic pain.

Operative steps

The lung is retracted from the posterior port with a short sponge stick or lung grasper. This manoeuver facilitates the exposure of the inferior pulmonary ligament. The ligament is incised with the hook diathermy up to the inferior edge of the inferior pulmonary vein. Care must be taken to apply the diathermy at the junction between the pleural reflection and the lung. Carrying out the dissection through some of the lung parenchyma will result in irritating bleeding throughout the procedure.

Once the inferior pulmonary vein is visualized, we continue the dissection anteriorly to identify the superior pulmonary vein. After confirming normal venous anatomy, the inferior pulmonary vein is dissected, encircled with a vessel loop and divided with a 30 mm vascular stapler. According to the anatomy, the stapler can be inserted either through the utility incision or the posterior port.

The inferior pulmonary vein is a rather robust structure, away from other major hilar structures. Take care during VATS procedures not to dissect too much into the lung which can result in the division of only a few branches of the inferior pulmonary vein, rather than the whole vein. It can also lead to catastrophic bleeding when removing the specimen from unidentified venous vessels.

Once the vein is divided, there are two possibilities:

1. Fissureless technique: next structure to be divided is the bronchus which lies just superiorly to the vein. It is important to identify the middle lobe bronchus and avoid narrowing it with the stapler. Try to avoid injuring the interlobar PA that lies just superiorly to the bronchus.
   Once the bronchus has been divided, then the artery lies just superiorly and is easily seen. The anterior portion of the fissure is completed with staplers keeping the interlobar pulmonary artery under direct view. Then it is easy to divide the pulmonary artery and the posterior fissure with a series of staplers running front to back.
2. If the fissure is relatively complete it is possible to dissect it to identify the interlobar PA. We suggest using two peanuts used simultaneously to open the fissural plane and then the endo-dissector to open the adventia of the PA. Once the PA is seen, and before division, it is useful to divide the anterior portion of the oblique fissure. We use a right angle dissector placed inferiorly on the pericardium between the superior and inferior pulmonary veins. Dissection is then carried out by maintaining the tip of the dissector anterior to the previously identified PA. Once the tunnel is created, the fissure is divided with a stapler inserted from the posterior port. This manoeuver allows a better visualization of the interlobar artery. Care must be taken during dissection, not to injury the superior segmental artery. Sometime it is advisable to take the common basal trunk first and then divide the superior segmental artery. Once the artery is divided, it is easy to complete the fissure front to back with a stapler inserted through the utility incision.

The lobe is then extracted through a specimen retrieval bag.

Preference cards

1. 30° scope with HD camera. We tried several 3D systems, but we don't think they add much in VATS
2. Specifically designated VATS instruments (Scanlan)
3. LigaSure device
4. Covidien stapler with the tip at the end 30mm for vessels
5. Alexis soft tissue retractor
6. Silicone vessel loops

Tips

1. A sponge on a stick should be mounted at all times throughout the procedure, to be used in any case of sudden bleeding.
2. There is a controversy on whether it is better to use a silk tie to retract vessels before transection instead of a vessel loop. The advocates of the silk tie believe that it does not need to be removed before staple firing. We believe that having a string attached to a vessel's stump potentially could create a point for inadvertent traction during surgery with subsequent bleeding. If removed before firing, we worry that the harsh material could saw through the back wall of delicate vessels. There are also surgeons that prefer to pass the stapler directly. While this is possible most of the time, we believe that using a vessel loop provides improved visualization and control and reduces the number of vascular injuries.
3. When performing open surgery, emphasis is not often placed on removal of N1 nodes prior to obtaining vascular or bronchial control. As these nodes are often included with the specimen, they are typically not taken out separately before planned lobectomy. In VATS lobectomy, performance of regional lymphadenectomy often facilitates dissection. Arterial branch points and lobar bronchial origins are often signaled by clusters of lymph nodes. Removal of these lymph nodes creates obvious anatomic pathways for circumferential dissection and subsequent surgical control. This is particularly true with regard to surrounding the upper lobe bronchus on the right. One or two nodes are typically present at the angle created by the inferior aspect of the upper lobe origin and the bronchus intermedius.

LEFT UPPER VATS LOBECTOMY

Port and patient positioning is standard as previously described.

We start the dissection incising the inferior pulmonary ligament with hook diathermy. Care must be taken not to injure the descending aorta which lies immediately behind.

The dissection then proceeds anteriorly to identify the superior pulmonary vein and the truncus anterior. There is usually a station 10 lymph node which needs to be removed to facilitate the subsequent division of the vessel.

Once the inferior and superior border of the upper lobe vein is visible, a dissector is passed behind the vein and then the vein it is encircled with a silicone vessel loop. To facilitate the retraction of the lung it is possible to divide, if grossly incomplete, the fissure between upper and lower lobe.

Once the vein has been divided, the first portion of the PA becomes more visible. At this point, if the fissure is easy to dissect, we prefer to expose the lingula branch and divide it with stapler.

Then we divide the truncus anterior. The division of the lingula and the truncus allow extra mobility of the PA, which reduces the risk of accidental injury during dissection of the bronchus.

Division of the upper lobe bronchus is the most dangerous manoeuver in a left upper lobectomy as it is done partially blindly dissecting behind the interlobar PA. Care must be taken to dissect along the bronchial wall, without being too harsh as there is a risk of injuring the membranous part of the bronchus. Lymph nodes, if present, are swiped toward the specimen. The bronchus is eventually encircled and divided with a stapler.

Retraction on the bronchial stump facilitates exposure of the remaining vessels of the PA. We prefer to dissect them individually and use a stapler to divide them. There are reports of division with hemlock clips and/or energy devices, although such method should, in our opinion, be only reserved to small branches.

Eventually, once all the branches have been divided, the fissure is complete front to back with multiple stapler loads. Care must be taken to stay always above the interlobar PA. Moreover, it is advisable to pull the lung into the stapler rather than push the stapler through, to avoid the risk of accidental damage to the PA.

The lobe is then extracted with an endo-bag.

LEFT LOWER VATS LOBECTOMY

Patient positioning and port positioning as previously described.

We start the dissection incising the inferior pulmonary ligament with diathermy. Care must be taken not to injure the descending aorta which lies immediately behind.

The inferior pulmonary vein is dissected and encircled with a vessel loop. Before division we check that the venous drainage of the upper lobe is present. The inferior vein is then divided with staler.

At this point there are two options:

1. If the fissure is relatively complete, we expose the PA and divide it with stapler after dissection and encircling with a vessel loop. There are several ways to expose the PA, but we think that the safest and most effective is the 'kissing peanuts' technique. Basically two peanuts are used in conjunction and the thin lung tissue above the PA is gently separated. Once the PA is seen, the fascia is opened with an endo-dissector and the PA is dissected. Some surgeons use a hook diathermy. We feel, however, that the endo-dissector offers the advantage of no poking with the hot tip of the diathermy onto the PA trying to lift the fascia. Care must be taken when passing the stapler as the superior segmental branch is often separate from the main basal trunk and is not always immediately visible. Passing a stapler blindly might risk damaging the PA. Once the basal trunk is divided we divide any other branch that lies more posteriorly with stapler.
2. If the fissure is grossly incomplete, then we retract the lung upward and encircle the bronchus. This manoeuver offers the advantage of leaving the fissure intact, but is potentially quite dangerous as the PA is barely visible.

Once the PA is divided as in the previous option, the bronchus becomes visible. All lymph nodes are swiped toward the specimen and the bronchus is divided with a stapler. Care should be taken not to leave the bronchus too long as, especially in patients with COPD, there could be dehiscence of the stump due to infective reasons.

The fissure is then completed front to back with staplers and the lung extracted with an endo-bag.

Chapter 7 VATS mediastinal lymph node dissection

Kwhanmien Kim

INTRODUCTION

Lymph node dissection, including hilar and mediastinal lymph nodes, is an important procedure in non-small cell lung cancer surgery. Mediastinal lymph node dissection (MLND) is crucial to achieve completeness of lung cancer surgery. Whether MLND is associated improved survival rate of the patient with non-small cell lung cancer is still under discussion, but it can provide accurate pathological staging and better local control. Complete lymph node dissection can be defined as removal of all lymph nodes and fat tissues from each nodal station. Recent publications have shown the equivalent oncologic performance of MLND by video-assisted thoracic surgery (VATS) compared with open thoracotomy. The technique for thoracoscopic lymph node dissection is almost the same as that of an open thoracotomy, but it can vary according to the position of the thoracoscope, presence of the working window, the surgical instruments used, and the adequacy of surgical view provided by thoracoscope. However, the extent of lymhadenectomy and requirement of nodal stations for removal in relation to lung cancer locations are still controversial.

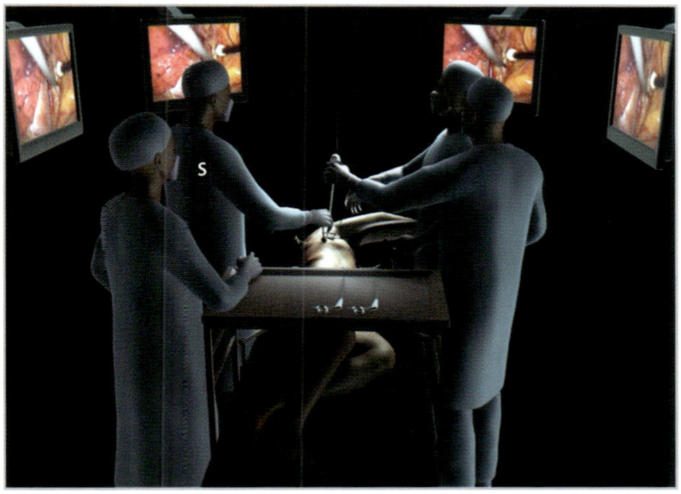

Figure 7.1 Surgeon stands at the right side of the patient, trying to avoid competing with assistants' instruments. S, surgeon.

PORT PLACEMENT

There are many different port placements for VATS lobectomy according to surgeon's preference. Before thoracoscopic port placement, it is important to consider ergonomically appropriate locations for these ports which allow: easy handling of the instruments, the ability to convert to an open thoracotomy in an emergency situation, a better cosmetic outcome, and minimal postoperative pain. My standard approach includes two ports and one utility incision (working window). The first port for the initial thoracoscopic exploration is placed at the 7th or 8th intercostal space (ICS) in the mid-axillary line. A working window of about 4 cm in length is placed at the 4th or 5th ICS in the mid-clavicular line. Specially-designed wound retractors are commercially available to enhance instrument handling and prevent wound contamination. An additional 5 mm or 10 mm port is made at the 5th or 6th ICS in below the scapular tip. This port configuration guarantees safe and prompt conversion to open thoracotomy in emergent situations by connecting the working window and the posterior port. Simply by changing the thoracoscope port and applying appropriate maneuvers, all lung lobes can be resected and MLND can be achieved by this three-port configuration without major modifications. However, it depends on the surgeon's preference to decide where to stand, where to place the thoracoscope, and whether to change the thoracoscope port or use a fixed-port. It is important that the surgeon's instruments are not liable to crossover with the assistant's instruments (the 'no hand cross-over' technique). I recommend standing at the right side of the operating table as it allows smooth right-hand maneuvers (**Figure 7.1**).

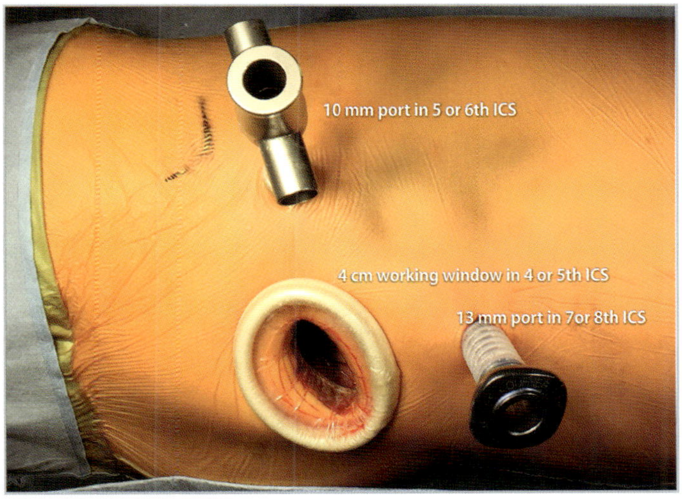

Figure 7.2 Port placement for VATS lobectomy and mediastinal lymph node dissection in the left side. ICS, intercostal space.

When performing a left-sided VATS lobectomy, a 10-mm port for the thoracoscope is placed in the 5th or 6th ICS in the anterior scapular line, as it can provide better fissure development and subcarinal exposure (**Figure 7.2**).

TECHNIQUE OF VATS MEDIASTINAL LYMPH NODE DISSECTION

Right

2R, 3, and 4R (right paratracheal and pretracheal nodes)

The mediastinal pleural is opened from the junction of the azygos vein and the superior vena cava (SVC). From below the azygos vein to the right brachiocephalic artery, between the trachea and the SVC, a longitudinal incision is made on the parietal pleura. It is easy to dissect all the mediastinal fat tissue including lymph nodes from below the azygos vein to the level of the innominate artery in upward direction.

By elevating the azygos vein and gently retracting the right pulmonary artery trunk, the mediastinal fat pad between the right main bronchus (RMB) and anterior carinal area is well visualized and dissected first, then dissection continues to the pericardium around the aortic arch. The azygos vein is retracted caudally and the SVC is retracted anteriorly with an endoscopic retractor and peanut, the mediastinal fat pad is dissected from the trachea and the SVC, and from the caudal border of the innominate artery (**Figure 7.3**). All mediastinal fat tissues including lymph nodes are removed en bloc. Small veins draining from the mediastinal fat tissues directly into the SVC are ligated with hemoclips or divided with ultrasonic device. At the apex, the right recurrent laryngeal nerve can be damaged by thermal injury. Because there are many small lymphatic channels in this area, those should be ligated or treated safely to avoid postoperative chylothorax. I prefer to use an ultrasonic device (Harmonic ACE, Ethicon), as it is easy to dissect mediastinal fat tissues with less bleeding and it may help to prevent postoperative lymphatic leak.

7 (subcarinal nodes, right-sided approach)

After tilting the operating table to the left ward and retracting the right lung anteriorly, the right subcarinal area is easily exposed. The parietal pleural is then opened, avoiding injury to the vagus nerve. Although the small vagal branches running into the bronchus are usually divided, it is better to save those branches to decrease dry cough after operation. The subcarinal fat pad is dissected en bloc, beginning inferiorly and moving upwards to the carina with electrocautery or ultrasonic devices. Dissection starts from the inferior border of the bronchus intermedius and the inferior pulmonary vein, then moving upwards. The subcarinal lymph nodes are then dissected from the esophagus, and the left and right main bronchi. The anterior subcarinal space can be reached by an anterior approach if clear dissection is difficult from behind (**Figure 7.4**).

Left

5 and 6 (aortopulmonary window and paraaortic nodes)

The mediastinal pleura is opened between the phrenic and the vagus nerves at the level of the aortopulmonary window. The incision is extended along the vagus nerve in a cephalad direction and horizontally above the left main pulmonary artery (LMPA). Care should be taken to avoid the phrenic nerve and the left recurrent laryngeal nerve injuries. Level 6 lymph nodes are located in the area medial to the ligamentum arteriosum and level 5 lymph nodes are between the lower border of the aortic arch and the upper rim of the LMPA. The aortopulmonary fat pad containing level 5 and 6 lymph nodes is removed en bloc (**Figure 7.5**).

4L (left paratracheal nodes)

The left paratracheal lymph nodes are located between the upper margin of the aortic arch and the upper rim of the LMPA. After pushing down the main left pulmonary artery with a peanut and retracting the

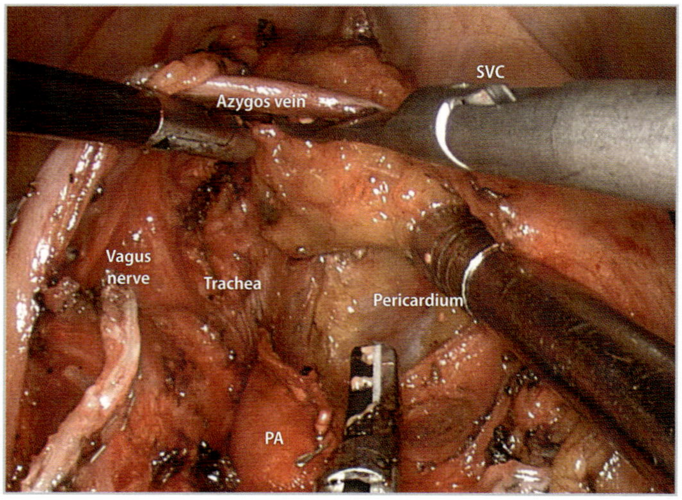

Figure 7.3 Dissection of lymph node levels 2R, 3R, and 4R. With elevation of the azygos vein and pushing down the right pulmonary artery trunk, and retraction of the SVC anteriorly, mediastinal fat pad between the RMB and anterior carinal area is dissected first. SVC : superior vena cava; PA, pulmonary artery.

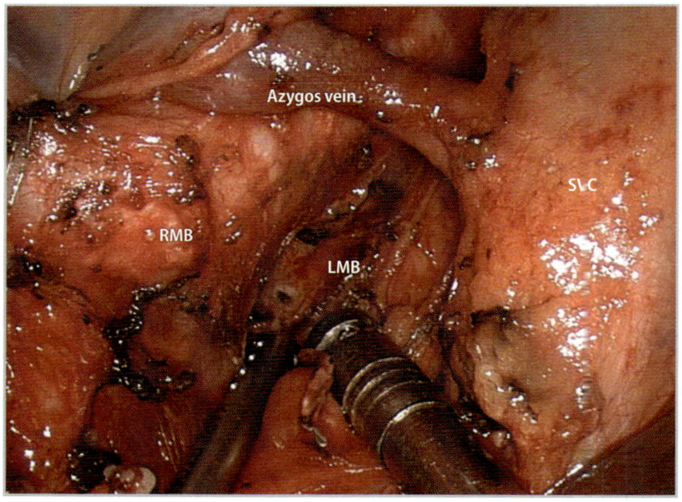

Figure 7.4 The anterior subcarinal space can be reached by an anterior approach if clear dissection is difficult from behind, pushing down the right pulmonary artery trunk and retracting the RMB posteriorly. LMB, left main bronchus; RMB, right main bronchus; SVC, superior vena cava.

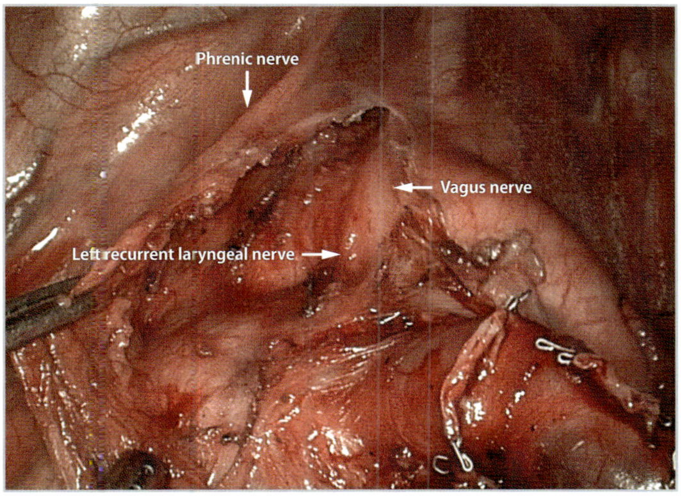

Figure 7.5 Dissection of lymph nodes level 5 and 6. Attention should be paid to avoid the phrenic and left recurrent laryngeal nerve injuries.

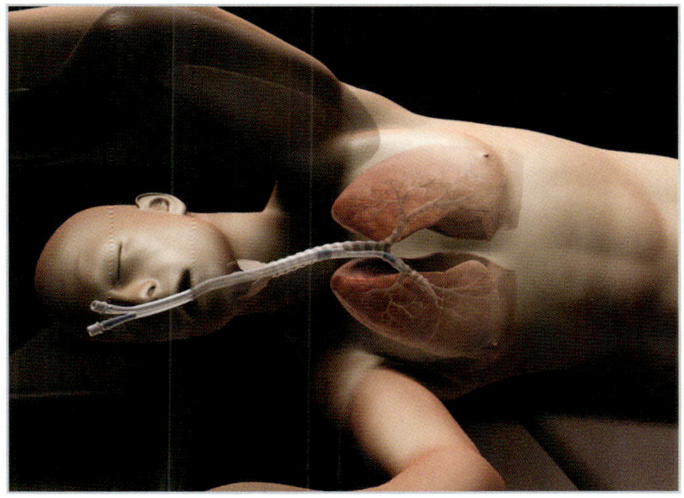

Figure 7.7 Endotracheal intubation of the right-sided double-lumen tube may facilitate the left side subcarinal lymph node dissection.

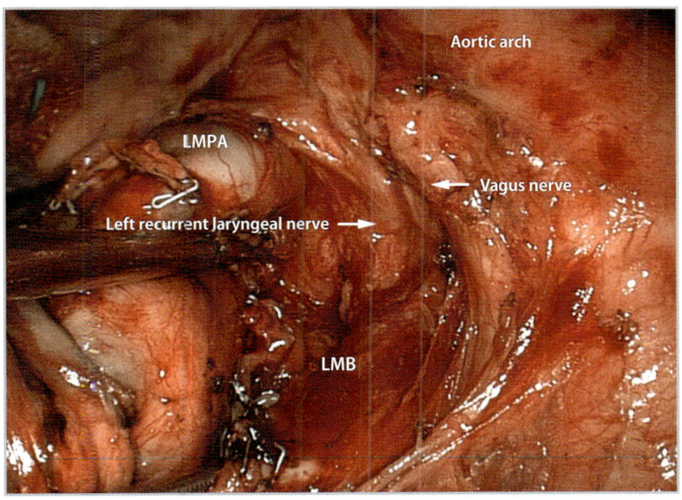

Figure 7.6 Dissection of 4L lymph nodes. Pushing down and retracting the LMPA trunk and the LMB, level 4L lymph nodes are exposed. Attention should be paid to avoid the left recurrent laryngeal nerve injury. LMPA, left main pulmonary artery; LMB, left main bronchus.

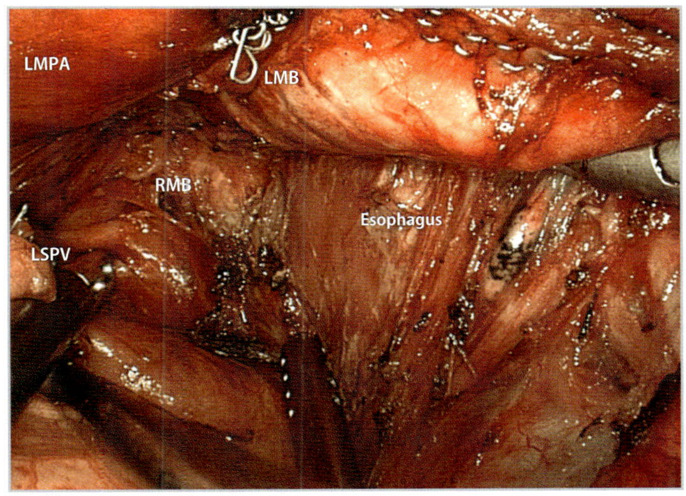

Figure 7.8 Dissection of left subcarinal lymph nodes by anterior approach. With elevation of the LMB and the left pulmonary artery trunk upward, and pushing down the LSPV, the left subcarinal space can be approached anteriorly, especially after VATS left upper lobectomy. LMPA, left main pulmonary artery; LMB, left main bronchus; RMB, right main bronchus; LSPV, left superior pulmonary vein.

aortic arch upward with an endoscopic retractor, 4L lymph nodes are dissected along the left main bronchus (LMB) to the trachea. The 4L lymph nodes are close to the left recurrent laryngeal nerve. To avoid left vocal cord palsy, the left recurrent laryngeal nerve and the proximal vagus nerve must be carefully preserved (**Figure 7.6**).

7 (subcarinal nodes, left-sided approach)

It is more difficult to expose the left subcarinal space because of the longer LMB, the descending aorta, and the spine. A right-sided double-lumen endotracheal intubation is necessary to facilitate the elevation of the LMB during the left subcarinal lymph node dissection (**Figure 7.7**). The left subcarinal space can be approached anteriorly with the lung retracted posteriorly while elevating the LMB and the LMPA, especially after left upper lobectomy (**Figure 7.8**). When the left lower lobectomy is performed, the left subcarinal space is approached posteriorly. The mediastinal pleura is opened anterior to and along the descending aorta. The small branches of the vagus nerve supplying the lung are divided. To expose the left subcarinal space, the LMB is retracted anteriorly with an endoscopic fan retractor or endoscopic peanut, the descending aorta and the esophagus are retracted posteriorly with an endoscopic esophageal retractor. The subcarinal fat pad is dissected from the LMB to the carina. Then, lymph node dissection is carried out from the esophagus and the RMB. The small arterial branches entering the lymph nodes from the anterior border of the trachea at the level of the carina should be treated appropriately to avoid postoperative bleeding (**Figure 7.9**).

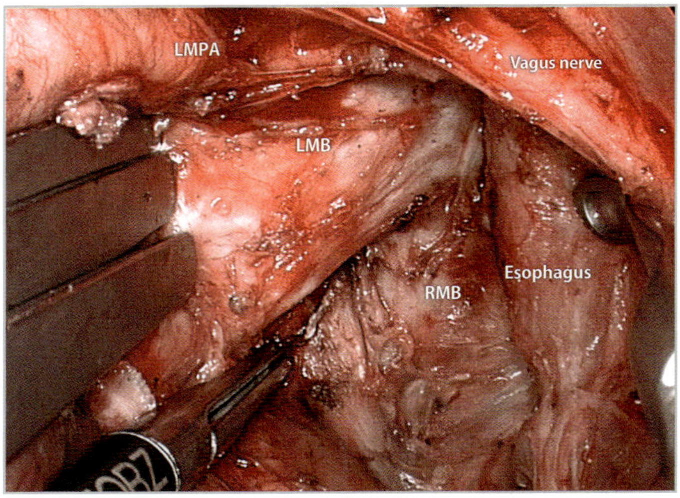

Figure 7.9 Dissection of left subcarinal lymph nodes by posterior approach. With the retraction of the left main bronchus anteriorly with a fan-retractor, retracting the esophagus and the descending aorta posteriorly with an endoscopic retractor, the left subcarinal space can be exposed widely. LMPA, left main pulmonary artery; LMB, left main bronchus; RMB, right main bronchus.

FURTHER READING

D'Amico TA. Videothoracoscopic mediastinal lymphadenectomy. Thorac Surg Clin 2010; 20:207–213.

Darling GE, Allen MS, Decker PA, et al. Number of lymph nodes harvested from a mediastinal lymphadenectomy: Results of the randomized, prospective American College of Surgery Oncology Group Z0030 trial. Chest 2011; 139:1124–1129.

Khalid A. Thoracoscopic mediastinal lymph node dissection for lung cancer. Semin Thoracic Surg 2012; 24:74–78.

Kim HK, Choi YS, Kim J, Shim YM, Kim K. Outcomes of unexpected pathologic N1 and N2 disease after video-assisted thoracic surgery lobectomy for clinical stage I non-small cell lung cancer. J Thorac Cardiovasc Surg 2010; 140:1288–1293.

Kim K, Kim HK, Park JS, et al. Video-assisted thoracic surgery lobectomy: single institutional experience with 704 cases. Ann Thorac Surg 2010; 89:S705–S709.

Kim K. Video-assisted thoracic surgery lobectomy. Korean J Thorac Cardiovasc Surg 2011; 44:1–8.

Lee HS, Jang HJ. Thoracoscopic mediastinal lymph node dissection for lung cancer. Semin Thoracic Surg 2012; 24:131–141.

Sagawa M, Sato M, Sakurada A, et al. A prospective trial of systematic nodal dissection for lung cancer by video-assissted thoracic surgery: can it be perfecto? Ann Thorac Surg 2002; 73:900–904.

Swanson SJ, Herndon JE, D'Amico TA, et al. Video-assisted thoracic surgery lobectomy: Report of CALGB 39802-A prospective, multi-institutional feasibility study. J Clin Oncol 2007; 25:4993–4997.

Watanabe A, Koyanagi T, Ohsawa H, et al. Systematic node dissection by VATS is not inferior to that through an open thoracotomy: a comparative clinicopathologic retrospective study. Surgery 2005; 138:510–517.

Watanabe A, Nakazawa J, Miyajima M, et al. Thoracoscopic mediastinal lymph node dissection for lung cancer. Semin Thoracic Surg 2012; 24:68–73.

Chapter 8 Thoracoscopic pneumonectomy

Hanghang Wang, Thomas A D'Amico

INTRODUCTION

Thoracoscopic lobectomy, also termed video-assisted thoracic surgery (VATS) lobectomy, is the less invasive alternative to open lobectomy via thoracotomy for the treatment of lung cancer. The advantages of VATS, compared to open lobectomy have been well established and include decreased post-operative pain, shorter length of stay, fewer postoperative complications,[1,2] superior compliance with adjuvant chemotherapy,[3] and preserved lung function.[4-7] The application of VATS techniques has also evolved over the last decade from treating small peripheral tumors to major pulmonary resections, including pneumonectomy.[8-10] VATS pneumonectomy, defined as pneumonectomy via completely thoracoscopic approaches without rib-spreading, has been described previously and is currently performed by a limited number of centers.[3,9,11-13] Part of the reason for its slow dissemination may be due to the belief that the morbidity of pneumonectomy is mainly a product of the extent of lung resection and its impact on pulmonary physiology, rather than the operative trauma associated with thoracotomy. Thus, the benefits of VATS pneumonectomy over open pneumonectomy seem less clear than those of VATS lobectomy. However, there is emerging evidence showing that VATS pneumonectomy is an oncologically equivalent treatment as open pneumonectomy and may offer benefits of decreased postoperative pain and shorter length of stay similar to VATS lobectomy.[8,10,11,13] In this chapter, we review the patient selection, preoperative evaluation, anesthesia, operative techniques, and potential complications of VATS pneumonectomy. Both the existing literature and our institutional experience in VATS pneumonectomy are summarized.

PATIENT SELECTION

Similar to pneumonectomy using the open approach, VATS pneumonectomy is the treatment of choice for locally advanced but resectable lung cancer or granulomatous lung disease that cannot be treated with lobectomy or sleeve lobectomy alone. Specific oncologic indications for VATS pneumonectomy include involvement of the central structures [e.g. main pulmonary artery (PA), mainstem bronchus], synchronous ipsilateral tumors, and hilar lesions not amenable to a sleeve resection.[11,14,15] Patient-specific factors include the ability to tolerate one-lung ventilation and adequate pulmonary reserve to survive the loss of the resected lung. Absolute contraindications to VATS pneumonectomy include the presence of N3 disease, extrathoracic disease, inability to achieve complete resection with pneumonectomy, inability to tolerate single-lung ventilation and inadequate pulmonary reserve. Relative contraindications (related to the difficulty of completing the procedure thoracoscopically) include large tumor mass (although there is no absolute size criteria), preoperative chemotherapy or chemoradiation therapy, and previous ipsilateral lobectomy.

The role of pneumonectomy as a treatment option for N2 disease remains controversial, owing to the heterogeneity of N2 disease and inconclusive results from clinical trials.[16-19] At our institution, patients are routinely evaluated by a dedicated multidisciplinary team in thoracic oncology comprised of thoracic surgeons, radiation oncologists and medical oncologists. Treatment plans are individualized for each patient in order to offer the best chances of survival.

PREOPERATIVE EVALUATION

Preoperative evaluation for patients undergoing VATS pneumonectomy for suspected lung cancer begins with a thorough clinical assessment. Clinical findings that suggest metastatic disease include constitutional symptoms (e.g. weight loss, anorexia, fatigue), neurological symptoms (e.g. headache, syncope, changes in mental status) and physical abnormalities (e.g. supraclavicular lymphadenopathy, bone tenderness, hepatomegaly).[20] Extrathoracic staging is attained through computed tomography (CT) scan, positron emission tomography (PET) imaging, tissue biopsy, and brain magnetic resonance imaging (MRI). Mediastinal staging may require CT scan, PET imaging, needle biopsy [endobronchial ultrasound (EBUS) – fine needle aspiration (FNA), endoscopic ultrasound (EUS) – FNA or combined EBUS/EUS-FNA], and/or surgical staging via a Chamberlain procedure, VATS or mediastinoscopy.[20]

Preoperative evaluation for VATS pneumonectomy also includes a complete history and physical examination, preoperative laboratory testing, and optimization of medical comorbidities.[21] Laboratory tests include complete blood counts, serum chemistries, liver function tests, coagulation assays, and blood typing and cross matching. Cardiovascular evaluation and management are based on functional capacity and risk stratification.[22] Pulmonary-specific assessments may include history of smoking, symptoms of chronic obstructive pulmonary disease (COPD), pulmonary function testing, and ventilation-perfusion scan or exercise testing.[21] Postoperative pulmonary function can be predicted using several methods, including the segment method, ventilation-perfusion scan and quantitative CT scanning.[23]

ANESTHESIA

VATS pneumonectomy is performed under general anesthesia with the one-lung ventilation technique to provide adequate surgical exposure.[24] General anesthesia is provided through intravenous and inhalational anesthetic agents. Ventilation and oxygenation are monitored by capnography and pulse oximetry.[24] After induction of anesthesia, a double-lumen endobronchial tube (directed into the contralateral bronchus) is used to collapse the operated lung and allow selective ventilation to the contralateral side.[25] Other intraoperative monitoring modalities include electrocardiogram, arterial pressure measurement, intermittent arterial blood gas (ABG) sampling, nasopharyngeal temperature monitoring and urinary output measurement.

One special anesthesia consideration in VATS pneumonectomy is the approach to intraoperative hypoxemia.[24] While the application of continuous positive airway pressure by oxygen insufflation to the non-ventilated lung is frequently used to improve oxygenation in open pneumonectomy, its use is limited in VATS pneumonectomy due to potential obstruction of the surgical field.[24] Therefore, alternative recruitment techniques need to be employed, such as adding PEEP to the ventilated lung or intermittent two-lung ventilation.[26] In addition, the surgeon and anesthesiologist must attempt to restrict the inspired oxygen concentration in patients who have undergone induction therapy to minimize the risk of postoperative lung injury.[27]

Postoperative analgesia for VATS pneumonectomy is routinely provided through thoracic epidural analgesia with a local anesthetic and/or opioid infusions.[24] Other forms of analgesia include patient controlled analgesia, paravertebral block and systemic analgesia (e.g. opioids, non-steroidal anti-inflammatory medications).

OPERATIVE TECHNIQUE

Overview

While the decision to perform VATS pneumonectomy is often determined during preoperative evaluation by tumor histology and anatomy, there are occasions when the need for pneumonectomy is established on the basis of intraoperative findings. In either case, care should be taken to avoid committing the patient to a VATS pneumonectomy if there is a possibility of parenchymal preservation by performing a lesser resection (VATS sleeve resection or lobectomy) without compromising the oncologic outcome. One advantage of the VATS approach over open pneumonectomy is that the extent of the disease and its resectability are determined early with VATS exploration, which obviates the morbidity of thoracotomy without resection and associated delay in appropriate treatment.

The number of incisions, location of the access site and sequence of dissection and division vary among different institutions that perform VATS pneumonectomy (**Table 8.1**). Specifically, some centers dissect the pulmonary veins (PVs) but delay division due to concerns of pulmonary congestion from continued arterial flow into the ligated venous segment.[13] Other studies advocate early division of the PV, citing evidence that surgical manipulation during pulmonary resection could stimulate the occurrence of micrometastasis in the circulation.[28] Both laboratory and clinical studies to date have shown that early venous ligation does not affect the amount of blood retained in the lungs during major pulmonary resections.[29,30] At the same time, despite experimental evidence of increased tumor marker expressions in delayed PV ligation,[28] this delay did not appear to play a role in tumor recurrence in a prior retrospective study.[31] Without evidence from any prospective randomized trials, the sequence of vessel dissection and division remains controversial and is currently determined by surgeon's preference and the intraoperative situation.

Patient positioning

Similar to VATS lobectomy, patients are placed in full lateral decubitus position in VATS pneumonectomy with the distal half of the operating table lowered at the level of the hip. This position widens the intercostal spaces and improves thoracoscopic access and exposure.[4]

Incision

We use two incisions in similar locations as in the VATS lobectomy technique described previously.[4] The first 1 cm incision is placed in the 8th intercostal space in the midaxillary line and serves as the primary port access for the thoracoscope. A 10 mm, 30° angled thoracoscope is inserted through the incision to optimize visualization. A second incision (4.5–6 cm) is made anteriorly in the 5th intercostal space without rib-spreading and functions as both the access and specimen retrieval site.

Exposure

Thoracoscopic exploration is performed after the first two incisions to confirm the tumor location and assess any contraindications to resection, including the presence of pleural disease. Additional incisions may be needed after inspection for better visualization or retraction. Lysis of pleural adhesions is also performed at this point if indicated.

Circumferential hilar dissection is then undertaken through the access incision using a combination of sharp and blunt dissection. This exposes the inferior PV, superior PV, bronchus, and main PA. Mediastinal lymph node dissection may be performed (preferred) at this time or deferred until pneumonectomy is completed.

Pulmonary veins

The inferior pulmonary ligament is then divided. The inferior PV is dissected free and encircled with a curved clamp. Division of the inferior PV is achieved using a linear reticulating stapling device.

This exposes the superior pulmonary vein, which is in close proximity to the PA anteriorly on both sides. The superior PV is similarly encircled, stapled and divided using the stapling device.

Pulmonary artery

The main PA is then dissected free from any adhesions, encircled, stapled and divided. (**Figure 8.1**). The nature of the dissection is to dissect directly on the bronchus, minimizing the retraction of, and any dissection close to, the artery itself. As all other hilar dissection has already been completed and only these two structures remain – the artery and the bronchus – this dissection should always be performed with no risk of PA injury. In cases where the tumor is close to the origin of the PA, obtaining enough room to apply the stapler may be impossible and an intrapericardial pneumonectomy may be indicated. These cases may require conversion to thoracotomy and intrapericardial dissection.

Table 8.1 Summary of operative techniques of VATS pneumonectomy at different institutions. PV, pulmonary vein; PA, pulmonary artery.

Institution	No. of incisions	Access site	Sequence of dissection
City Hospital, Edinburgh, UK[8]	3	Submammary incision (6 cm)	PV → main bronchus → PA
UMass Memorial Healthcare, MA, USA[14]	3	5th intercostal space anterior, three fingerbreadth	PV → main bronchus → PA
Roswell Park Cancer Institute, NY, USA[9,11,13,15]	3	3rd–4th interspace, 4 cm	PV → PA → main bronchus, delayed PV division
Himeji Medical Center, Japan[12]	3	4th intercostal space anterior, 3–5 cm	PV → PA → main bronchus
Duke University Medical Center, NC, USA[32]	2	5th intercostal space anterior, 4.5–6 cm	PV → PA → main bronchus

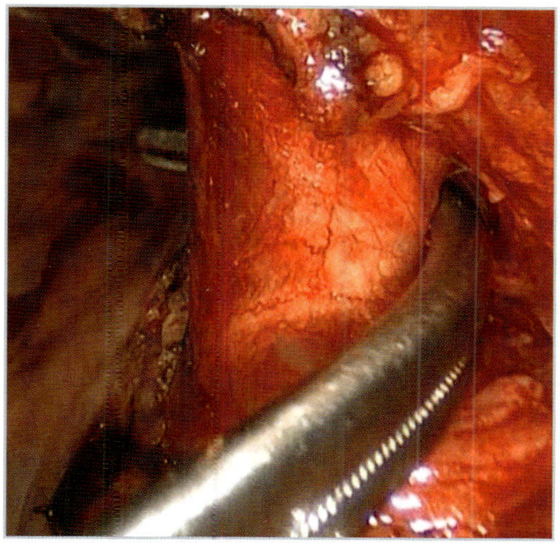

Figure 8.1 Safe dissection of the left pulmonary artery.

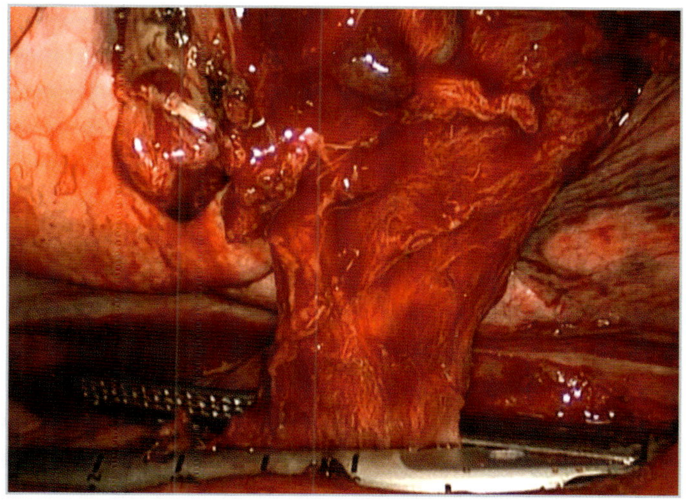

Figure 8.2 Bronchial dissection with an adequate length of left main bronchus.

Bronchus

Next, full bronchial mobilization is undertaken by circumferential bronchial dissection to optimize the bronchial stump. This dissection includes all the lymphatic tissue within the peribronchial space. Complete subcarinal lymphadenectomy is recommended prior to bronchial division for both oncological and technical advantages. For left pneumonectomy, extensive proximal dissection of the entire left main bronchus under the aortic arch is recommended in order to optimize the length of the resected bronchus and minimize the length of the bronchial stump. Division of the main bronchus is performed with the linear stapler as close as possible to the carina to avoid a long bronchial stump (**Figure 8.2**). Care should be taken to visualize the contralateral main bronchus, especially during left VATS pneumonectomy. The bronchus is usually the last structure divided to avoid single attachment by the PA and inadvertent injury due to excessive torque. In cases where the tumor is anterior making the hilar dissection difficult, the bronchus may be dissected and divided prior to division of the PA, allowing for better exposure.

The specimen is removed through the anterior incision using a protective bag to prevent tumor implantation in the incision. The specimen is sent for frozen section analysis of the resection line to assure negative margins. Additional resection may be required if frozen section reveals positive margins.

Mediastinal lymph node dissection is then undertaken to include the remaining mediastinal lymph node compartments not resected en bloc with VATS pneumonectomy.

Closure

The chest is copiously irrigated with warm bacitracin-containing normal saline and aspirated dry. The bronchial stump is inspected to rule out any air leak. If an air leak is encountered, repeat stapling or intracorporeal suturing may be employed and the bronchial stump may be covered with adjacent vascularized tissue, including pleural flaps, pericardial fat pad and intercostal muscles. We do not routinely cover the bronchial stump with the exception of patients who undergo right pneumonectomy after induction chemoradiation therapy.

Techniques for drainage of the postpneumonectomy space remain controversial. We routinely leave a single chest tube, which is exteriorized through the medial port incision; it is connected to a balanced drainage device. This chest tube is left in place to achieve stabilization of the mediastinum and to monitor postoperative drainage. The anterior incision is closed with absorbable sutures and sterile dressings are applied.

CONVERSION TO THORACOTOMY

The reported conversion rate from VATS pneumonectomy to thoracotomy ranges from 2.1% to 25% at different institutions (**Table 8.2**).[9,11,12] Reasons for conversion include tumor extension precluding thoracoscopic dissection, adhesions, bleeding and difficult anatomy. In our institutional experience, indications for conversion included proximal nature of the tumor requiring an intrapericardial pneumonectomy, PA bleeding, severe adhesions from previous thoracic surgery, and difficult hilar dissection not amenable to VATS. Patients who required conversion in our institution were more likely to have poorer pulmonary function, more medical comorbidities, and have received neoadjuvant chemotherapy. Patients who required conversion also tended to have a longer operative time and higher intraoperative blood loss than patients who underwent either thoracotomy or complete VATS pneumonectomy, likely reflective of the difficult situations associated with conversion. As opposed to conversion for lobectomy, conversion for pneumonectomy carries short-term consequences; the decision to convert to open pneumonectomy should be made early to prevent catastrophic blood loss from the proximal PA, an issue that is usually not a significant concern during lobectomy.

MORTALITY AND MORBIDITY

Thirty-day mortality of VATS pneumonectomy is reported to be 2–7.5% and comparable to open pneumonectomy (**Table 8.2**).[11-13,15] Complications after VATS pneumonectomy are similar to open pneumonectomy and include atrial fibrillation, myocardial infarction, pneumonia, empyema and bronchopleural fistula.[8,11-13,15] Atrial fibrillation remains the most common complication with incidence of up to 24% in our experience.

Table 8.2 Outcomes of VATS pneumonectomy in previous studies

Author (Year)	No. of attempted VATS pneumonectomy	Conversion rate (%)	30-day mortality (%)
Craig & Walker[8]	6	0	0
Nwogu; Sahai et al.[9,11,15]	32	25	3
Nagai et al.[12]	47	2.1	2.1
Battoo et al.[13]	67	15.9	7.5

VATS VERSUS OPEN PNEUMONECTOMY

Several groups have reported increased operative time in VATS compared to open pneumonectomy.[11,15] In our experience, the median operative time of complete VATS pneumonectomy (excluding conversions) is not significantly different from open pneumonectomy. In general, we recommend developing advanced thoracoscopic skills with VATS lobectomy before attempting VATS pneumonectomy.

Similar to VATS lobectomy, VATS pneumonectomy has been shown to have the advantage of decreased postoperative pain and shorter length of stay (LOS) over open pneumonectomy. In their initial experience of VATS pneumonectomy, Craig et al. found that patients had less mean morphine consumption per hour than open pneumonectomy patients during the first 36 hours after surgery.[8] A significant benefit of VATS versus open pneumonectomy was also observed with respect to chronic post-thoracotomy pain at 1-year follow-up in a recent study.[13] A shorter LOS (median LOS = 4.5 versus 6 days) was reported by Nwogu et al. in their initial experience with VATS pneumonectomy[11] and confirmed in our experience (median LOS = 4 versus 5 days).

Existing evidence indicates equivalent oncologic outcomes between VATS and open pneumonectomy.[11] In their study of patients with stage I, II and III disease, Nwogu et al. showed equivalent survival of VATS and open pneumonectomy patients at a median follow-up of 47 months.[11] In the study by Battoo et al. of 30 patients with p-stage 0, I, and II disease who underwent successful VATS pneumonectomy, there was a trend towards improved median survival compared with open pneumonectomy.[13] Our institutional study of propensity-matched VATS versus open pneumonectomy patients showed similar recurrence rate and survival.

CONCLUSION

VATS pneumonectomy is currently only performed in a limited number of centers, despite early experiences that have established its feasibility and efficacy. Similar to VATS lobectomy, to be considered an alternative to open pneumonectomy, VATS pneumonectomy needs to be applied with the same oncologic principles.[4] As experience accumulates with VATS pneumonectomy and more outcome data become available, we expect increased adoption of this technique in the treatment of locally advanced lung cancers in the near future.

REFERENCES

1. Villamizar NR, Darrabie MD, Burfeind WR, et al. Thoracoscopic lobectomy is associated with lower morbidity compared with thoracotomy. J Thorac Cardiovasc Surg 2009; 138:419–425.
2. Paul S, Altorki NK, Sheng S, et al. Thoracoscopic lobectomy is associated with lower morbidity than open lobectomy: A propensity-matched analysis from the STS database. J Thorac Cardiovasc Surg 2010; 139:366–378.
3. Petersen RP, Pham D, Burfeind WR, et al. Thoracoscopic lobectomy facilitates the delivery of chemotherapy after resection for lung cancer. Ann Thorac Surg 2007; 83:1245–1250.
4. Burfeind WR DT. Thoracoscopic lobectomy. Oper Tech Thorac Cardiovasc Surg 2004; 9:98–114.
5. Daniels LJ, Balderson SS, Onaitis MW, D'Amico TA. Thoracoscopic lobectomy: a safe and effective strategy for patients with stage I lung cancer. Ann Thorac Surg 2002; 74:860–864.
6. Swanson SJ, Herndon JE, D'Amico TA, et al. Video-assisted thoracic surgery lobectomy: Report of CALGB 39802 - a prospective, multi-institution feasibility study. J Clin Oncol 2007; 25:4993–4997.
7. Demmy TL, James TA, Swanson SJ, McKenna RJ, D'Amico TA. Troubleshooting video-assisted thoracic surgery lobectomy. Ann Thorac Surg 2005; 79:1744–1752.
8. Craig SR, Walker WS. Initial experience of video assisted thoracoscopic pneumonectomy. Thorax 1995:392–395.
9. Nwogu CE, Glinianski M, Demmy TL. Minimally invasive pneumonectomy. Ann Thorac Surg 2006; 82:e3–4.
10. Villamizar NR, Darrabie M, Hanna J, et al. Impact of T status and N status on perioperative outcomes after thoracoscopic lobectomy for lung cancer. J Thorac Cardiovasc Surg 2013; 145:514–521.
11. Nwogu CE, Yendamuri S, Demmy TL. Does thoracoscopic pneumonectomy for lung cancer affect survival? Ann Thorac Surg 2010; 89:S2102–S2106.
12. Nagai S, Imanishi N, Matsuoka T, et al. Video-assisted thoracoscopic pneumonectomy: retrospective outcome analysis of 47 consecutive patients. Ann Thorac Surg 2014:3–8.
13. Battoo A, Jahan A, Yang Z, et al. Thoracoscopic pneumonectomy. Chest 2014; 146:1300.
14. Conlan AA, Sandor A. Total thoracoscopic pneumonectomy: indications and technical considerations. J Thorac Cardiovasc Surg 2003; 126:2083–2085.
15. Sahai RK, Nwogu CE, Yendamuri S, et al. Is thoracoscopic pneumonectomy safe? Ann Thorac Surg 2009; 88:1086–1092.
16. Higgins KA, Chino JP, Ready N, et al. Persistent N2 disease after neoadjuvant chemotherapy for non-small-cell lung cancer. J Thorac Cardiovasc Surg 2011; 142:1175–1179.
17. Yanagawa J, Rusch VW. Current surgical therapy for stage IIIA (N2) non-small cell lung cancer. Semin Thorac Cardiovasc Surg 2011; 23:291–296.
18. Martins RG, D'Amico TA, Loo BW, et al. The management of patients with stage IIIA non – small cell lung cancer with N2 mediastinal node involvement 2012; 10:599–613.
19. Tanaka S, Aoki M, Ishikawa H, Otake Y. Pneumonectomy for node-positive non-small cell lung cancer: can it be a treatment option for N2 disease? Gen Thorac Cardiovasc Surg 2014; 62:370–375.
20. Silvestri GA, Gonzalez AV, Jantz MA, et al. Methods for staging non-small cell lung cancer: diagnosis and management of lung cancer, 3rd edn: American college of chest physicians evidence-based clinical practice guidelines. Chest 2013; 143:211–250.
21. Datta D, Lahiri B. Preoperative evaluation of patients undergoing lung resection surgery. Chest 2003; 123:2096–2103.
22. Fleisher LA, Fleischmann KE, Auerbach AD, et al. 2014 ACC/AHA guideline on perioperative cardiovascular evaluation and management of patients undergoing noncardiac surgery. J Am Coll Cardiol 2014; 64:e77–137.

23. Poonyagariyagorn H, Mazzone PJ. Lung cancer: preoperative pulmonary evaluation of the lung resection candidate. Semin Respir Crit Care Med 2008; 29:271–284.
24. Fischer GW, Cohen E. An update on anesthesia for thoracoscopic surgery. Curr Opin Anaesthesiol 2010; 23:7–11.
25. Brodsky JB, Cohen E. Video-assisted thoracoscopic surgery. Curr Opin Anaesthesiol 2000; 13:41–45.
26. Kitabjian L, Bordi S, Elisha S, et al. Anesthesia case management for video-assisted thoracoscopic surgery. AANA J 2013; 81:65–75.
27. Grichnik KP, D'Amico TA. Acute lung injury and acute respiratory distress syndrome after pulmonary resection. Semin Cardiothorac Vasc Anesth 2004; 8:317–334.
28. Du J. Effects of different sequences of pulmonary artery and vein ligations during pulmonary lobectomy on blood micrometastasis of non-small cell lung cancer. Oncol Lett 2012:463–468.
29. Miller GE, Smeloff EA. Physiologic basis of preliminary venous ligation in the surgery of pulmonary neoplasms. Am J Surg 1969; 118:921–924.
30. Yellin A, Sadetzki S, Simansky DA, et al The sequence of vessel interruption during lobectomy – does it affect the amount of blood retained in the lobe? Eur J Cardiothorac Surg 2007; 31:711–713.
31. Refaely Y, Sadetzki S, Chetrit A, et al. The sequence of vessel interruption during lobectomy for non-small cell lung cancer: Is it indeed important? J Thorac Cardiovasc Surg 2003; 125:1313–1320.
32. Burfeind WR, D'Amico TA. Thoracoscopic Lobectomy. Operative Techniques in Thoracic and Cardiovascular Surgery 2004; 9:98-114.

Chapter 9 Thoracoscopic sleeve lobectomy

David N Ranney, Thomas A D'Amico

INTRODUCTION

Minimally invasive surgery has attracted significant attention in the thoracic surgical community with the goal of providing surgical outcomes at least equivalent to open approaches, and with reduced operative morbidity. With respect to oncologic outcomes, the integrity of complete tumor resection must be maintained to justify these less invasive techniques. With the advent of video-assisted thoracic surgery (VATS), surgical approaches continue to evolve and thus necessitate further study to identify patients who will benefit from these approaches without sacrificing long-term oncologic outcomes.

It has been well established that VATS offers reduced postoperative pain, decreased length of stay, improved postoperative pulmonary mechanics, fewer postoperative complications, and superior compliance with adjuvant chemotherapy.[1-3] In retrospective reviews, VATS lobectomy has been found to be comparable in terms of oncologic outcomes to traditional thoracotomy.[4] As such, VATS has been the preferred approach in those patients who are without contraindication.[5]

A subset of patients with lesions residing at the lobar bronchial orifice were once deemed unsuitable for VATS given the technical difficulty of a bronchial anastomosis via thoracoscopy and concern for an associated increased risk of complications. However, as experience with minimally invasive techniques has improved, VATS sleeve lobectomy has emerged as an alternative approach. This particular method achieves lobectomy with bronchial re-anastomosis; a technique that spares the need for thoracotomy or pneumonectomy and their associated morbidities.[6]

Sleeve lobectomy by thoracotomy was first reported in 1947 by Sir Prince Thomas, when he treated a patient with a carcinoid tumor located at the right mainstem bronchus.[7] As VATS techniques became increasingly utilized, the first sleeve lobectomy by thoracoscopy was described in 2002 by Luigi Santambrogio when treating a patient who had a mucoepidermoid carcinoma.[8] The first case series of VATS sleeve lobectomy patients was published by Ali Mahtabifard in 2008, which included 13 patients with various pulmonary malignancies. Since then only a paucity of case series have been published from a multitude of centers around the world.[9] In addition, there have been case reports of uniportal VATS sleeve lobectomy.[10]

PATIENT CHARACTERISTICS

Patients with clinical stage I known or suspected lung cancer located at the lobar bronchial orifice are the intended candidates for VATS sleeve resection, including non-small cell lung cancer as well as benign to low grade malignant neoplasms. Clinical data suggest approximately 80% of these malignant lesions are carcinoid. Benign lesions eligible for resection include stenoses related to prior infection or trauma. Tumor visualization via bronchoscopy is essential for operative planning and provides visual information that is unavailable with cross-sectional imaging alone, including both the location and extent of tumor invasion.[11]

The thoracoscopic approach to sleeve lobectomy was initially thought to be an alternative only for patients who lacked the cardiopulmonary reserve for more extensive resections. In time, however, this technique has been found to be advantageous for patients with minimal or absent pre-existing pulmonary dysfunction as well.

Patients in whom sleeve lobectomy is likely to be deferred include those with N2 nodal disease and T4 disease. Involvement of N1 nodes should not be considered a contraindicaton to sleeve resection.[12] Chest wall invasion is not necessarily a contraindication and has been reported in the literature. In this instance, the thoracoscope can be used to better visualize the extent of tumor geometry intracorporally which may aide in dissection. Tumors with vertebral involvement or particular size and orientations may not be suitable for this approach.[8]

TECHNIQUE

Set-up

The patient should be placed in the lateral decubitus position similar to standard VATS lobectomy. Double lumen endotracheal intubation can be used to isolate each mainstem; for left sided sleeve resection, a right dual lumen endotracheal tube is preferred. Multiple arrangements of port placements have been described in the literature. Typically, three to four ports are used, although VATS sleeve lobectomies have also been performed using only two ports. Some studies have described single-port techniques, although these are less common.[13] A 10 mm port can be used for the thoracoscope in the 7th to 8th intercostal space in the mid-axillary line. A second access port in the 5th intercostal space in the anterior axillary line is placed next.[2] Additional ports can be added depending on the operative field, affected bronchus, and tumor orientation.

TECHNICAL CONSIDERATIONS

Once access into the chest is achieved, thorough inspection should follow. The upper lobes offer more favorable anatomy for the VATS approach in regard to efficiency of retraction, manipulation, and visualization.[11] Prior to resection, a complete hilar and mediastinal lymph node dissection should be performed first. This strategy accomplishes excellent hilar mobilization required for sleeve reconstruction and it may identify patients in whom sleeve resection is inappropriate either in patients who are oncologically inoperable or who require pneumonectomy. This is especially important in patients that have undergone induction therapy.[14]

For upper lobe sleeve resections, it may be beneficial to open the fissure (either stapling or energy source is preferred, to minimize postoperative air leaks). While not mandatory, opening the fissure allows more thorough hilar inspection prior to committing to the resection.

The lobar pulmonary vessels are then mobilized. For right upper lobectomy, division of the upper lobe branches of the superior vena cava is usually accomplished first, followed by division of the anterior trunk and posterior branch of the pulmonary artery. For a left upper lobe sleeve resection, division of the lingular and posterior vessels is easily accomplished as soon as the fissure is opened, followed by the superior pulmonary vein and the truncal artery.

Care should be taken to minimize manipulation of the bronchial vessels as these will provide blood supply to the upcoming bronchial anastomosis.[11] Avoiding skeletonization of the remaining bronchi is essential for this same reason.[15]

The lobe to be resected is isolated after all vascular structures have been ligated by first dividing the bronchus proximally as this margin is most straightforward based on preoperative bronchoscopy (**Figure 9.1A**). Subsequently, the bronchus is divided distally (**Figure 9.1B**) to aide in tumor visualization.[8] For left upper lobe sleeve resection, it may be helpful to secure the proximal bronchus with a retention suture to avoid retraction into the mediastinum.

Frozen section specimens from both margins should be sent intraoperatively. In general, 5 mm margins for high grade lesions and 3-mm margins for low grade lesions are the preferred minimum values,[11] although it is frequently not possible to determine more than whether the margin is positive or negative with an intraoperative frozen section. The remaining bronchial ends should be assessed for size mismatch; upper lobe sleeve resections are associated with minimal mismatch; lower lobe sleeve resections may be more problematic. While waiting for frozen section results, it is sometimes beneficial to perform a hilar release by opening the pericardium around the inferior pulmonary vein (**Figure 9.2**).[8]

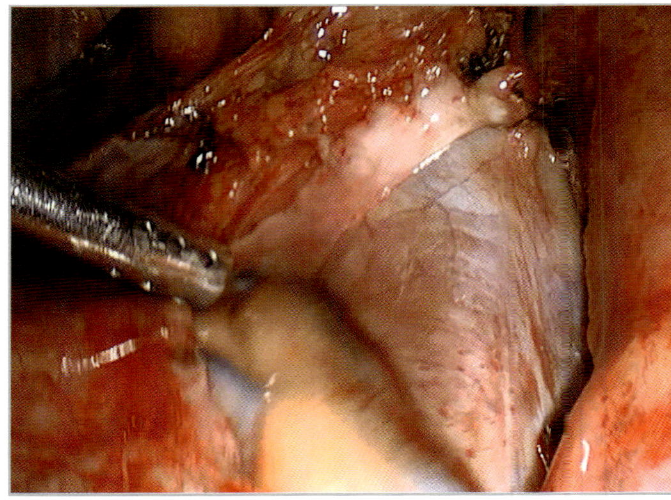

Figure 9.2 Pericardial release.

Methods of bronchial anastomosis vary in the literature. Interrupted, continuous, and combination methods have been described.[16,13,2] Zero-silk stay sutures can be used to assist in aligning bronchial ends if necessary at the initiation of the anastomosis (**Figure 9.3**). In general, the posterior membranous portion should be aligned and anastomosed first, given it is more technically difficult. Anastomosis of the remaining anterior cartilaginous portion should follow. Our preference is for the use of a continuous 4-0 absorbable monofilament suture for the anastomosis (**Figure 9.4**). Additionally, mediastinal fat flaps have been used to cover the anastomosis, although we do not perform this adjunct routinely.[17]

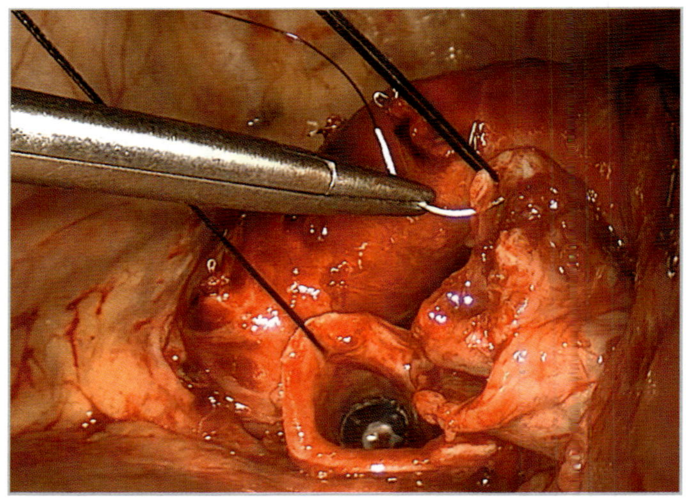

Figure 9.3 Starting the anastomosis with stay sutures in place.

Following completion of the anastomosis, it should be submerged in water to assess for air leak during pulmonary reinflation. A positive test warrants oversewing of the suspected anastomotic gap. The

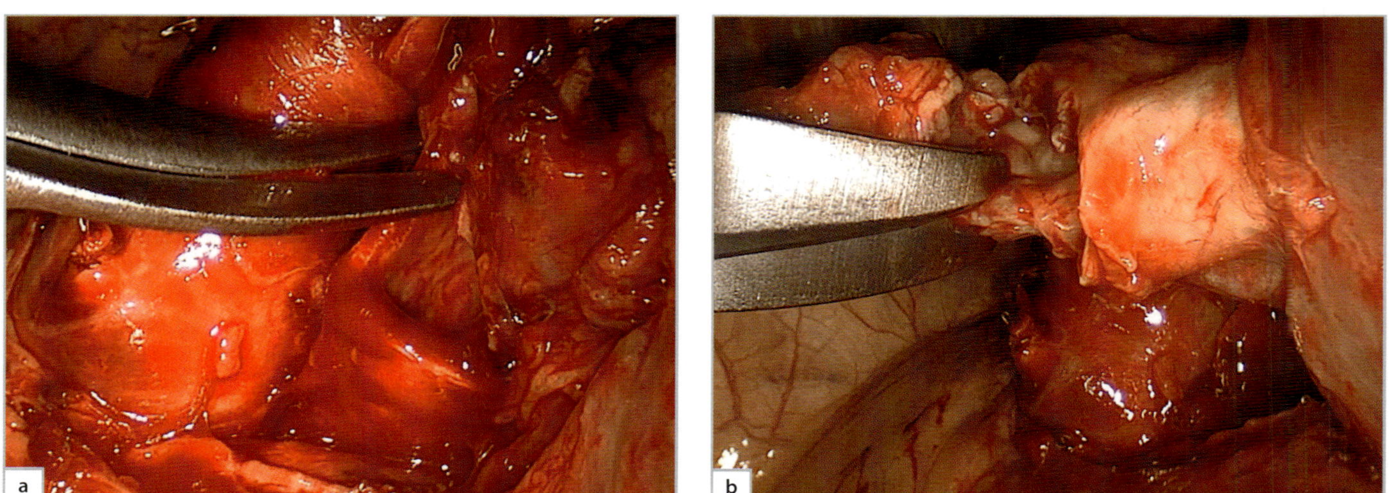

Figure 9.1 (a) Transection of the proximal left bronchus. (b) Transection of distal left bronchus.

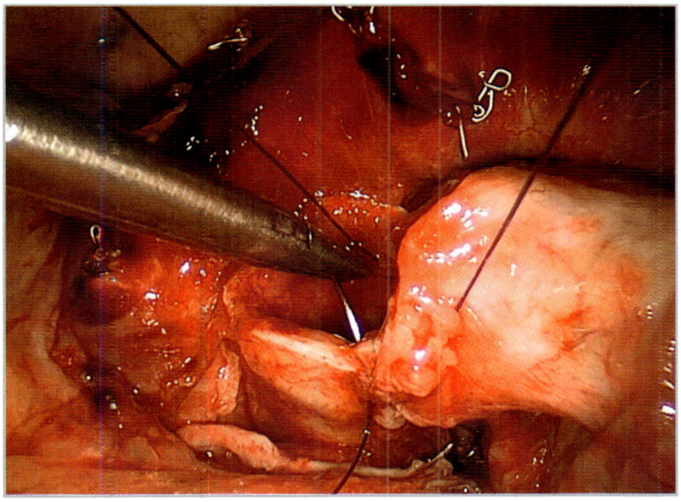

Figure 9.4 Completing the anastomosis with a continuous suture.

procedure should conclude with flexible bronchoscopy in order to inspect the airways for blood and secretions. This is especially important distal to the anastomosis given the reduction in ciliary function following transection of the bronchi.[8] Most patients are eligible for extubation prior to leaving the operating room, and do not routinely require intensive care immediately after surgery.

POSTOPERATIVE CARE

Postoperative pulmonary toilet and clearance of secretions are of utmost importance following this procedure as is the case with any thoracic surgical procedure. At our institution, each patient is given an incentive spirometer to use immediately after surgery. Patients should be encouraged to achieve early ambulation. To maintain adequate pulmonary mechanics and ventilation, adequate analgesia should be highly prioritized. This can be achieved with traditional narcotic and non-narcotic analgesia as well as the use of thoracic epidural, intercostal nerve block, or intercostal anesthetic infusions. Judicious use of postoperative fluid administration is believed to prevent postoperative pulmonary edema, particularly during the postsurgical inflammatory phase.

Chest tube management is an important component of any VATS surgical case. Quantity and quality of drainage should be noted, which typically consists of a transition from postoperative frank blood to decreasing amounts of serosanguinous fluid. The presence of air leaks should be identified and monitored. Small air leaks are not infrequent following lobectomy and typically seal in time as bronchial and parenchymal tissue heals. Larger or clinically significant air leaks with or without worsening subcutaneous emphysema may suggest anastomotic dehiscence or technical complication and should warrant more aggressive management. We typically remove our chest tubes when daily drainage is less than 300 mL of serosanguinous fluid and the absence of an air leak is verified. Small residual pneumothoraces should be monitored with serial radiographs to ensure stability in addition to routine clinical monitoring. Patients are typically discharged on postoperative day 5 assuming chest tube removal, ambulation at baseline levels, adequate analgesia, tolerance of a diet and oral medications, and demonstration of adequate pulmonary function.

COMPLICATIONS

Few studies exist that directly compare VATS sleeve lobectomy to traditional thoracotomy. Mahtabifard and colleagues examined a series of 13 patients undergoing VATS sleeve resection. This series reported zero postoperative deaths and nine patients free of complications. One patient had an anastomotic stricture which required stenting on the eighth postoperative day. A second patient had an anastomotic dehiscence which required the patient returning to the operating room for repair of what was found to be a separation on the posterior membranous portion of the anastomosis. Other complications in this series included atrial fibrillation with successful pharmacological cardioversion and one patient who required reintubation.

General complications not specific to sleeve resection may be encountered perioperatively. Numerous sources of bleeding may occur. In particular, care should be taken during hilar dissection to minimize the frequency of larger vessel injuries. At the conclusion of the case, port sites should be visualized from inside the chest to identify any intercostal vessel bleeding. Postoperatively, chest tube drainage may appear as frank blood temporarily. Persistence of this, however, should raise suspicion for ongoing bleeding, particularly if the quantity is not decreasing and the patient has already ambulated. It has been suggested that the VATS approach results in less bleeding compared to thoracotomy, which may result in less pulmonary edema and ongoing blood losses into the pleural cavity.[18] However, these statistics are widely variable among studies and their specificity to sleeve resections in particular have not been demonstrated.

Infectious sequelae of VATS are related to postoperative pneumonia. Although theoretical improvements in pulmonary mechanics may suggest better pulmonary toilet and a reduced incidence of pneumonia, this correlation has not been well demonstrated for sleeve resection in particular.

CLINICAL OUTCOMES

Few reports are available which specifically compare VATS sleeve lobectomy to pneumonectomy via thoracotomy for similar lesions. The benefits of VATS sleeve lobectomy are two-fold as this approach offers the advantages of VATS over thoracotomy as well as the advantages of lobectomy over pneumonectomy. Thus, the data related to these differences are worth addressing. It is recognized, however, that patients who undergo sleeve resection or undergo pneumonectomy are not directly comparable.

A 2011 study compared open sleeve lobectomy in 19 patients to open pneumonectomy in 20 patients. Three-year disease free and overall survival rates were statistically equivalent between groups. The sleeve resection group, however, incurred a lower rate of mortality, lower incidence of anastomotic complications, and better postoperative pulmonary function defined by quantitative pulmonary function tests.[19] A meta-analysis in 2010 also addressed these two study groups including thousands of patients from multiple treatment centers. The study suggested that sleeve lobectomy carried higher 5-year survival (50% versus 30%), lower perioperative mortality (3% versus 6%), and lower recurrence rates (17% versus 30%).[20] Although patients undergoing pneumonectomy may be confounded by a greater proportion of patients with advanced disease, several individual studies suggested similar results. A subsequent meta-analysis by Shi and colleagues in 2012 reiterated a lower postoperative mortality in those undergoing sleeve resection versus pneumonectomy with no difference in complication rate or locoregional recurrence rate.[21]

The advantages of VATS over thoracotomy have been well described in a single institution series,[3] multi-institutional series,[5,1] and meta-analyses.[6,22] It is evident that randomized trials may be useful to provide better comparisons between these patient populations. Studies directly comparing VATS sleeve lobectomy to the alternatives of open sleeve lobectomy and pneumonectomy are lacking.

CONCLUSION

As with the adoption of any new surgical technique, there is an associated learning curve required to provide the intended advantages of the new technique without causing a higher incidence of complications or adverse outcomes. VATS sleeve lobectomy is no exception and is regarded as perhaps one of the most difficult procedures to perform in VATS surgery. One study attempted to quantify the learning curve for VATS lobectomy by retrospectively analyzing the medical record at set time intervals. A lower incidence of complications was noted 6 months following implementation of the VATS method.[23] The study suggested 6–12 months or 30–60 operations as the benchmark for technical proficiency. Given that sleeve resection presents an additional technical challenge by adding a bronchial anastomosis, it is unclear to what degree this time frame and learning curve apply to the VATS sleeve technique. We recommend sufficient case volume in both open sleeve and general VATS techniques in order to prepare for the inherent challenges of VATS sleeve resections. One study suggested at least 200 VATS lobectomy cases and 30 open sleeve resection cases to prepare adequately for VATS sleeve resection.[24]

An alternative approach to sleeve lobectomy performed entirely thoracoscopically is the hybrid approach. This technique combines mini-thoracotomy with video assisted ports to provide an intermediate form of minimally invasive surgery. This remains a viable technique and has been described in the literature. In a single-center prospective study in 2011, 148 patients underwent the hybrid approach for sleeve resection of a non-small cell lung cancer. Of these, 90.5% did not require conversion to open thoracotomy and did not succumb to significant perioperative morbidity or mortality.[25] In addition, this technique has been shown to provide comparable results in regard to long term and perioperative outcomes whether performed at a community facility or a higher volume center.[25] This feature may not be transferrable to VATS sleeve resections given that arguably higher case volumes may be necessary in order to achieve proficiency.

In addition to thoracoscopic approaches for various lung resections, robotic surgery has emerged as the next era in minimally invasive surgery. As skills in robotic surgery are acquired by trainees and attending surgeons, its use has been expanded to operations that were not previously thought to benefit from such an approach. The first such case study is from 2010 and reports the use of a robotic system for VATS sleeve lobectomy.[26] This particular patient had a low grade neuroendocrine tumor located at the right upper lobe bronchial orifice. With the exception of prolonged chest tube duration due to persistent pleural effusion, the patient did well and was discharged on post-operative day fifteen following adequate bronchoscopic evaluation of an intact anastomosis.

In conclusion, VATS sleeve lobectomy remains as an alternative technique for patients with lobar bronchial orifice tumors. Although technically more challenging, this technique offers the perioperative advantages of thoracoscopy over thoracotomy as well as the long term and functional advantages of lobectomy over pneumonectomy. As case series continue to appear in the literature, it is evident that this technique is a viable technique at many more centers than are currently offering this approach. Separate experience with VATS procedures and open sleeve lobectomy will aide in expediting the learning curve associated with this challenging yet rewarding technique.

REFERENCES

1. Paul S, Altorki NK, Sheng S, Lee PC, et al. Thoracoscopic lobectomy is associated with lower morbidity than open lobectomy: a propensity-matched analysis from the STS Database. J Thorac Cardiovasc Surg 2010; 139:366–378.
2. Sabiston D, Sellke F, del Nido P, Swanson S. Lung cancer: minimally invasive approaches. In: Sabiston and Spencer's Surgery of the Chest. Philadelphia: Saunders 2010.
3. Villamizar NR, Darrabie MD, Burfeind WR, et al. Thoracoscopic lobectomy is associated with lower morbidity compared to thoracotomy. J Thorac Cardiovasc Surg 2009; 138: 419–425.
4. Berry MF, D'Amico TA, Onaitis MW, Kelsey CR. Thoracoscopic approach to lobectomy for lung cancer does not compromise oncologic efficacy. Ann of Thorac Surg 2014; 98:197–202.
5. Ceppa DP, Kosinski AS, Berry MF, Tong BC, et al. Thoracoscopic lobectomy has increasing benefit in patients with poor pulmonary function: A Society of Thoracic Surgeons database analysis. Ann Surg 2012; 256:487–493.
6. Cao C, Zhu ZH, Yan TD, et al. Video-assisted thoracic surgery versus open thoracotomy for non-small cell lung cancer: a propensity score analysis based on a multi-institutional registry. Eur J Cardiothorac Surg 2013; 44:849–854.
7. Pena E, Blanco M, Ovalle JP. Two-incision approach for video-assisted thoracoscopic sleeve lobectomy. Asian Cardiovasc Thorac Ann 2014; 22:371–373.
8. Kara HV, Balderson SS, D'Amico TA. Challenging cases: thoracoscopic lobectomy with chest wall resection and sleeve lobectomy – Duke experience. J Thorac Dis 2014; 6:S637–S640.
9. Mahtabifard A, Fuller CB, McKenna RJ. Video-assisted sleeve lobectomy: a case series. Ann Thorac Surg 2008; 85:S729–732.
10. Gonzalez-Rivas D, Fieira E, Delgado M, et al. Uniportal video-assisted thoracoscopic sleeve lobectomy and other complex resections. J Thorac Dis 2014; 6:S674–S681.
11. Predina JD, Kunkala M, Aliperti LA, Singhal AK, Singhal S. Sleeve Lobectomy: Current Indications and Future Directions. Ann Thorac Cardiovasc Surg 2010; 16:310–318.
12. Berry MF, Worni M, Wang X, et al. Sleeve lobectomy for non-small lung cancer with N1 nodal disease does not compromise survival. Ann Thorac Surg 2013; 97: 230–235.
13. Gonzalez-Rivas D, Delgado M, Fieira E, Pato O. Left lower sleeve lobectomy by uniportal video-assisted thoracoscopic approach. Interac Cardiovasc Thorac Surg 2014; 18:237–239
14. Burfeind Jr. WR, D'Amico TA, Toloza EM, et al. Low morbidity and mortality for bronchoplastic procedures with and without induction therapy. Ann Thorac Surg 2005; 80:418–422.
15. Bertolaccini L, Viti A, Terzi A. Moving beyond the boundary: the emerging role of video-assisted thoracic surgery for bronchoplastic resections. J Thorac Dis 2014; 6:1170–1172.
16. Fan J, Yao J, Chang Z, et al. Left lower sleeve lobectomy and systematic lymph node dissection by complete video-assisted thoracic surgery. J Thorac Dis 2014; 6:1826–1830.
17. McKenna RJ, Mahtabifard A, Swanson SJ. Sleeve lobectomy, right upper lobe; sleeve lobectomy: right middle lobe superior segment. In Atlas of Minimally Invasive Thoracic Surgery. Philadelphia: Elsevier, 2011.
18. Dylewdki MR, Lazzaro RS. Robotics – The answer to the Achilles' heel of VATS pulmonary resection. Chin J Cancer Res 2012; 24:259–260.
19. Lee HK, Lee HS, Kim KI, et al. Outcomes of sleeve lobectomy versus pneumonectomy for lung cancer. Korean J Thorac Cardiovasc Surg 2011; 44:413–417.
20. Stallard J, Loberg A, Dunning J, Dark J. Is a sleeve lobectomy significant better than a pneumonectomy? Interac Cardiovasc Thorac Surg 2010; 11:660–666.

21. Shi W, Zhang W, Sun H, Shao Y. Sleeve lobectomy versus pneumonectomy for non-small cell lung cancer: a meta-analysis. World J Surg Oncol 2012; 10:265.
22. Yan TD, Cao C, D'Amico TA, et al. Video-assisted thoracoscopic surgery lobectomy at 20 years: a consensus statement. Eur J Cardiothorac Surg 2014; 45:633–639.
23. Arad T, Levi-Faber D, Nir RR, Kremer R. The learning curve of video assisted thoracoscopic surgery (VATS) for lung lobectomy–a single Israeli center experience. Harefuah 2012; 151:261–265.
24. Han Y, Zhou S, Yu D, et al. Video-assisted left upper bronchial sleeve lobectomy. J Thorac Dis 2013; 5:S304–S306.
25. He J, Shao W, Cao C, et al. Long-term outcome of hybrid surgical approach of video-assisted minithoracotomy sleeve lobectomy for non-small cell lung cancer. Surg Endosc 2011; 25:2509–2515.
26. Schmid T, Augustin F, Kainz G, et al. Hybrid video-assisted thoracic surgery – robotic minimally invasive right upper lobe sleeve lobectomy. Ann Thorac Surg 2011; 91:1961–1965.

Chapter 10 VATS en bloc chest wall resection

Todd Demmy, Peter Smit, Mark Hennon

INTRODUCTION

Primary non-small cell lung carcinoma with chest wall invasion represents approximately 5% of all resected lung cancers.[1] For patients with potentially resectable disease, defined by the absence of mediastinal nodal disease and distant metastases, lung resection with en bloc chest wall resection carries a three-fold higher risk of mortality compared to standard lobectomy. In large database series, 90-day perioperative mortality for lobectomy with en bloc chest wall resection is surpassed only by pneumonectomy.[2] This is primarily a result of acute respiratory insufficiency postoperatively.[3] Nevertheless, patients with node negative disease who receive complete resection for locally advanced non-small cell lung cancer (NSCLC) experience improved long-term survival compared to those managed without surgery. The survival benefit is even observed among older patients and those with resectable nodal disease.[4]

Surgical management of locally advanced NSCLC with chest wall involvement has traditionally required a thoracotomy for tumor and en bloc chest wall resection. However, growing experience with thoracoscopic pulmonary resections for early stage lung cancer has allowed surgeons to safely approach more complex tumor pathology by minimally invasive approaches. Challenges to extending thoracoscopic resection for more advanced stage lung cancers include concern for achieving a sound oncologic resection, the inherent technical challenges associated with chest wall reconstruction, and potential lack of perioperative benefit due to the violation of chest wall integrity that occurs regardless of approach. Potential benefits do exist and include more accurate rib selection based on the interior view, maintaining the external musculature of the chest wall, avoiding the physiologic/neurogenic effects associated with spreading other ribs throughout the duration of the case, and improved visualization with high definition viewing scopes to aid with dissection. Thoracoscopic surgical approaches for these tumors now exist, allowing for the possible benefits of a minimally invasive approach while maintaining the principles of a complete oncologic resection.[5,6]

The first report of video-assisted thoracoscopic surgery (VATS) for treatment of lung cancer with chest wall invasion was published in 2000. Widmann et al. described the successful application of a minimally invasive VATS approach for surgical resection of a stage-IIB NSCLC with chest wall invasion in a 60-year-old man who had completed neoadjuvant radiotherapy. Lung resection and chest wall dissection were completed thoracoscopically. A long-handled osteotome was used to transect the anterior rib margins of ribs 3 and 4, while elevation of the specimen disarticulated the rib heads from the vertebral bodies. No reconstruction was required due to the posterior location of the affected rib segments. Negative margins over 1-cm were achieved. Their patient experienced a rapid recovery with return to baseline physical activity without restrictions by the second postoperative week.[7]

While there is a paucity of large series data for VATS en bloc chest wall resections for locally advanced lung cancer, published reports over the last two decades demonstrate that this approach is both safe and feasible, expanding the pool of patients eligible for surgical resection who might otherwise not tolerate an open approach.

PATIENT SELECTION

Favorable features for thoracoscopic en bloc chest wall resection include tumors invading the chest wall adjacent to the access incision, those that require removal of four or fewer ribs, and that do not need postresection chest wall reconstruction as with subscapular tumors. Although explicit criteria have not been defined for selecting appropriate patients, this minimally invasive approach may be particularly attractive for treating frail patients with significant comorbid conditions or neoadjuvant therapies. In older patients with low BMI and impaired pulmonary function, 60-day mortality can reach 47%.[8] Such patients are frequently deemed high risk for resection and often do not tolerate an open thoracotomy with rib-spreading and the associated extensive soft tissue trauma.[9]

Relative contraindications to a thoracoscopic approach to chest wall resection have been described. Posterior tumors abutting the spine that require rib disarticulation are more challenging than lateral or anterior tumors. Large tumors (those > 7 cm in diameter) can limit visualization and may not be adequately approached by VATS without significant risk of injury to adjacent structures. This is especially true for large superior sulcus tumors that may impair suitable camera views of the thoracic outlet. Limited mobility of hilar structures due to extensive adenopathy or neo-adjuvant radiation therapy can also impede a minimally invasive approach.[7]

TECHNICAL CHALLENGES AND SOLUTIONS

Technical challenges associated with thoracoscopic chest wall resection are being overcome by increasing surgeon experience coupled with evolving technology. Division of ribs and bone is now facilitated by use of thoracoscopic bone shears or high-speed burr-style drills adopted from other surgical subspecialties such as neurosurgery. Thoracoscopic energy devices aid in dividing chest wall muscle and neurovascular structures. Access incision placement relative to the area of tumor invasion is also now understood to be a key maneuver that facilitates dissection and extraction of the specimen.

SURGICAL APPROACH

Positioning

Patients are placed in the standard lateral decubitus position with adjustments as necessary to facilitate chest wall resection if an open procedure is required. Ensure the patient is well secured to the operative field to allow for table tilting to approach extreme anterior or posterior tumors.[10]

Incision placement

When planning for VATS chest wall resection, traditional placement of incisions may be altered to allow for easier tumor extraction. The first incision (1–2 cm) is generally made over the 7th or 8th intercostal space perpendicular to the mid-axillary line. An open, flexible port for the camera through this incision helps prevent lens-smearing and reduces inadvertent intercostal nerve injury. We prefer to use a flexible-tip, high definition thoracoscope for multi-angle viewing and superb video clarity. From this initial incision, a thorough survey of the pleural cavity is possible to identify the lung and chest wall tumor location and plan for additional port placement.

In contrast to the traditional thoracoscopic lobectomy, the larger access incision (4–8 cm) may vary according to tumor location. Placing this incision close to or overlying the involved chest wall section is generally avoided as it may result in impaired wound healing or increased infection risk secondary to factors associated with chest wall reconstruction including but not limited to prosthetic mesh placement. A more anteriorly located access incision relative to the involved segment facilitates medial/anterior rib division, and provides a wider intercostal space for specimen extraction.

En-bloc tumor resection

Once the port site incisions are created, the parietal pleura surrounding the area of tumor invasion is scored by unipolar electrocautery to define the planned area of chest wall resection (**Figure 10.1**). Standard rib cutting tools are then used to divide the ribs closest to the access incision (**Figure 10.2**). Mobilization of the chest wall segment proceeds using a thoracoscopic energy-sealing or cutting device to dissect in the extra-thoracic subcutaneous and muscular planes, followed by division of the intercostal muscles and neurovascular bundles. A right-angled instrument can assist with hooking the intercostal bundle for division (**Figure 10.3**). The lateral or posterior rib resections are completed using thoracoscopic bone shears or a high-speed drill (**Figure 10.4**). If need be, dividing the tumor from the remaining lung by wedge resection can be performed to facilitate the chest wall resection prior to performing any hilar dissection. As a general rule, the chest wall tumor dissection should be completed prior to performing the hilar dissection.

After mobilizing the rib block, the pulmonary and hilar dissections are performed to complete the tumor resection. A sturdy nylon sac is placed through the access incision and deployed within the pleural cavity to extract the specimen. Orienting the ribs perpendicular to the access incision facilitates specimen removal. Care must be taken to prevent bone fragments from tearing the extraction sac as the specimen is removed. If significant difficulty is encountered with extracting the specimen, then an alternate site should be considered, such as through a separate subxiphoid incision.

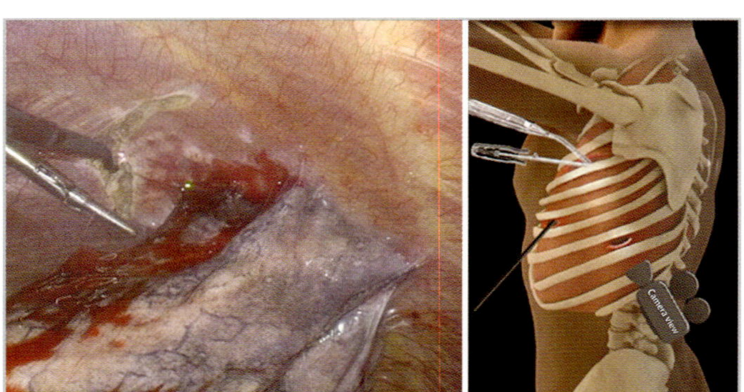

Figure 10.1 The parietal pleura is scored around the periphery of the area of tumor invasion.

Chest wall reconstruction

Chest wall defects underneath the scapula (apical and posterior rib resections) do not usually require additional support as the overlying muscles have been preserved. However, certain locations are at higher

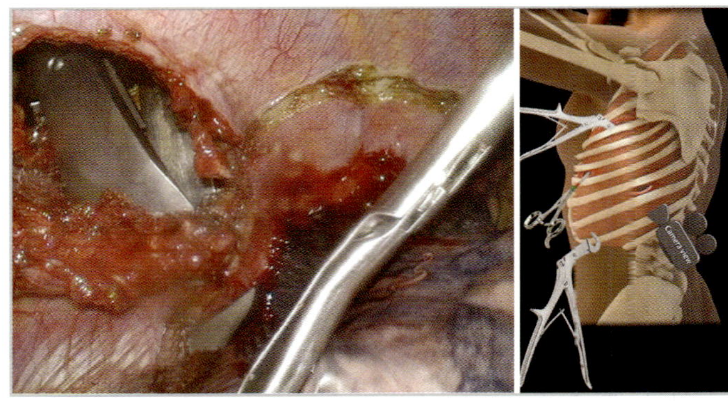

Figure 10.2 Anteromedial rib division through the access incision with a standard rib shear.

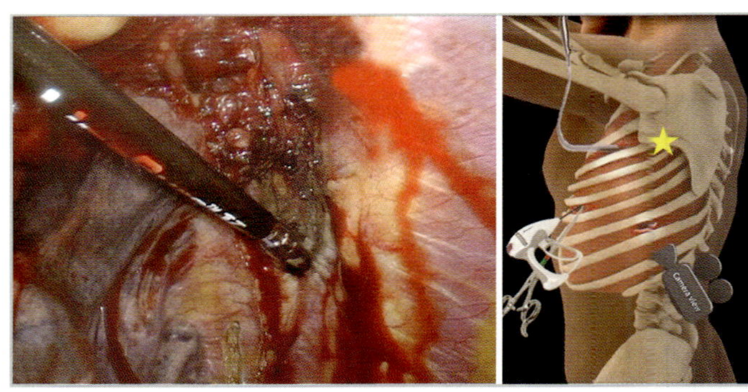

Figure 10.3 Intercostal muscle division with a sealant energy device. The star indicates the area of chest wall invasion.

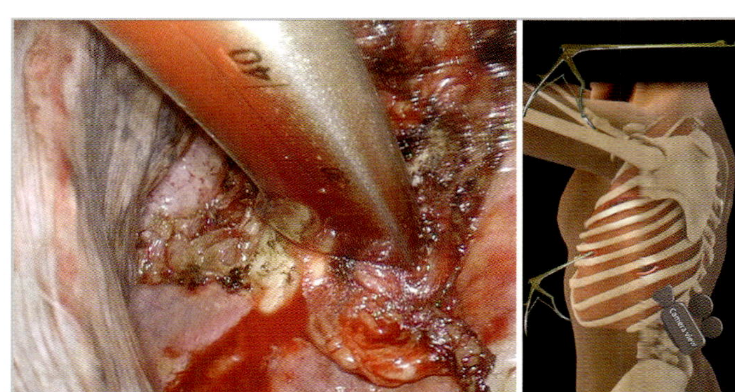

Figure 10.4 Posterolateral rib division using endoscopic rib cutters.

risk for herniation or paradoxical respiratory motion, particularly high lateral chest wall resections involving three or more ribs, which makes adequate postoperative chest wall stability imperative.[11]

Large defects without overlying bony support can be addressed using prosthetic patches or muscle flap coverage. A prosthetic mesh (polypropylene or polytetrafluoroethylene) is chosen with sufficient overlap to prevent port site herniation. Measurements are made based upon the extracted specimen with a 1-cm overlap allowed for on all sides. Anchoring holes are punched in the mesh prior to intracorporeal placement. Once the mesh is placed within the chest cavity and unfurled, anchoring sutures are delivered by a needle passer through 2 mm incisions. These sutures are then tied externally with the knots retracted below the skin. Alternately, the sutures can be secured by an intracorporeal tied knot or suture fixation device. Additional reconstruction options include tensor fascia latae muscle in place of synthetic mesh, rib or fibula grafts in combination with synthetic mesh for added stability, or thick myocutaneous flaps (latissimus dorsi or rectus abdominis).

OUTCOMES

As experience grows with minimally invasive approaches to locally advanced lung cancer, a growing body of publications supports its safety. Long term benefits are not clearly defined yet. Berry et al. looked retrospectively at 10 years of their patient data for primary NSCLC, comparing 93 patients who underwent a traditional thoracotomy versus 12 patients who had resection performed by a hybrid thoracoscopic approach utilizing a two-incision VATS approach to complete the lung resection and chest wall dissection. The two incisions include a mid-axillary, 1 cm incision in the 8th intercostal space for the camera and a 4–5 cm access incision anteriorly placed in the 5th intercostal space. A counter incision over the involved rib spaces completes the resection and tumor removal.[12] Patient demographics, tumor characteristics, and resection details were comparable between the two groups with negative chest wall margins achieved in all patients. Perioperative mortality and morbidity also did not differ between the groups. However, patients who underwent a hybrid VATS approach had a shorter median length of stay by 0.5 days ($p = 0.03$).[9]

Our initial experience with the feasibility of an entirely thoracoscopic approach to en bloc chest wall resection has been described. In a case series of three patients with pathologies ranging from stage IIA to IIIB primary NSCLC with chest wall invasion, complete resection was achieved thoracoscopically. At 3 weeks post-procedure, all patients had minimal or no pain medication requirements. No evidence of recurrence or deaths occurred with follow-up at 6, 16, and 26 months postoperative.[8]

With growing experience, we analyzed and compared all VATS and open chest wall resections from 2007 to 2013. Forty-seven chest wall resections were performed during this study period, among which 17 (36%) were performed by VATS without open conversion. Fifteen VATS procedures were performed for NSCLC. In a subset analysis of VATS versus open chest wall resection for NSCLCs, patients treated by VATS were older (76 versus 56 years, $p < 0.01$) and experienced shorter intensive care unit and hospital lengths of stay. Only 7% of VATS resections required chest wall reconstruction compared to 56% for open resection ($p < 0.001$). Operative time, amount of blood less, and number of resected ribs did not significantly differ between the two groups. With a median follow-up of 18 months, no significant differences in perioperative morbidity or 90-day mortality were observed, although both groups suffered significant morbidity and mortality. We concluded that VATS is an acceptable surgical strategy for locally advanced NSCLC, but a completely thoracoscopic approach for elderly, frail patients did not offer the same protective effects observed previously with VATS lobectomy alone.[13]

Additional refinements to the VATS approach for chest wall invasion are already being reported. Gonzalez-Rivas and colleagues have described their technique for a single-site thoracoscopic approach for non-small cell lung tumors with chest wall invasion.[14] The procedure begins with placement of a single incision through the 5th intercostal space (large enough to accommodate 3 to 4 instruments and a 10-mm 30° high definition videoscope), followed by a survey of the chest cavity to determine lobe mobility and the extent of chest wall invasion, which dictates the order of resection. A small counter incision over the involved chest wall is placed for the costal resection, which can be performed with conventional rib cutters, forgoing the need for specialized thoracoscopic instruments.[15] A touted advantage to this technique is the direct visualization of the target lesion by the camera in coordination with parallel, bimanual instrumentation that mimics maneuvers performed with an open approach.[16]

Refinements to the thoracoscopic approach for chest wall resection of locally advanced lung cancers will come with newer technologies and greater surgeon experience. In addition, both perioperative and long-term outcomes analyses are ongoing in effort to better define those patients who would most benefit from this minimally invasive approach.

REFERENCES

1. McCaughan BC, Martini N, Bains MS, McCormack PM. Chest wall invasion in carcinoma of the lung. Therapeutic and prognostic implications. J Thorac Cardiovasc Surg 1985; 89:836–841.
2. Hu Y, McMurry TL, Wells KM, et al. Postoperative mortality is an inadequate quality indicator for lung cancer resection. Ann Thorac Surg 2014; 97:973–979.
3. Stoelben E, Ludwig C. Chest wall resection for lung cancer: indications and techniques. Eur J Cardiothorac Surg 2009; 35:450–456.
4. Speicher PJ, Englum BR, Ganapathi AM, et al. Outcomes after treatment of 17,378 patients with locally advanced (T3N0-2) non-small-cell lung cancer. Eur J Cardiothorac Surg 2015; 47:636–641.
5. Hennon MW, Demmy TL. Video-assisted thoracoscopic surgery (VATS) for locally advanced lung cancer. Ann Cardiothorac Surg 2012; 1:37–42.
6. Battoo A, Demmy TL, Yendamuri S. Complex thoracoscopic pulmonary resections for the treatment of lung cancer-a review. Indian J Surg Oncol 2013; 4:142–147.
7. Widmann MD, Caccavale RJ, Bocage JP, Lewis RJ. Video-assisted thoracic surgery resection of chest wall en bloc for lung carcinoma. Ann Thorac Surg 2000; 70:2138–2140.
8. Demmy TL, Nwogu CE, Yendamuri S. Thoracoscopic chest wall resection: what is its role? Ann Thorac Surg 2010; 89:S2142–2145.
9. Berry MF, Onaitis MW, Tong BC, et al. Feasibility of hybrid thoracoscopic lobectomy and en-bloc chest wall resection. Eur J Cardiothorac Surg 2012; 41:888–892.
10. Demmy TL, Yendamuri S, Hennon MW, et al. Thoracoscopic maneuvers for chest wall resection and reconstruction. J Thorac Cardiovasc Surg 2012; 144:S52–S27.
11. Tukiainen E. Chest wall reconstruction after oncological resections. Scand J Surg 2013; 102:9–13.
12. Kara HV, Balderson SS, D'Amico TA. Challenging cases: thoracoscopic lobectomy with chest wall resection and sleeve lobectomy-Duke experience. J Thorac Dis 2014; 6:S637–640.

13. Hennon MW, Dexter EU, Huang M, et al. Does thoracoscopic surgery decrease the morbidity of combined lung and chest wall resection? Ann Thorac Surg 2015; 99:1929–1934.
14. Gonzalez-Rivas D, Fieira E, Delgado M, et al. Uniportal video-assisted thoracoscopic sleeve lobectomy and other complex resections. J Thorac Dis 2014; 6:S674–6781.
15. Gonzalez-Rivas D, Fernandez R, Fieira E, Mendez L. Single-incision thoracoscopic right upper lobectomy with chest wall resection by posterior approach. Innovations 2013; 8:70–72.
16. Bertolaccini L, Rocco G, Viti A, Terzi A. Geometrical characteristics of uniportal VATS. J Thorac Dis 2013; 5:S214–216.

Chapter 11 Segmental resections

Luis Angel Hernandez-Arenas, Yang Yang, Robert S George

INTRODUCTION

Developments in computed tomography technology in recent years mean that the diagnosis of small lung nodules, ground glass lesions and non-solid lung cancers has been on the rise.[1-3] Segmentectomy is an alternative procedure when the lesions are deeply located in the lung and it is necessary to secure an adequate surgical margin.[4]

In this chapter, we will describe the surgical technique of the most common segmental resections performed using the uniportal approach.

INDICATIONS

- Benign process
- Congenital lesion
- Lung metastasis
- Possible second tumors
- Ground glass lesions (GGOs)
- Carcinoid tumors
- Non-small cell lung cancer < 2 cm (still in debate)

RECOMMENDATIONS

- Segmentectomy is feasible in tumors < 2 cm when the preoperative CT scan shows the lesion completely contained within the anatomic boundaries of the segment with no lymph node involvement
- Sub-lobar resections can be offered to a high-risk patient with poor lung function or marginal performance status
- GGO lesions can be safety managed with segmentectomy
- Achieve surgical margins > 1 cm to avoid local tumors recurrences
- There is still a lack of evidence in patients with early stage NSCLC < 2 cm in size, caution should be taken when a sub-lobar resection is indicated in this kind of patient

Position and incision technique:

- Following the induction of general anesthesia and double-lumen endotracheal intubation, the patient is placed in decubitus position of 90°. If available, the operating table is flexed between the iliac crest and the costal margin. Alternatively, a pillow is placed beneath the chest at the level of the xiphoid process to widen the intercostal spaces on the operative side. The arms are extended and the upper arm is supported with pillows or a padded arm-rest and soft rolls or a beanbag is used to secure the patient on the table
- The surgeon is positioned in front of the patient. An assistant and a scrub nurse stands at the back and a screen is placed at the head of the patient
- A 3–4 cm incision is placed between the middle and posterior axillary lines in the 5th or 4th intercostal space

SURGICAL TECHNIQUE: RIGHT SIDE

Uniportal VATS right upper lobe apical segmentectomy (S1)

Retract the lung with a thoracoscopic grasper or a sponge on a stick to expose the anterior mediastinal pleura. With bimanual instrumentation dissect the hilar structures adequately. The first step is to identify the mediastinal trunk of the artery and the upper vein (**Figure 11.1**).

- Identify, dissect and divide the apical segmental vein with vascular endostapler, tie with silk or ligate using Click'a V Endoscopic Polymer Clip Appliers 45° (Grena 170 Ltd. Brentford, England) and then resect with energy device (**Figure 11.2**)

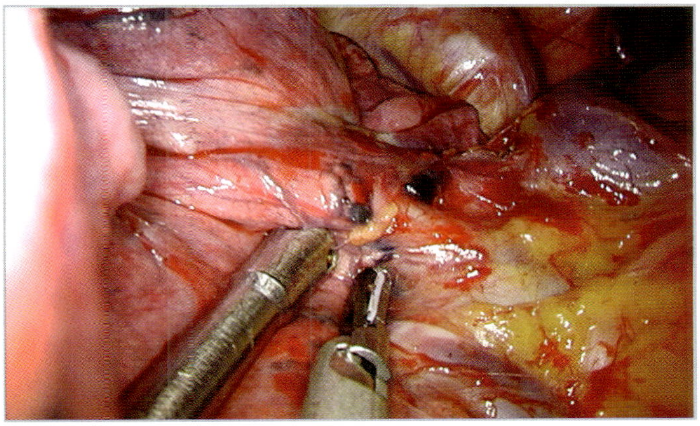

Figure 11.1 Expose of the anterior mediastinal pleura. Trunk of the artery and upper vein are both exposed.

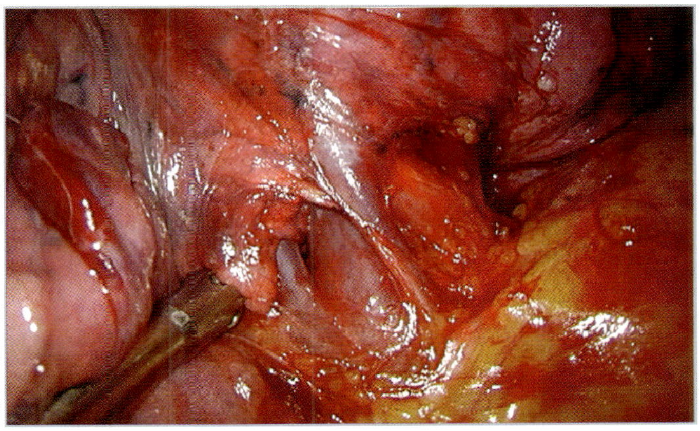

Figure 11.2 Dissection of the right apical vein.

- Identify, dissect and divide the apical artery with vascular endostapler or tied with silk or ligate using Click'a V Endoscopic Polymer Clip Appliers 45° (Grena 170 Ltd. Brentford, England) and resected with energy device (**Figure 11.3**)
- Identify, dissect and divide the apical bronchus with articulated endostapler. Before you transect the bronchus always identify the anterior and posterior bronchus and ask your anesthetist to insufflate the lung to check you are transecting the correct segmental bronchus (in some cases a curved-tip stapler technology was used to facilitate the passage around the structures) (**Figure 11.4**)
- During insufflation the portion that remains collapsed is the apical segment
- Pull up the upper lobe with thoracoscopic grasper and complete the intersegmental fissure created after the insufflation with endostapler. Always include in the segmental resection the stump of the artery, the vein and the segmental bronchus (**Figure 11.5**)
- Retrieve the resected lung with an Endocatch bag

Uniportal VATS right upper lobe posterior segmentectomy (S2)

- Retract the lung with thoracoscopic grasper or a sponge on a stick to expose the fissure. The first step is to identify the posterior segmental artery or vein. If the fissure is incomplete then open the posterior mediastinal pleura and find the posterior segmental bronchus (**Figure 11.6**)
- Identify, dissect and divide the posterior segmental vein with a vascular endostapler or tie with silk, or ligate using Click'a V Endoscopic Polymer Clip Appliers 45° (Grena 170 Ltd. Brentford, England) and then resect with an energy device
- Identify, dissect and divide the posterior artery with a vascular endostapler or tie with silk or ligate using Click'a V Endoscopic Polymer Clip Appliers 45° (Grena 170 Ltd. Brentford, England) and then resect with energy device (**Figure 11.7**)
- Identify, dissect and divide the posterior bronchus with articulated endostapler. Before you transect the bronchus always ask the anesthetist to insufflate the lung to check you are transecting the correct segmental bronchus (in some cases a curved-tip stapler technology is used to facilitate the passage around the structures) (**Figure 11.8**)
- During insufflation the portion that remains collapsed is the posterior segment
- Pull up the upper lobe with a thoracoscopic grasper and complete the intersegmental fissure created after the insufflation with endostapler. Always include the stump of the artery, the vein and the segmental bronchus in the segmental resection (**Figure 11.9**)
- Retrieve the resected lung with an Endocatch bag

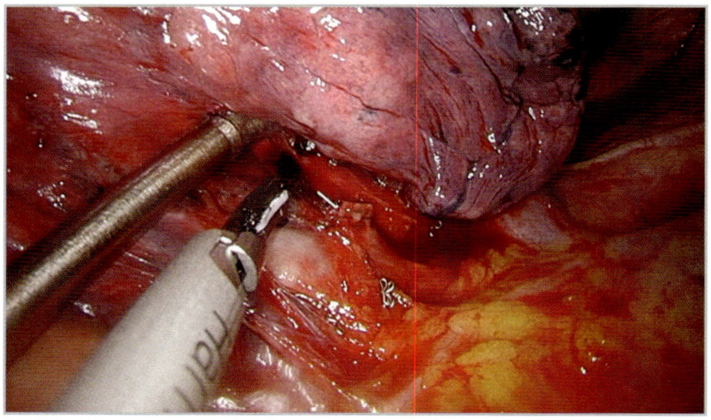

Figure 11.3 Apical artery dissected and divided with endovascular stapler.

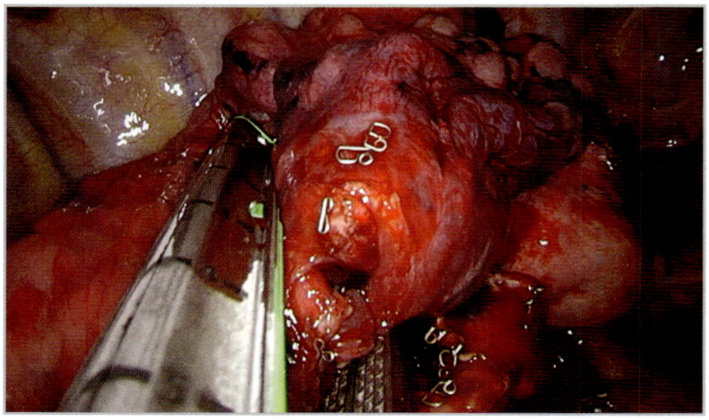

Figure 11.5 Completion of the intersegment fissure of apical segment after insufflation of the lung ensuring the stumps of the vein, artery and segmental bronchus are included within the specimen.

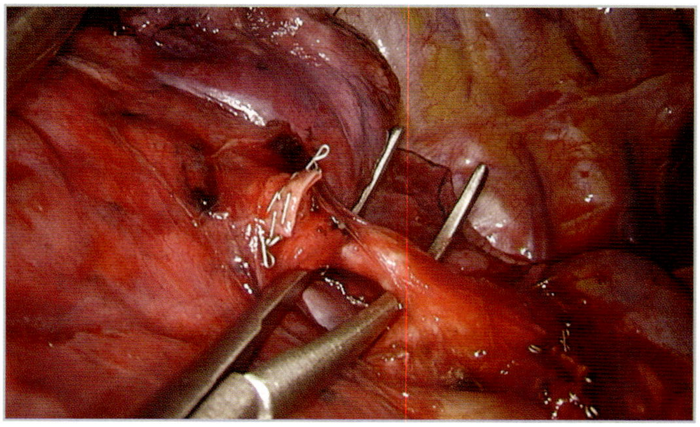

Figure 11.4 Dissection of right apical bronchus.

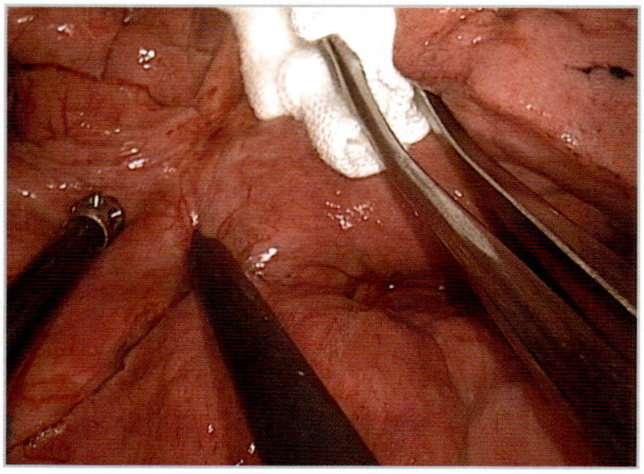

Figure 11.6 Bimanual instrumentation with sponge on a stick and suction to expose the fissure.

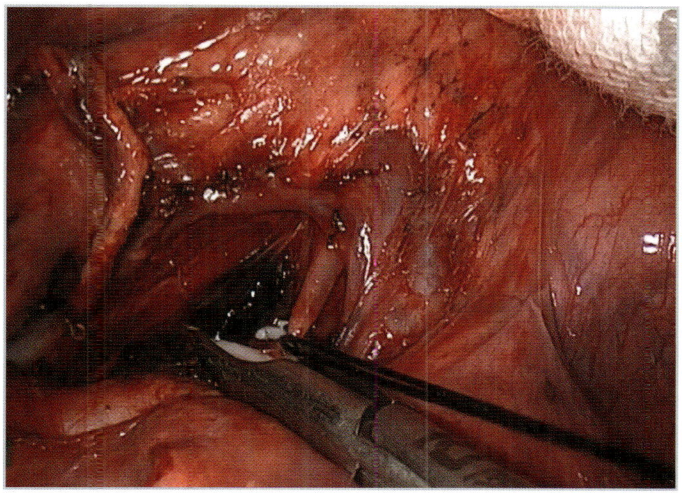

Figure 11.7 Posterior segmental artery are dissected and ligated using Click'a V Endoscopic Polymer Clip Appliers 45° (Grena 170 Ltd. Brentford, England) and then resected with energy device.

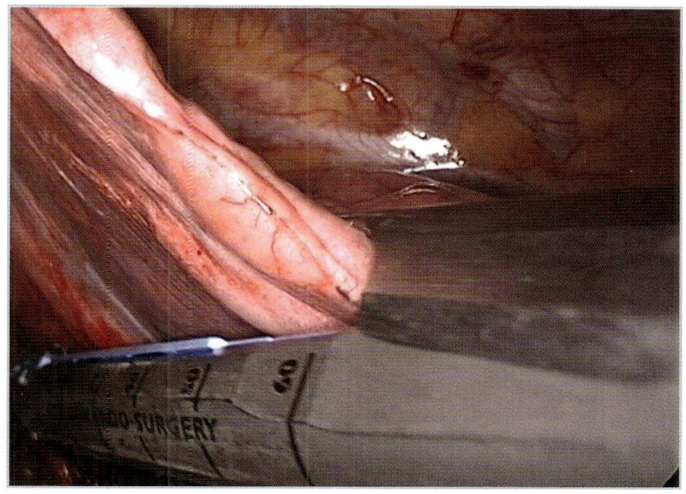

Figure 11.9 Following insufflation, the intersegmental fissure is created with endostapler Included in the segmental resection are the stumps of the artery, the vein and the segmental bronchus.

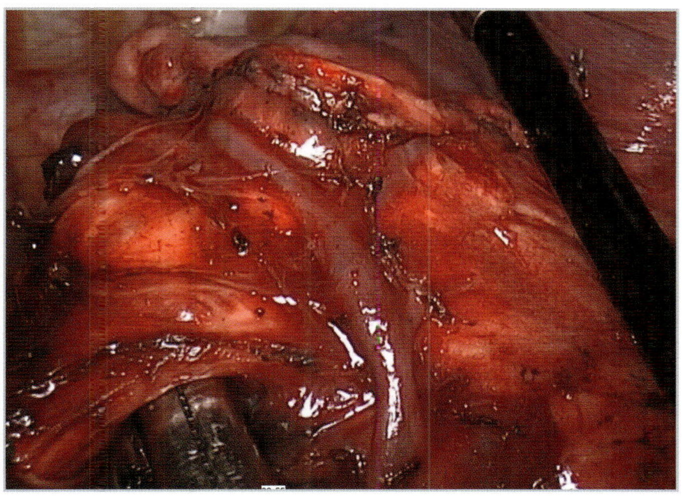

Figure 11.8 Dissection of right posterior segmental bronchus.

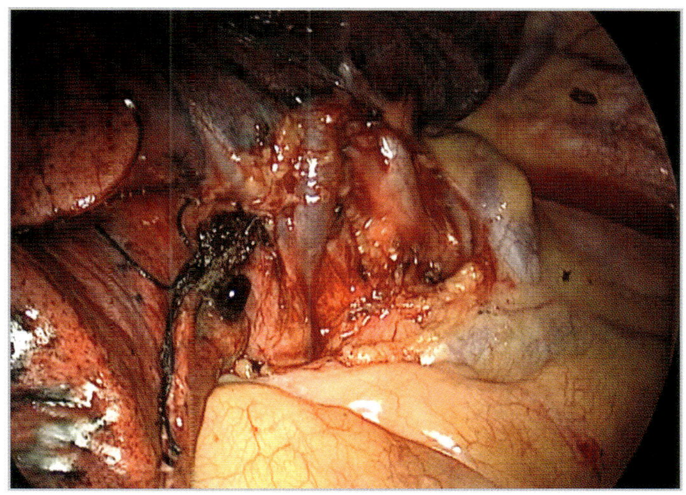

Figure 11.10 Retracting the lung with thoracoscopic grasper exposing the anterior mediastinal pleura with bimanual instrumentation. Identification of the mediastinal trunk of the artery and the upper vein

Uniportal VATS right upper lobe anterior segmentectomy (S3)

- Retract the lung with thoracoscopic grasper or a sponge on a stick to expose the anterior mediastinal pleura and with bimanual instrumentation dissect the hilar structures adequately. The first step is to identify the mediastinal trunk of the artery and the upper vein (**Figure 11.10**)
- Identify, dissect and divide the anterior segmental vein with vascular endostapler, tie with silk or ligate using Click'a V Endoscopic Polymer Clip Appliers 45° (Grena 170 Ltd. Brentford, England) and then resect with energy device (**Figure 11.11**)
- Identify, dissect and divide the anterior artery with vascular endostapler. tie with silk or ligate using Click'a V Endoscopic Polymer Clip Appliers 45° (Grena 170 Ltd. Brentford, England) and then resect with energy device (**Figure 11.12**).
- Identify, dissect and divide the anterior bronchus with articulated endostapler. Before transecting the bronchus always ask the anesthetist to insufflate the lung to check you are transecting the correct segmental bronchus. (in some cases a curved-tip stapler technology was used to facilitate the passage around the structures) (**Figure 11.13**).
- During insufflation the portion that remains collapsed is the anterior segment (**Figure 11.14**)
- Pull up the upper lobe with thoracoscopic grasper and complete the intersegmental fissure created after the insufflation with endostapler. Always include the stump of the artery, the vein and the segmental bronchus in the segmental resection (**Figure 11.15**)
- Retrieve the resected lung with an Endocatch bag.

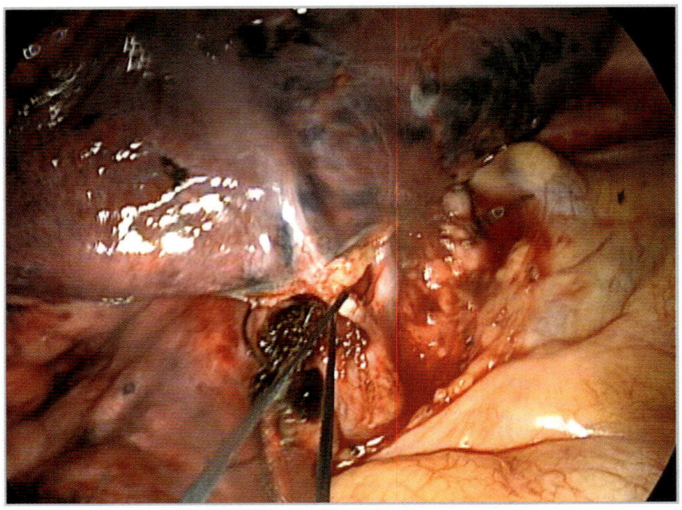

Figure 11.11 Dissection of right anterior segmental vein.

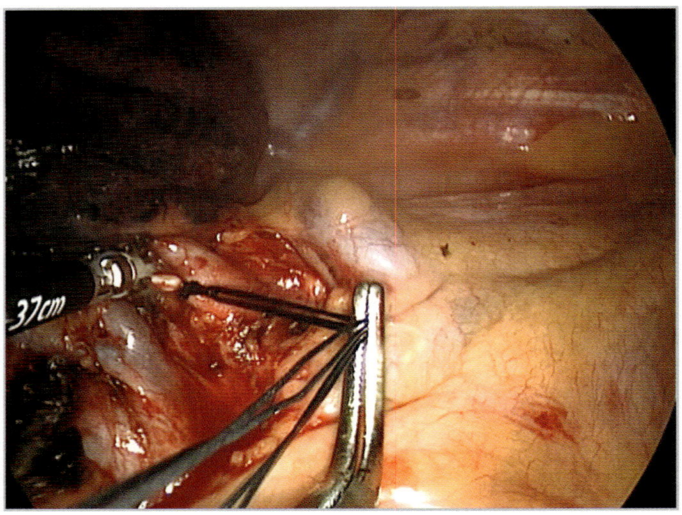

Figure 11.12 Dissecting and dividing the anterior artery following tying and resection with energy device.

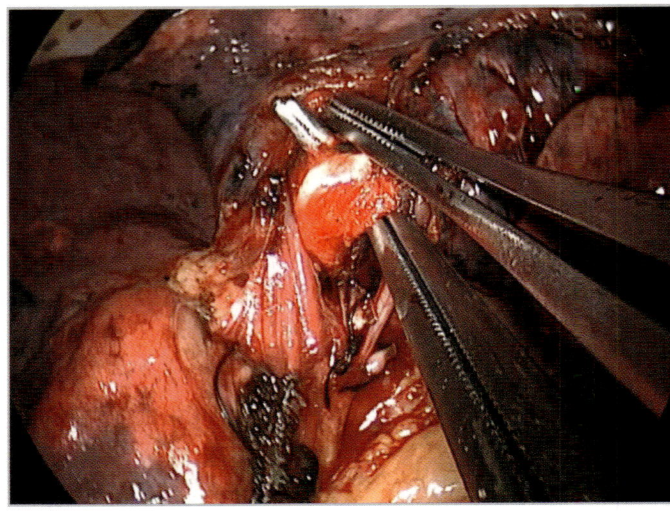

Figure 11.13 Dissection of right anterior segmental bronchus.

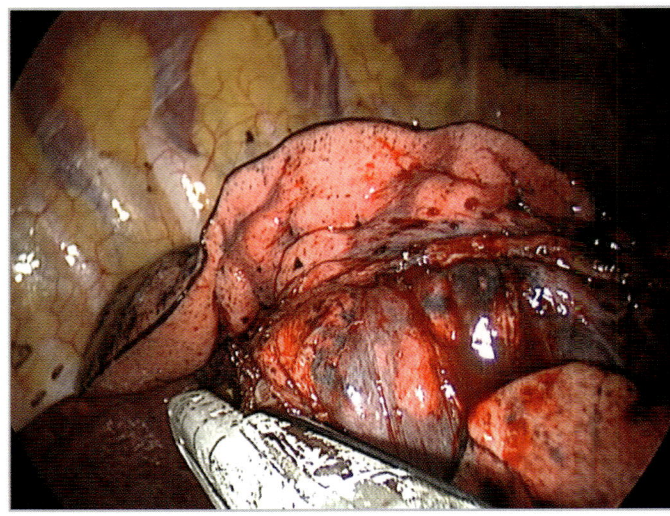

Figure 11.14 Anterior segmental bronchus clamped with endostapler curve technology and insufflating the lung before the division of the segmental bronchus confirms the segment.

Uniportal VATS right lower lobe dorsal segmentectomy (S6)

- Retract the lung with a thoracoscopic grasper or a sponge on a stick to expose the fissure. The first step is to identify the dorsal segmental artery or vein. In case of an incomplete fissure open the posterior mediastinal pleura and find the dorsal segmental bronchus.
- Identify, dissect and divide the dorsal segmental vein with vascular endostapler, tie with silk or ligate using Click'a V Endoscopic Polymer Clip Appliers 45°(Grena 170 Ltd. Brentford, England) and then resect with energy device.
- Identify, dissect and divide the dorsal artery with vascular endostapler, tie with silk or ligate using Click'a V Endoscopic Polymer Clip Appliers 45° (Grena 170 Ltd. Brentford, England) and then resect with energy device (**Figure 11.16**)
- Identify, dissect and divide the dorsal bronchus with articulated endostapler (**Figure 11.17**). Before transecting the bronchus always ask the anesthetist to insufflate the lung to check you are transecting the correct segmental bronchus. (in some cases a curved-tip stapler technology is used to facilitate the passage around the structures)
- During insufflation the portion that remains collapsed is the dorsal segment
- Pull up the upper lobe with thoracoscopic grasper and complete the intersegmental fissure created after the insufflation with endostapler. Always include the stump of the artery, the vein and the segmental bronchus in the segmental resection
- Retrieve the resected lung with an Endocatch bag

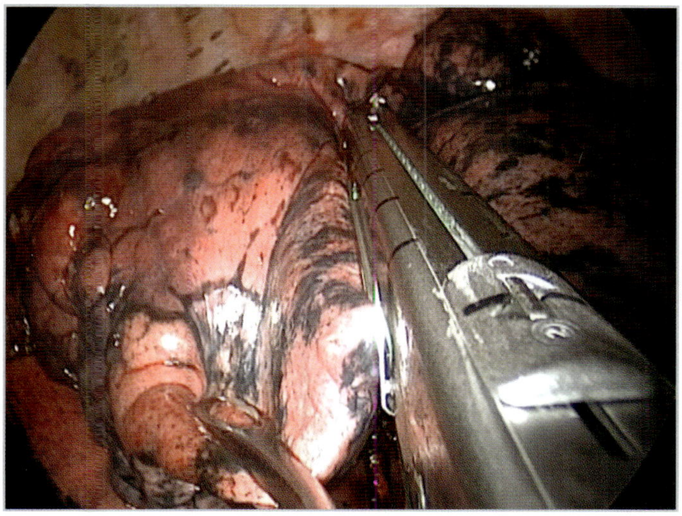

Figure 11.15 Completing the intersegmental fissure created after the insufflation with endostapler. Included in the specimen are the stumps of the artery, the vein and the segmental bronchus.

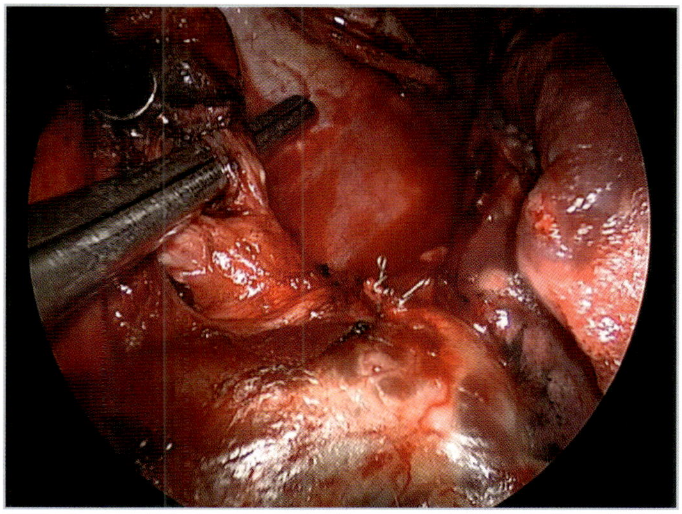

Figure 11.17 Dissection of the dorsal segmental bronchus, after dissecting the artery.

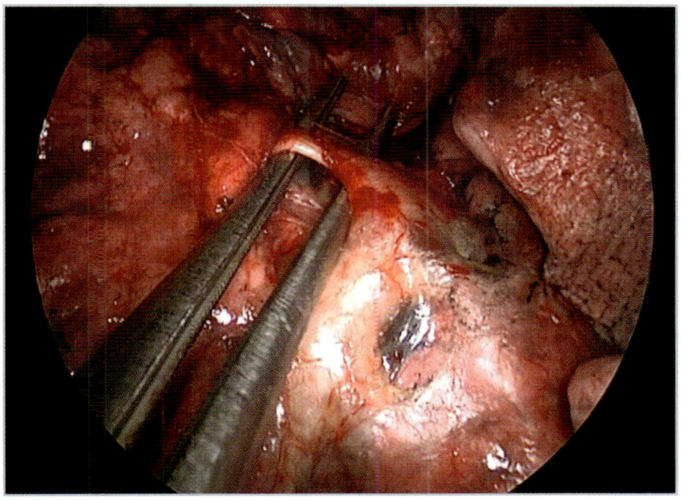

Figure 11.16 Dissection of the right dorsal segmental artery.

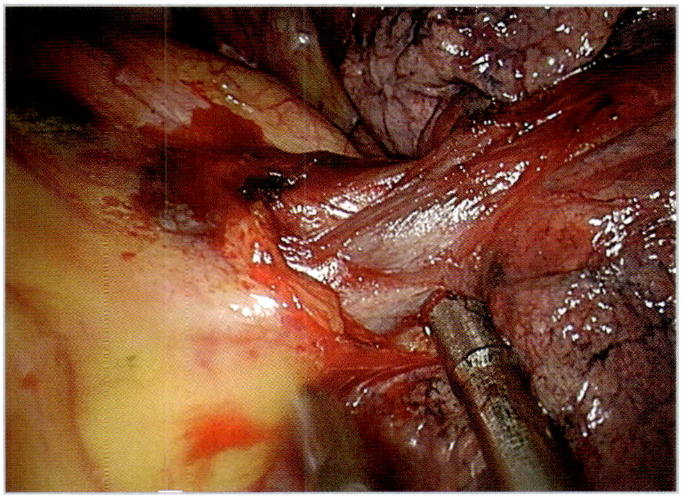

Figure 11.18 Retracting the lung with thoracoscopic grasper to expose the anterior mediastinal pleura. Bimanual instrumentation dissecting the hilar structures, mediastinal trunk of the left artery and the left upper vein.

SURGICAL TECHNIQUE: LEFT SIDE

Uniportal VATS left upper lobe apical segmentectomy (S1)

Technical highlights

- Retract the lung with thoracoscopic grasper or a sponge on a stick to expose the anterior mediastinal pleura and with bimanual instrumentation dissect the hilar structures adequately. The first step is to identify the mediastinal trunk of the artery and the upper vein (**Figure 11.18**)
- Identify, dissect and divide the left apical segmental vein with vascular endostapler, tie with silk or ligate using Click'a V Endoscopic Polymer Clip Appliers 45° (Grena 170 Ltd. Brentford, England) and then resect with energy device (**Figure 11.19**)
- Identify, dissect and divide the left apical artery with vascular endostapler, tie with silk or ligate using Click'a V Endoscopic Polymer Clip Appliers 45° (Grena 170 Ltd. Brentford, England) and then resect with energy device (**Figure 11.20**)
- Identify, dissect and divide the left apical bronchus with an articulated endostapler. Before you transect the bronchus always identify the anterior and posterior bronchus and ask your anesthetist to insufflate the lung to check you are transecting the correct segmental bronchus; in some cases a curved-tip stapler technology was used to facilitate the passage around the structures (**Figure 11.21**)
- During insufflation the portion that remains collapsed is the apical segment.
- Pull up the upper lobe with thoracoscopic grasper and complete the intersegmental fissure created after the insufflation with endostapler. Always include the stump of the artery, the vein and the segmental bronchus in the segmental resection
- Retrieve the resected lung with an Endocatch bag

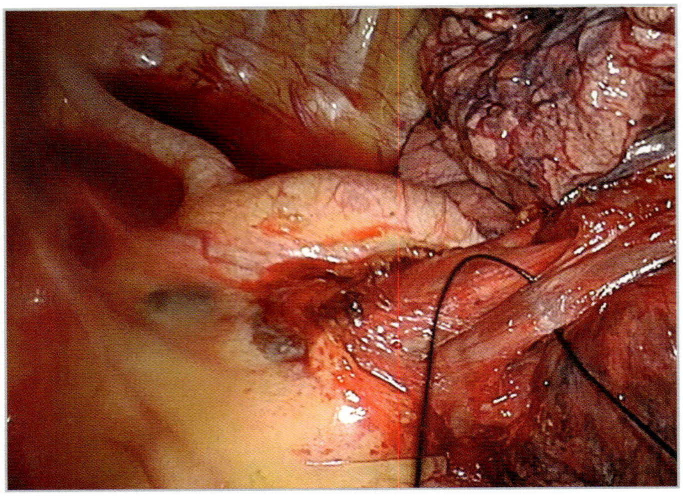

Figure 11.19 Dissecting the apical segmental vein.

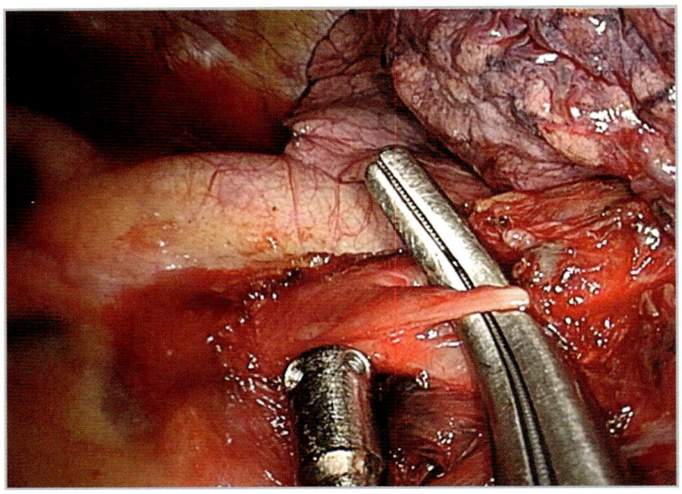

Figure 11.20 Dissecting the left apical segmental artery.

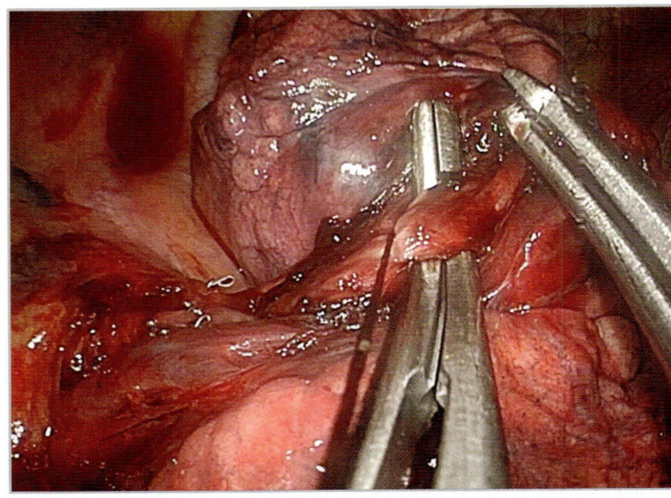

Figure 11.21 Dissection of the left apical segmental bronchus.

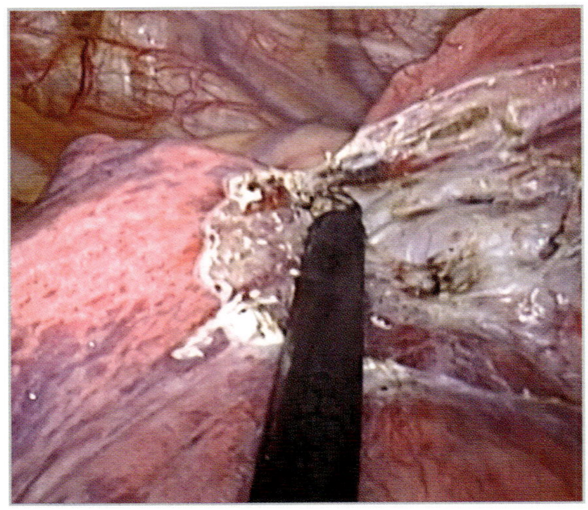

Figure 11.22 Retracting the lung with sponge on a stick to expose the fissure, identifying the left posterior segmental artery.

Uniportal VATS left upper lobe posterior segmentectomy (S2)

- Retract the lung with thoracoscopic grasper or a sponge on a stick to expose the fissure. The first step is to identify the posterior segmental artery or vein. In case of an incomplete fissure the first step is to open the posterior mediastinal pleura and find the posterior segmental bronchus (**Figure 11.22**)
- Identify, dissect and divide the posterior segmental vein with vascular endostapler, tie with silk or ligate using Click'a V Endoscopic Polymer Clip Appliers 45° (Grena 170 Ltd. Brentford, England) and then resect with energy device.
- Identify, dissect and divide the posterior artery with vascular endostapler, tie with silk or ligate using Click'a V Endoscopic Polymer Clip Appliers 45° (Grena 170 Ltd. Brentford, England) and then resect with energy device. From the anterior approach identify and divide the second posterior artery arising from the common trunk of the apical segmental artery. Sometimes you can obviate this branch and divide it with the fissure (**Figure 11.23**)
- Identify, dissect and divide the posterior bronchus with articulated endostapler. Before transecting the bronchus always ask the anesthesist to insufflate the lung to check you are transecting the correct segmental bronchus; in some cases a curved-tip stapler technology is used to facilitate the passage around the structures (**Figure 11.24**)
- During insufflation the portion that remains collapsed is the posterior segment
- Pull up the upper lobe with thoracoscopic grasper and complete the intersegmental fissure created after the insufflation with endostapler. Always include the stump of the artery, the vein and the segmental bronchus in the segmental resection (**Figure 11.25**)
- Retrieve the resected lung with an Endocatch bag

Uniportal VATS left upper lobe trisegmentectomy (S1+S2+S3)

- Retract the lung with thoracoscopic grasper or a sponge on a stick to expose the anterior mediastinal pleura and with bimanual instrumentation dissect the hilar structures adequately. The first

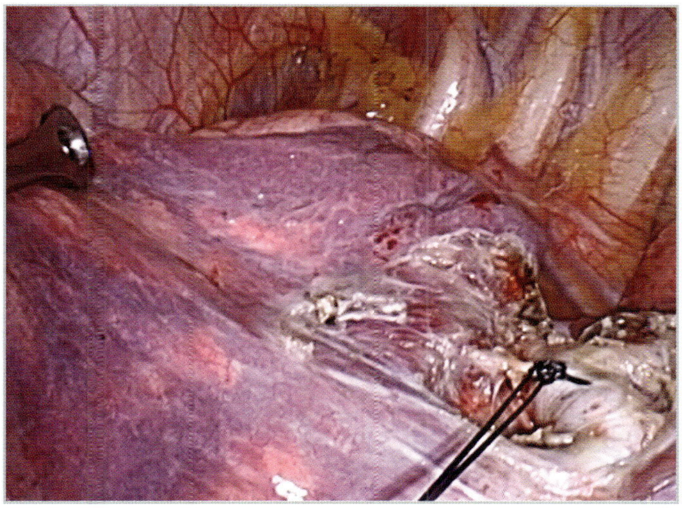

Figure 11.23 Disesection of the left posterior segmental artery with silk.

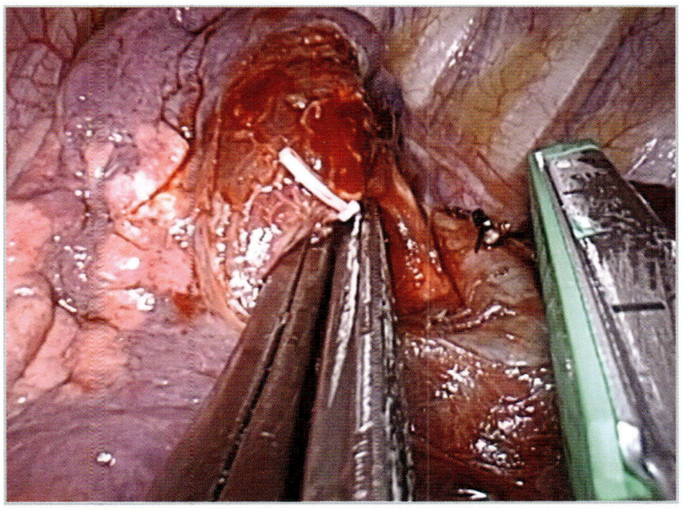

Figure 11.24 Identifying, dissecting and dividing the posterior bronchus with articulated endostapler.

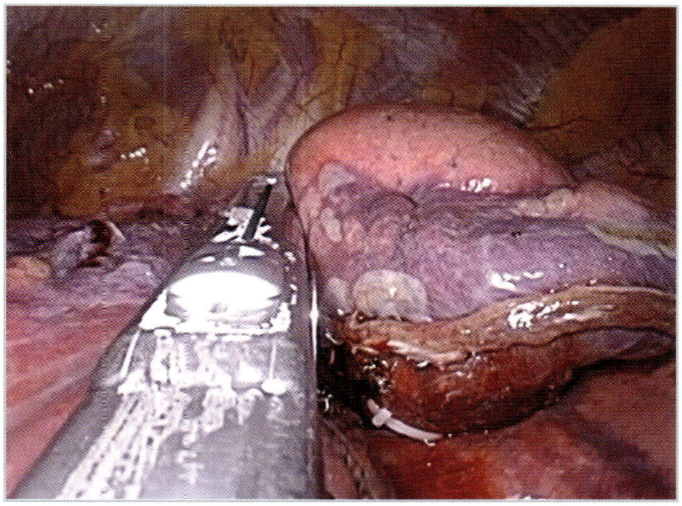

Figure 11.25 Completing the intersegmental fissure created after the insufflation with endostapler. The staple line includes the stump of the artery, the vein and the segmental bronchus.

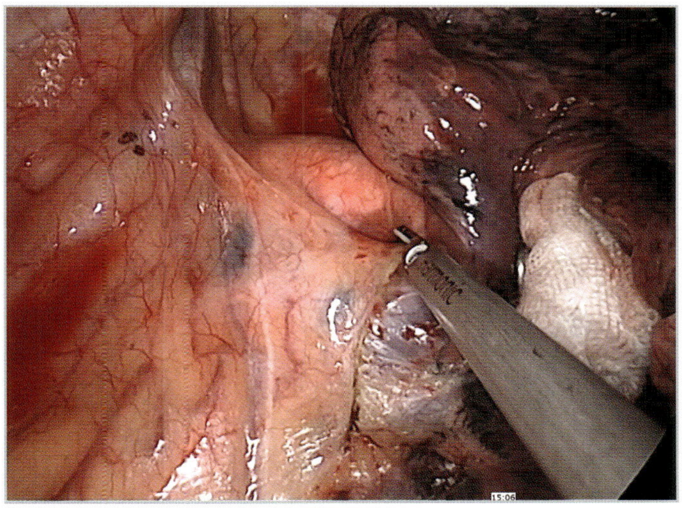

Figure 11.26 Exposure of the anterior mediastinal pleura with bimanual instrumentation. Pleura opened and part of the left upper vein is exposed.

step is to identify the mediastinal trunk of the left artery and the left upper vein (**Figure 11.26**)

- Identify, dissect and divide the trisegmental vein with vascular endostapler, tie with silk or ligate using Click'a V Endoscopic Polymer Clip Applier 45° (Grena 170 Ltd. Brentford, England) and then resect with energy device (**Figure 11.27**)
- Identify, dissect and divide the trisegmental artery with vascular endostapler, tie with silk or ligate using Click'a V Endoscopic Polymer Clip Applier 45° (Grena 170 Ltd. Brentford, England) and then resect with energy device (**Figure 11.28**)
- Following the vein is possible to identify the trisegmental bronchus, dissect and divide the trisegmental bronchus with articulated endostapler (**Figure 11.29**). Before transect the bronchus always identify the lingular bronchus and ask your anesthetist to insufflate the lung to check you are transecting the correct segmental bronchus; in some cases a curved-tip stapler technology was used to facilitate the passage around the structures
- During insufflation the portion that remains collapsed is the trisegmental segment
- Pull up the upper lobe with thoracoscopic grasper and complete the intersegmental fissure created after the insufflation with endostapler. Always include the stump of the artery, the vein and the segmental bronchus in the segmental resection
- Retrieve the resected lung with an Endocatch bag

Uniportal VATS left upper lobe lingulectomy (S4-S5)

- Retract the lung with thoracoscopic grasper or a sponge on a stick to expose the anterior mediastinal pleura and with bimanual instrumentation dissect the hilar structures adequately. The first step is to identify the mediastinal trunk of the left artery and the left upper vein (**Figure 11.30**)

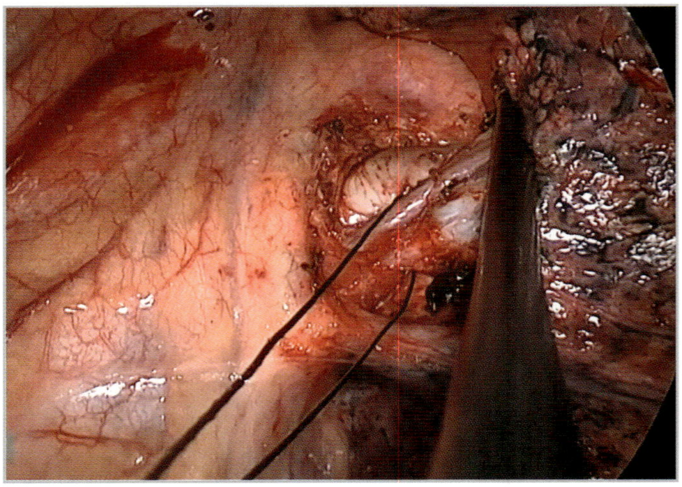

Figure 11.27 Shows the trisegmental vein dissected.

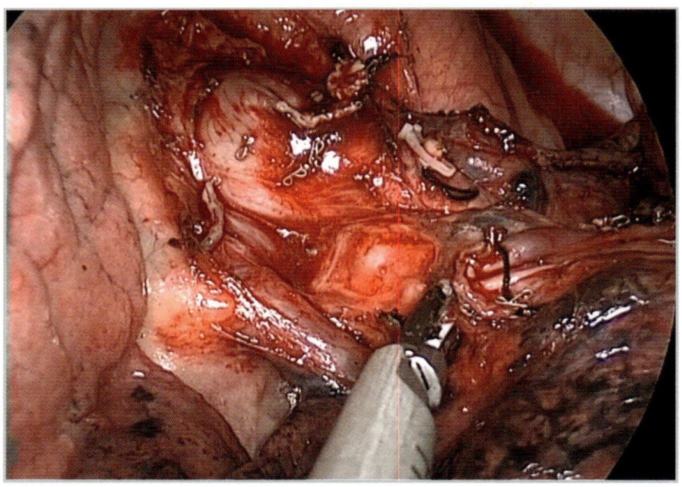

Figure 11.28 Shows the trisegmental artery and vein dissected and resected with endostapler V click.

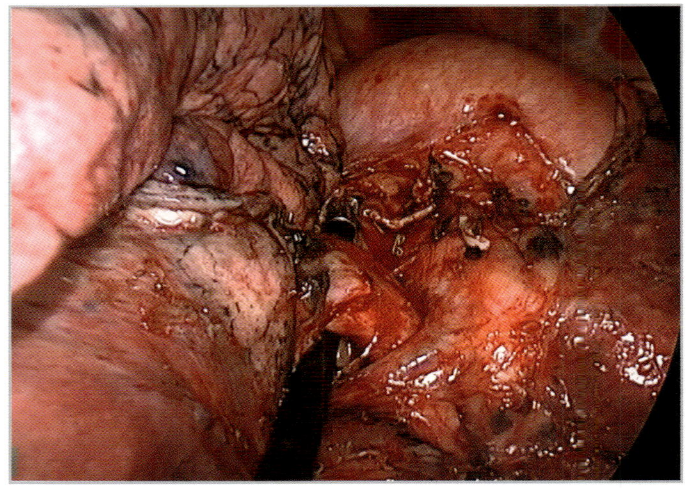

Figure 11.29 Fissure opened and trisegmental bronchus located and dissected ready to be resected with endostapler.

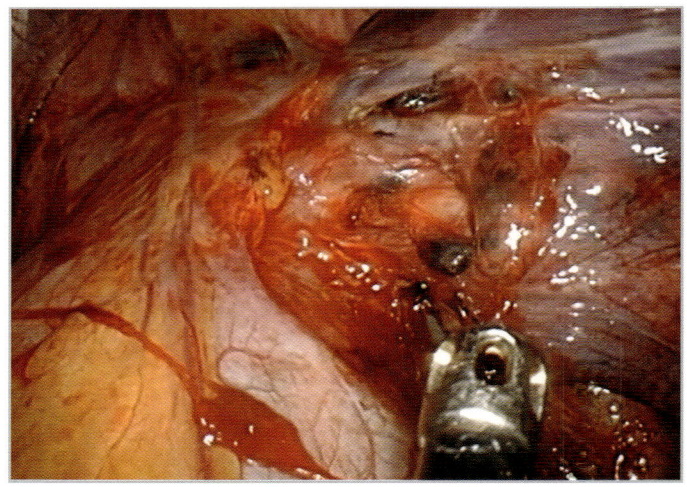

Figure 11.30 Retracting the lung with thoracoscopic grasper exposing the anterior mediastinal pleura. Using bimanual instrumentation dissect the mediastinal trunk of the left artery and the left upper vein.

- Identify, dissect and divide the lingular vein with vascular endostapler, tie with silk or ligate using Click'a V Endoscopic Polymer Clip Appliers 45° (Grena 170 Ltd. Brentford, England) and then resect with energy device (**Figure 11.31**)
- Identify, dissect and divide the lingular artery in the fissure with vascular endostapler, tie with silk or ligate using Click'a V Endoscopic Polymer Clip Appliers 45° (Grena 170 Ltd. Brentford, England) and then resect with energy device (**Figure 11.32**)
- Following the vein is possible to identify the lingular bronchus. Dissect and divide the lingular bronchus with articulated endostapler (**Figure 11.33**). Before transecting the lingular bronchus always identify the trisegmental bronchus and ask your anesthetist to insufflate the lung to confirm you are transecting the correct segmental bronchus; in some cases a curved-tip stapler technology was used to facilitate the passage around the structures
- During insufflation the portion that remains collapsed is the lingual
- Pull up the upper lobe with thoracoscopic grasper and complete the intersegmental fissure created after the insufflation with endostapler. Always include the stump of the artery, the vein and the segmental bronchus in the segmental resection
- Retrieve the resected lung with an Endocatch bag

Uniportal VATS left lower lobe dorsal segmentectomy (S6)

- Retract the lung with thoracoscopic grasper or a sponge on a stick to expose the fissure. The first step is to identify the left dorsal segmental artery or vein (**Figure 11.34**)
- Identify, dissect and divide the dorsal vein with vascular endostapler, tie with silk or ligate using Click'a V Endoscopic Polymer Clip Appliers 45° (Grena 170 Ltd. Brentford, England) and then resect with energy device. It is worth noting that sometimes the dorsal vein cannot be visualized and can be excluded

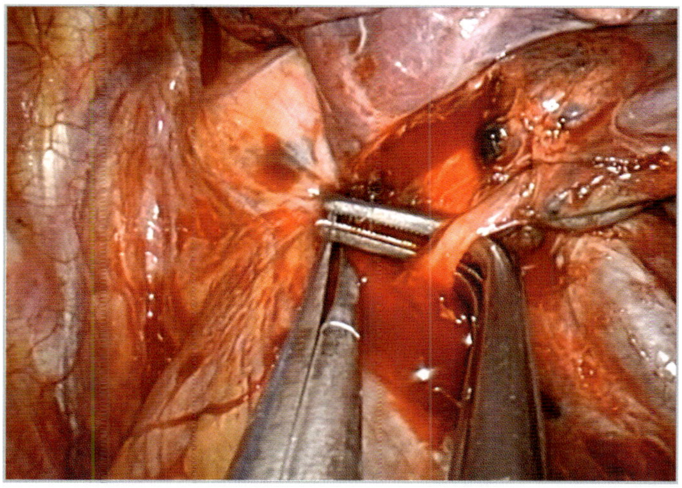

Figure 11.31 Dissecting the lingular vein.

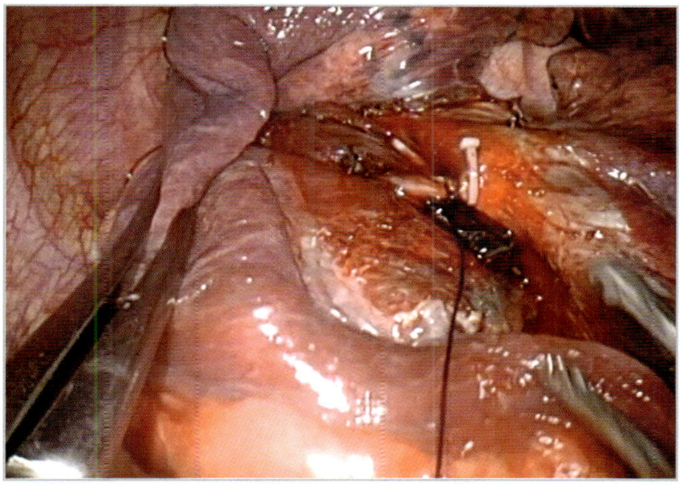

Figure 11.32 Dissecting the lingular artery with silk and Click'a V Endoscopic Polymer Clip Appliers 45° (Grena 170 Ltd. Brentford, England) and then resecting with energy device.

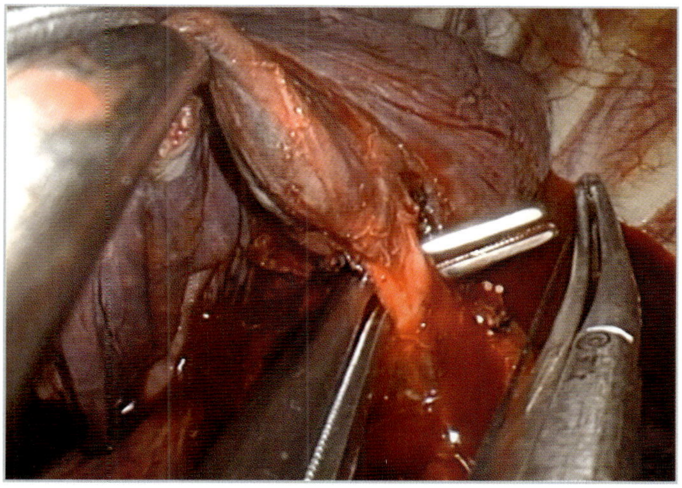

Figure 11.33 Dissecting the lingular bronchus.

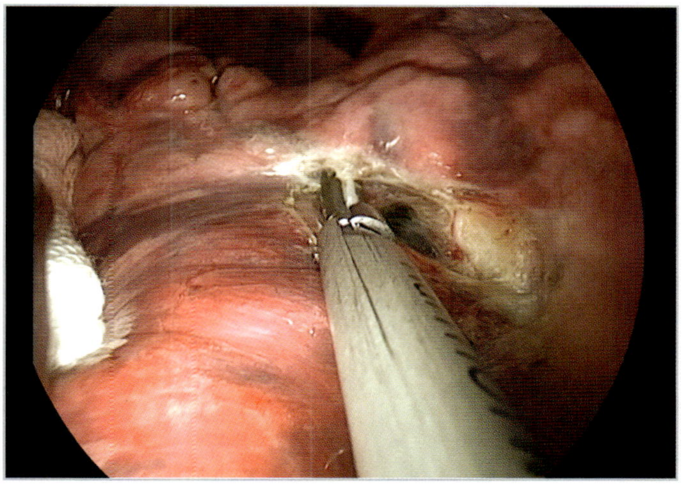

Figure 11.34 Retracting the lung with sponge on a stick to expose the fissure.

- Identify, dissect and divide the dorsal segmental artery with vascular endostapler, tie with silk or ligate using Click'a V Endoscopic Polymer Clip Appliers 45° (Grena 170 Ltd. Brentford, England) and then resect with energy device (**Figure 11.35**)
- Identify, dissect and divide the dorsal segmental bronchus with articulated endostapler (**Figure 11.36**). The place to find it is behind the stump of the dorsal segmental artery. Before transecting the bronchus always ask the anesthetist to insufflate the lung to confirm you are transecting the correct segmental bronchus; in some cases a curved-tip stapler technology is used to facilitate the passage around the structures
- During insufflation the portion that remains collapsed is the posterior segment
- Pull up the dorsal segment with thoracoscopic grasper and complete the intersegmental fissure created after the insufflation with endostapler. Always include the stump of the artery, the vein and the segmental bronchus in the segmental resection (**Figure 11.37**)
- Retrieve the resected lung with an Endocatch bag

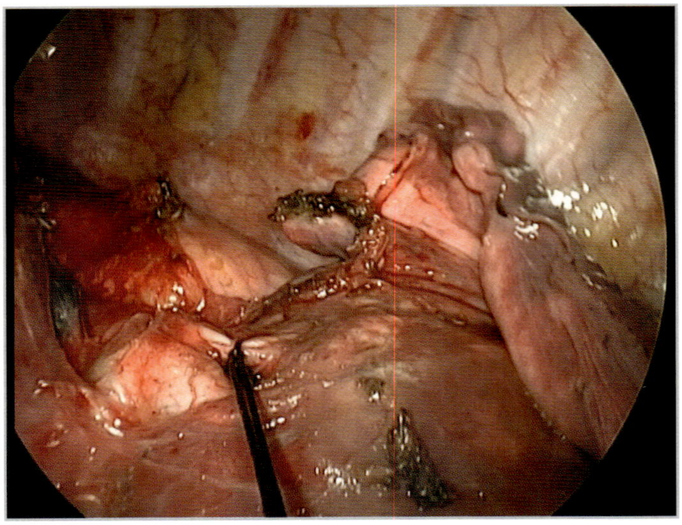

Figure 11.35 Dissection of the left dorsal segmental artery. The artery is marked with a silk.

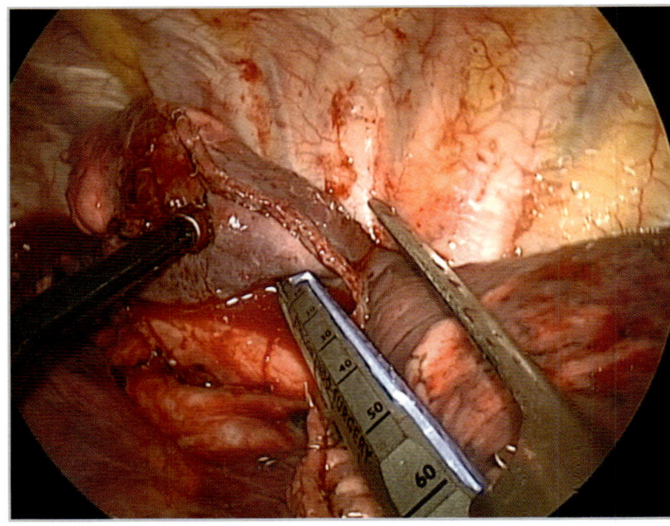

Figure 11.37 Pulling up the dorsal segment with suction to complete the intersegmental fissure created following after the insufflation using endostapler.

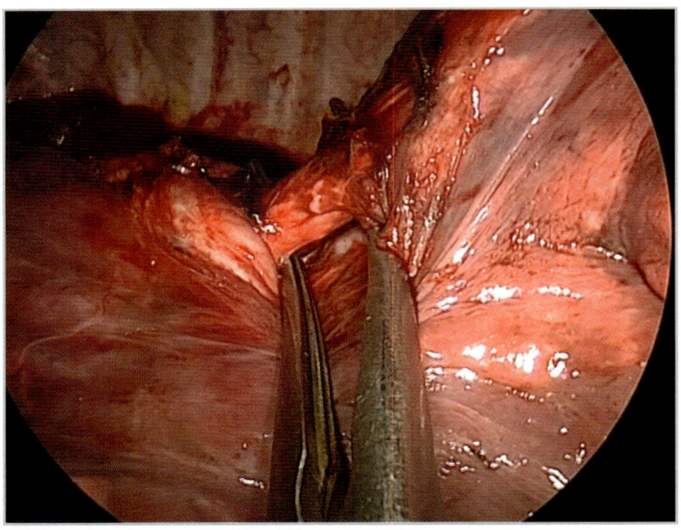

Figure 11.36 Dissection of the left dorsal segmental bronchus.

REFERENCES

1. Yoshida J, Nagai K, Yokose T, et al. Limited resection trial for pulmonary ground-glass opacity nodules: fifty-case experience. J Thorac Cardiovasc Surg 2005; 129:991–996.
2. Nakayama H, Yamada K, Saito H, et al. Sublobar resection for patients with peripheral small adenocarcinomas of the lung: surgical outcome is associated with features on computed tomographic imaging. Ann Thorac Surg 2007; 84:1675–1679.
3. Asamura H. Minimally invasive approach to early, peripheral adenocarcinoma with ground-glass opacity appearance. Ann Thorac Surg 2008; 85:S701–704.
4. Schuchert MJ, Pettiford BL, Keeley S, et al. Anatomic segmentectomy in the treatment of stage I non-small cell lung cancer. Ann Thorac Surg 2007; 84:926–932.

Chapter 12 Intraoperative complications and conversions

Liu Lunxu, Liu Chengwu

INTRODUCTION

Video-assisted thoracic surgery (VATS) has widely increased in popularity in the last few years.[1] Although the number of these procedures being performed has increased, complications have also risen at a similar rate, raising concerns about the safety of the procedure. Despite intraoperative issues being common, there is very little literature that has focused on detailed accounts of intraoperative complications, causes of conversion and management of intraoperative crisis. This chapter will discuss the most common intraoperative complications and potential causes of conversion, with an emphasis on potentially dangerous situations, and specific strategies for management.

Intraoperative complications and conversions can be classified into the following categories: equipment malfunction, anatomical problems (e.g. absent or fused fissure, diffuse or complete pleural adhesions, large tumor size, tumor location/invasion, lymph node issues), and intraoperative accidents (e.g. bleeding from either a vascular or airway injury).

ABSENT OR FUSED FISSURE

Traditionally, lobectomies were performed through a thoracotomy starting with the isolation of the pulmonary artery in the fissure. During the early stages of VATS lobectomy, this technique was transferred into a thoracoscopic lobectomy. However, when an absent or fused fissure was encountered, conversion was essential as there was no appropriate strategy for dissecting the pulmonary arteries buried deep in the pulmonary parenchyma. An absent or fused fissure became one of the main causes of conversion at that time. D'Amico and Ng et al. then proposed the fissureless technique by addressing the hilar structures first and then completing the fissure last to overcome this problem.[4,5] Then the authors developed the 'single-direction thoracoscopic lobectomy technique', which allowed all dissection to be performed at the pulmonary hilum without the need to dissect any pulmonary parenchyma or fissure (**Figure 12.1**).[6] The fissureless technique has also been proven to minimize the risk of postoperative air leaks.[4,5]

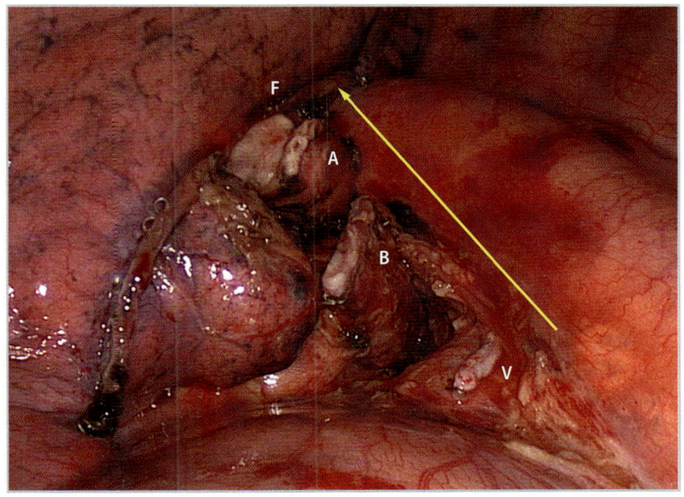

Figure 12.1 Single-direction thoracoscopic lobectomy. Dissection is initiated at the hilum and proceeds progressively in a single direction (yellow arrow) from the superficial to deep structures. For example, in a left lower lobectomy the inferior pulmonary vein (V), bronchus (B), pulmonary artery (A) were dissected and transected sequentially, with the fissure (F) divided last.

DIFFUSE OR COMPLETE PLEURAL ADHESIONS

Many different forms of pleural adhesion can be encountered during thoracoscopic lung surgery. On one hand, those loose, membranous, or cord-like adhesions can be easily dissected by a thoracoscopic approach. On the other hand, diffuse or complete pleural adhesions usually prevent lung collapse, increasing the risk of lung injury from the trocar or thoracoscope and, in severe cases, preventing access to the pleural space altogether, requiring conversion to thoracotomy. Diffuse or complete pleural adhesions were once considered a contraindication of VATS major lung resection. However, thoracoscopic adhesiolysis has now become feasible. The effect of thoracoscopic improved visualization and afforded a more accurate identification of the regional anatomy and a clearer plane of dissection between the visceral and parietal pleura. The key point in thoracoscopic adhesiolysis lies in the construction of 'tunnels' between working ports through blunt digital dissection at the beginning of the procedure (**Figure 12.2**).

Preoperative detection of adhesions is challenging. Computed tomography (CT) scans have been reported to have limited accuracy in predicting common diffuse or complete adhesions, except for those with severe pleural thickening and/or calcified adhesions.[7] However, transthoracic ultrasound has been reported to be effective in the detection of adhesions before surgery.[8]

COMPLICATED PULMONARY HILUM

Central tumor location and lymph node issues (metastatic lymph nodes invasion and inflammatory or calcified periarterial/peribronchial lymph nodes) may impede the progress of VATS lobectomy. These situations can be described as complicated pulmonary hilum or difficult pulmonary hilum. Cases with central tumor location that needed bronchial and/or arterial reconstruction were excluded from VATS lobectomy during the early days of thoracoscopic lobectomy. As surgical experience increased more complex surgical interventions, including partial or sleeve reconstruction of bronchus accompanied

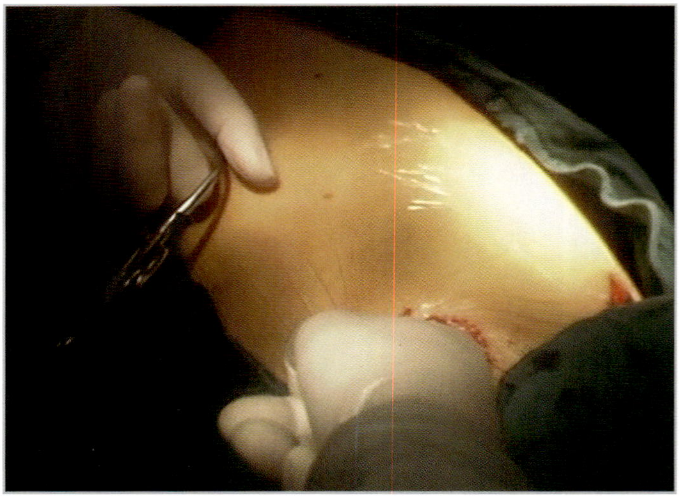

Figure 12.2 Constructing 'tunnels' between working ports through blunt dissection using fingers to troubleshoot pleural adhesions.

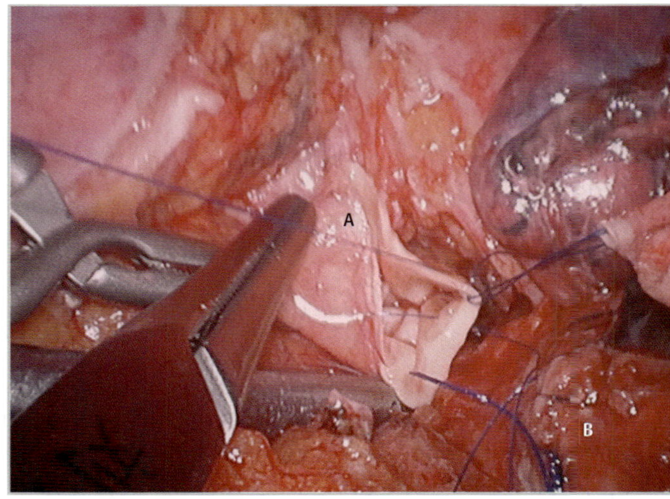

Figure 12.3 VATS bronchovascular upper double sleeve lobectomy. The left main bronchus and the left lower bronchus were first anastomosed, followed by the anastomosis of the left main pulmonary artery and the left lower pulmonary artery. (A) pulmonary artery, (B) bronchus.

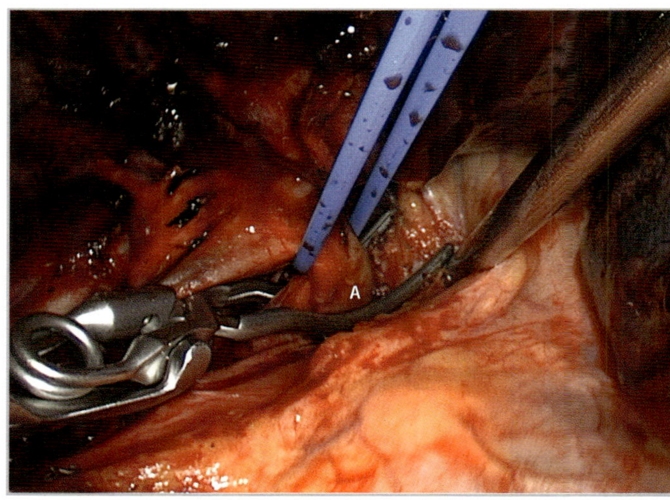

Figure 12.4 Cross-clamping the main pulmonary artery using a releasable endoscopic bulldog clamp in a right upper lobectomy complicated with severe hilar lymphadenopathy (the apico-anterior branch of the right upper pulmonary artery was enwrapped by calcified lymphadenopathy). After cross-clamping the right main pulmonary artery, dissection of the arterial branches was simple. A, right main pulmonary artery.

with or without partial or sleeve reconstruction of arteries, and pneumonectomy, became feasible. And in 1995, Craig et al. performed the first VATS pneumonectomy.[9] In 2002, Santambrogio et al. reportedly performed the first case of a VATS bronchial sleeve lobectomy.[10] Thereafter, accumulated experience revealed the feasibility and safety of VATS sleeve lobectomy in several experienced centers during the past decade.[11,12] More complicated central tumors requiring half carina resection and bronchial sleeve resection could also be approached with thoracoscopic techniques.[13]

A central tumor poses challenges in the dissection of the hilar structure. For example, it is very difficult to control sudden dramatic bleeding from the pulmonary artery, which may become life-threatening. Most thoracic surgeons opt to convert from a thoracoscopic approach to a thoracotomy when there is sudden bleeding or a risk of massive bleeding caused by severe adhesions between the pulmonary artery and the tissues (most of them are hilar lymph nodes) surrounding it. Inherited from open thoracotomy, the technique of cross-clamping the main pulmonary artery before starting any vascular dissection has become a recommended procedure. With the main pulmonary artery controlled, the surgeon can dissect the artery from surrounding tissues without worrying about massive bleeding or conversion. In 2007, Watanabe et al. described the method of controlling the main pulmonary artery using silk sutures, which avoided blocking the thoracoscopic view and an additional incision for clamping.[15] Kamiyoshihara et al. and Zhang et al. illustrated their technique to clamp the main pulmonary artery using open vascular clamps.[16,17] The author improved this clamping technique by using an endoscopic bulldog clamp (**Figure 12.4**). This technique has several advantages:

- Limited port space could be spared and it negates the need for further incisions
- Suturing is more ergonomic without the handle of the clamp sticking out through the wound
- The risk of pulmonary artery laceration is reduced when the lung is retracted for exposure, because the pulmonary artery trunk is still movable after clamping

BLEEDING

Intraoperative bleeding is considered the main reason for conversion to thoracotomy during thoracoscopic lung surgery.

Mild bleeding can usually be managed easily. However, oozing blood becomes irksome during dissection of anatomical structures. Traditionally, blunt dissection was mostly used when dissecting hilar structures. This method tends to cause consistent ooze, which would impair visualization, especially in cases with inflammatory adhesions. We recommend the use of energy devices instead of blunt dissection to reduce this oozing. In our institute, we use the method of 'suction-electrocoagulation' during dissection to ensure a clean operating field (**Figure 12.5**). There are several effective methods to deal with mild bleeding, such as the use of thrombostatic material, biological sealant, or discreet utilization of energy sources. Titanium or Hemlock clips may also be helpful to curb bleeding from some visible small blood vessels. Bleeding of the bronchial or vascular stumps after transecting the bronchus or vessels using endo-stapler can also occur. Compression with wetted gauze is sometimes useful. A quick electrocoagulation at the bleeding point of the stump is helpful, but care should be taken to avoid melting the staples and causing additional injury. Bothersome bleeding often happens during thoracoscopic mediastinal lymph node dissection, which can be caused by accidental injuries to the bronchial arteries crossing the field and damages to the nodes from directly grasping them during dissection. This bleeding is intractable because its location is often deep in the interspace between the vulnerable vital organs. Recently, the author developed the method of 'non-grasping en bloc thoracoscopic mediastinal lymph node dissection' (**Figure 12.6**), which enabled en bloc dissection of the mediastinal lymph nodes.[18]

Massive bleeding during thoracoscopic lung surgery is mostly caused by injury to the vessels, particularly the pulmonary artery, and can be catastrophic because managing it under thoracoscopy is challenging even for the experienced thoracic surgeon. Historically, the only way to control the bleeding was by compression or tamponade of the injured site while converting to thoracotomy. Any hand-held instruments such as endo-stapler, suction, ring forceps, gauze, vascular clamps, can be used to control the bleeding site and this should be performed as soon as possible, and carefully. Once the bleeding has been controlled, hemostatic materials, hemoclips, and endo-stapler can be used to manage the site of injury. In 2013, the author described a new method, the 'suction-compressing angiorrhaphy technique (SCAT)' for dealing with severe bleeding due to vascular injury during thoracoscopic lung surgery (**Figure 12.7**).[19] Bleeding control and angiorrhaphy were both achieved through thoracoscopy in most cases of vascular injury. Although most of the bleeding can be managed, in the author's experience emergent conversion to open thoracotomy is still sometimes unavoidable, e.g. when there is insufficient room to achieve a satisfactory proximal clamping of the injured vessel.[20]

Safety is always the top priority during thoracoscopic lung surgery, and precaution is always the most important issue especially in cases with high risk of vascular injury. If an accidental injury occurs, the surgeon should manage it either by the thoracoscopic technique or conversion to thoracotomy, depending on their own experience and skill.

EQUIPMENT MALFUNCTION

Equipment malfunction rarely happens, but it may cause serious complications. A failed staple line of the pulmonary vessels may cause severe bleeding, and a failed staple line of the bronchus may cause severe air leaks either with or without severe hemorrhage. Rescue repair can be performed either with thoracoscopy or conversion to thoracotomy. Absorbable polymer materials and autologous pleural or pericardial patches may be helpful to prevent postoperative bronchial fistula. Staple line failure of the incomplete fissure may also cause severe air leaks and bleeding. Reinforcement by suturing of the failed staple line can be performed easily under thoracoscopy.

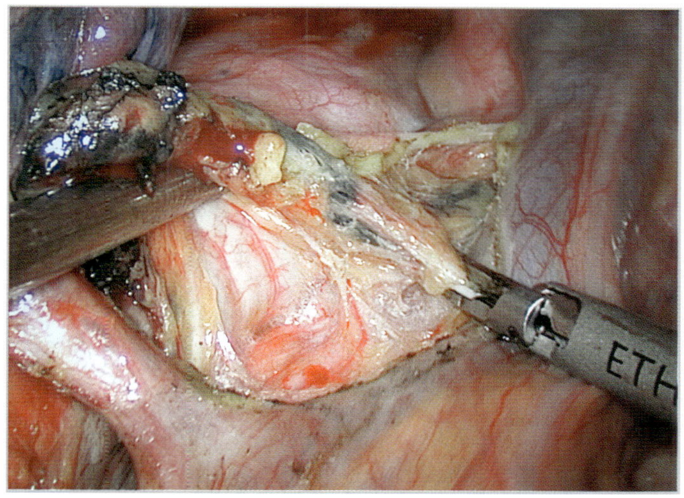

Figure 12.6 Non-grasping en bloc thoracoscopic mediastinal lymph node dissection.

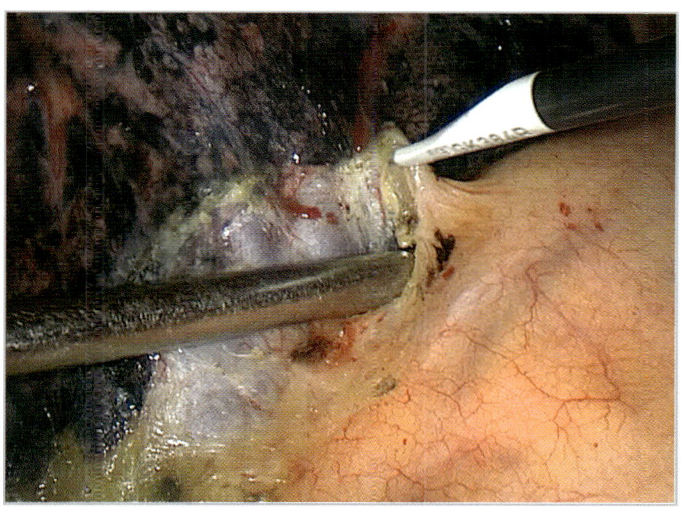

Figure 12.5 Suction-electrocoagulation collaborative dissection. A bloodless dissection technique in VATS lobectomy.

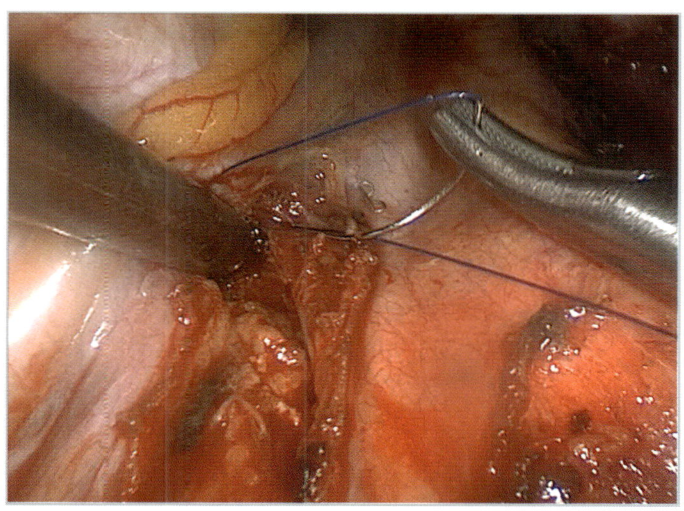

Figure 12.7 Suction-compressing angiorrhaphy technique (SCAT) in a rupture of the left subclavian vein. This was managed via a direct rotating suture after suction-compressing during dissection of the station 6 lymph nodes.

COMPLICATIONS DURING MEDIASTINAL LYMPHADENECTOMY

To achieve optimal exposure of deeply located lymph nodes most surgeons attempt to grasp them. However, tight grasping may cause damage to the target nodes, leading to bothersome bleeding and potential dissemination of cancer cells if the nodes are involved.

Chylothorax sometimes occurs due to leakage from draining the lymphatic vessels or direct injury to the ascending thoracic duct in the posterior mediastinum. The author has encountered several cases of injury to the thoracic duct, which crosses to the left just behind the ascending aorta, when performing dissection of paratracheal lymph nodes (station 4R/L). Ligation of the thoracic duct just above the diaphragm resulted in no postoperative chylothorax.

Recurrent laryngeal nerves are easily injured either by mechanical or thermal injuries when performing lymph node dissection. There is no need to expose the recurrent laryngeal nerves.

Injury to the membranous portion of the bronchi sometimes happens when dissecting the subcarinal lymph nodes (station 7). It is a serious complication which can require conversion to thoracotomy to repair.

CONCLUSION

The technical safety of VATS lung surgery is now widely accepted. Although there remains a range of situations that can cause intraoperative complications or unplanned conversions, most intraoperative complications or conversions can be either avoided or effectively managed; and no significant increase in mortality or morbidity has been observed.

REFERENCES

1. Yan TD, Cao C, D'Amico TA, et al. Video-assisted thoracoscopic surgery lobectomy at 20 years: a consensus statement. Eur J Cardiothorac Surg 2014; 45:633–639.
2. Hanna JM, Berry MF, D'Amico TA. Contraindications of video-assisted thoracoscopic surgical lobectomy and determinants of conversion to open. J Thorac Dis 2013; 5:S182–189.
3. Puri V, Patel A, Majumder K, et al. Intraoperative conversion from video-assisted thoracoscopic surgery lobectomy to open thoracotomy: a study of causes and implications. J Thorac Cardiovasc Surg 2015; 149: 55–61.
4. Balsara KR, Balderson SS, D'Amico TA. Surgical techniques to avoid parenchymal injury during lung resection (fissureless lobectomy). Thorac Surg Clin 2010; 20:365–369.
5. Ng T, Ryder BA, Machan JT, Cioffi WG. Decreasing the incidence of prolonged air leak after right upper lobectomy with the anterior fissureless technique. J Thorac Cardiovasc Surg 2010; 139:1007–1011.
6. Liu L, Che G, Pu Q, et al. A new concept of endoscopic lung cancer resection: Single-direction thoracoscopic lobectomy. Surg Oncol 2010; 19: e71–77.
7. Mason AC, Miller BH, Krasna MJ, White CS. Accuracy of CT for the detection of pleural adhesions: correlation with video-assisted thoracoscopic surgery. Chest 1999; 115:423–427.
8. Cassanelli N, Caroli G, Dolci G, et al. Accuracy of transthoracic ultrasound for the detection of pleural adhesions. Eur J Cardiothorac Surg 2012; 42: 813–818.
9. Craig SR, Walker WS. Initial experience of video assisted thoracoscopic pneumonectomy. Thorax 1995; 50:392–395.
10. Santambrogio L, Cioffi U, De Simone M, et al. Video-assisted sleeve lobectomy for mucoepidermoid carcinoma of the left lower lobar bronchus: a case report. Chest 2002; 121:635–636.
11. Mahtabifard A, Fuller CB, McKenna RJ. Video-assisted thoracic surgery sleeve lobectomy: a case series. Ann Thorac Surg 2008; 85:S729–732.
12. Ng CS. Thoracoscopic sleeve resection-the better approach? J Thorac Dis 2014; 6:1164–1166.
13. Xu X, Chen H, Yin W, et al. Thoracoscopic half carina resection and bronchial sleeve resection for central lung cancer. Surg Innov 2014; 21:481–486.
14. Liu L, Mei J, Pu Q, Ma L. Thoracoscopic bronchovascular double sleeve lobectomy for non-small-cell lung cancer. Eur J Cardiothorac Surg 2014; 46:493–495.
15. Watanabe A, Koyanagi T, Nakashima S, Higami T. How to clamp the main pulmonary artery during video-assisted thoracoscopic surgery lobectomy. Eur J Cardiothorac Surg 2007; 31:129–131.
16. Zhang Z, Huang J, Yin R, Xu L. A new technique for partial removal of the pulmonary artery in video-assisted thoracic surgical lobectomy. J Thorac Cardiovasc Surg 2012; 144:512–514.
17. Kamiyoshihara M, Nagashima T, Ibe T, Takeyoshi I. A tip for controlling the main pulmonary artery during video-assisted thoracic major pulmonary resection: the outside-field vascular clamping technique. Interact Cardiovasc Thorac Surg 2010; 11:693–695.
18. Liu C, Pu Q, Guo C, et al. Non-grasping en bloc mediastinal lymph node dissection for video-assisted thoracoscopic lung cancer surgery. BMC Surg 2015; 15:38.
19. Mei J, Pu Q, Liao H, et al. A novel method for troubleshooting vascular injury during anatomic thoracoscopic pulmonary resection without conversion to thoracotomy. Surg Endosc 2013; 27:530–537.
20. Xiao ZL, Mei JD, Pu Q, Liu LX. Technical strategy for dealing with bleeding during thoracoscopic lung surgery. Ann Cardiothorac Surg 2014; 3:213–215.

Chapter 13 VATS for minor procedures

Luca Bertolaccini, Alessandro Pardolesi, Piergiorgio Solli

INTRODUCTION

The advantages of video-assisted thoracoscopic surgery (VATS) are well known and include less postoperative pain, fewer postoperative complications, shortened hospital stay and reduced costs. The VATS approach was initially used for simple diagnostic and therapeutic procedures involving the pleura, lungs and mediastinum. However, VATS operations continue to replace many procedures that formerly required thoracotomies, such as lobectomies.

VATS RESECTION OF A SOLITARY PULMONARY NODULE

A solitary pulmonary nodule (SPN) is a radiographic spherical opacity in the lung, defined by the Fleishner Society < 3 cm in diameter.[1] A SPN is a common clinical problem; it may be accompanied by symptoms such as cough, loss of weight, physical discomfort, or hemoptysis. But, in most cases, the lesion is discovered incidentally on a chest roentgenogram or a computer tomography (CT) scan[2] obtained for various purposes such as screening programs, investigations for pulmonary embolism and other respiratory complaints, cardiac function evaluation and searches for metastases of malignancies other than lung cancer.[3] Although most nodules are incidental findings, the primary goal is to exclude their malignancy.[2] Subcentimetric nodules are often difficult to diagnose, mostly because lesions of this size linger below the resolution power of positron emission tomography (PET) and because they are difficult to biopsy with fine-needle aspiration (FNA). Once found, these small nodules should be periodically reassessed with serial scanning unless there is some other factor that increases the potential for malignancy, such as the history of the patient or the CT characteristics of the nodule. Highly suspicious peripheral nodules should undergo diagnostic procedures, such as a FNA biopsy, navigational bronchoscopy biopsy, or VATS.[2] VATS represents a minimally invasive tool to diagnose and potentially treat pulmonary nodules. Patients with lung nodules who are at high risk for lung cancer or pulmonary metastases from a tumor of another organ are good candidates for a diagnostic/therapeutic thoracoscopic wedge resection. If the frozen section shows a non-small cell lung cancer, these patients can immediately undergo a formal VATS lobectomy. While in cases of pulmonary metastases wedge resections are often all is needed, if an adequate resection margin can be obtained.[2] Localization is critical and can be difficult by VATS. There are several techniques to locate a 'difficult' SPN that cannot be detected by digital palpation. These techniques are preoperative or intraoperative injections of methylene blue dye at the site of an SPN, intraoperative ultrasound, CT-guided positioning of a metal wire, and radioguided detection. Each of these localization methods has its own advantages and drawbacks.[4] Due to over-infusion of the methylene blue dye or an error in nodule localization, the failure rate of the methylene blue injection is approximately 13%. Intraoperative ultrasound localization of SPN remains a highly operator-dependent procedure and requires a special flexible probe and complete collapse of the assessed lung.[5] As far as radioguided localization of SPN is concerned, the disadvantages of this technique rely essentially on the need of a preparatory procedure, consisting in the radionuclide injection that usually is performed by means of a spinal needle, placed near to the nodule under CT guidance.[6]

Technical notes

For VATS procedure, ipsilateral, single-lung ventilation with a double-lumen endotracheal tube is usually required. The patient is placed in most cases in the full lateral decubitus position. Dedicated VATS instrumentation is not necessary for most procedures, and standard open or laparoscopic instruments can be used to manipulate the lung. A 5-mm or 10-mm 30° thoracoscope is used for visualization. The 30° thoracoscope carries the advantage of increased visualization of the thorax, although the surgeon may need practice in order to acquaint him/herself with the scope orientation. Thoracoscopic port placement for the resection of peripheral SPN is standard, with the goal being to triangulate around the lesion. Port placement may vary slightly based on location of the lesion, and the ports may be placed higher or lower in the chest. The first port, usually used for the scope, is placed at the 8th or 9th intercostal space at the midaxillary line. The use of a thoracoport, either hard or soft, at this site assists in keeping the camera clear and allows fast and clean movements of the scope in and out the chest. Two additional ports are placed to triangulate around SPN. The anterior port is placed in the 5th interspace at the midclavicular line. A trocar is often not used in this location, and the incision must be large enough to allow entrance of instruments and finger palpation of the lung. An anterior incision is slightly preferable because interspaces are narrower posteriorly. The visualization of a subpleural nodule with the thoracoscope is sometimes favorite by an indentation on the visceral pleura. A finger can be placed through one of the access ports and a clamp placed through the other to manipulate the lung for palpation. Palpation of the lung is often essential in locating a subpleural SPN. The posterior port is placed at the 5th or 6th interspace, posterior to the midaxillary line. This access port is most often placed in line with the incision for a standard posterolateral thoracotomy, below the scapula. After the SPN is identified and localized, it is resected using an endoscopic stapler (**Figure 13.1**). Care must be taken to avoid manipulating or squashing the lesion, thereby hampering the pathologic interpretation. The stapler is often manoeuverd between both of the access ports to complete the wedge resection. Extraction of the specimen from the thoracic cavity is best accomplished with the assistance of a retrieval bag device so as not to contaminate the access port (**Figure 13.2**). A single chest tube is placed, usually thorough the inferior access, at the end of the procedure and connected to suction until the next day.

VATS FOR PNEUMOTHORAX

Spontaneous pneumothorax can occur at every age. Primary spontaneous pneumothorax occurs mainly in otherwise healthy people (mainly tall, young men) without lung disease. Secondary spontaneous pneumothorax occurs in patients with diagnosed and clinically overt lung disease (such as chronic obstructive lung disease) and is most frequent in older subjects.[7] The principles of pneumothorax

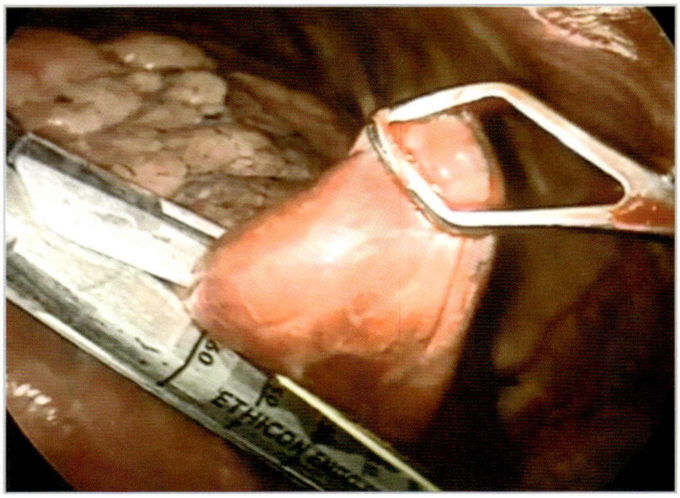

Figure 13.1 VATS in solitary pulmonary nodule management. After localization of the nodule a wedge resection is performed.

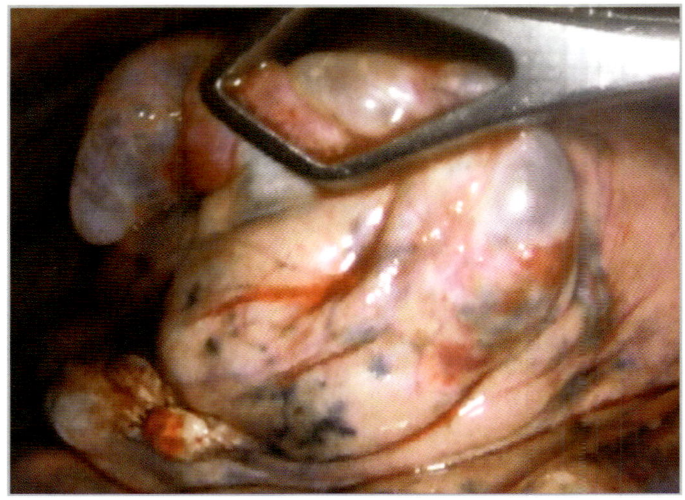

Figure 13.3 VATS for spontaneous pneumothorax. After visualization, the blebs or bullae are resected.

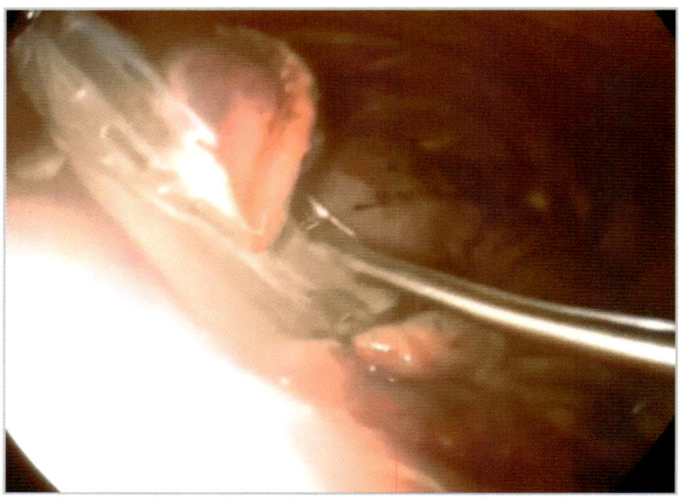

Figure 13.2 VATS in solitary pulmonary nodule management. The specimen containing the solitary pulmonary nodule is extracted from the thoracic cavity in a retrieval bag device so as not to contaminate the access port.

treatment rely in drainage of the pleural cavity, reduction of air leakage, pursuit of lung re-expansion and, prevention of future recurrences. Possible complications of pneumothorax include effusion, hemorrhage, empyema, respiratory failure, pneumomediastinum, arrhythmias, and hemodynamic instability and they need to be managed accordingly.[8] A surgical procedure, both via thoracotomy or VATS, can effectively reduce the recurrence rate of primary spontaneous pneumothorax after the first episode, from 23–50% to 3–7%. VATS seemed to have a higher postoperative recurrence rate than thoracotomy, but with the gradual development of instrumentation and the improvement of surgeon skill, results from both approaches are comparable.[9] VATS is now performed in most of patients undergoing surgery for pneumothorax and is recognized as a routine operation. Therefore, VATS should be considered the first-choice approach for most patients undergoing pneumothorax surgery. VATS is clearly less invasive than traditional thoracotomic approach, with minimal postoperative pain and a short chest tube and hospitalization time. Enhanced recovery ensures prompt and complete return to everyday activities, and it shows a trend toward early realization of social integration. VATS required post-operative administration of small doses of analgesic agents. The postoperative complication rate in patients undergoing VATS is reported to be 4.1–7.9%, with the most common complication being persistent air leaks while no fatal complications occurred.[10] While bleb resection by VATS has become the standard procedure, the method to obtain pleurodesis remains controversial. Various forms of pleurodesis are considered to reduce recurrences. Parietal pleurectomy, pleural abrasion, and talc poudrage were performed in the most highly ranked evidence-based studies focusing on attempts to reduce the recurrence rate.[10] Studies concerning the treatment of spontaneous pneumothorax have not been able to state the superiority of a pleurodesis method or another.[9]

Technical notes

After a placement of a double lumen endotracheal tube, patients are positioned in lateral decubitus. A 5 mm or 10 mm camera port is inserted through the 6th or 7th intercostal space along the mid-axillary line after lung deflation. Two working ports are inserted at the 3rd intercostal space on the anterior axillary line and at the 5th intercostal space at the posterior axillary line, respectively. The order of the steps of the operation usually goes on as follows: lysis of adhesions, visualization, and resection of the blebs or bullae (**Figure 13.3**), and pleurodesis. Adhesions may be present due to previous pneumothoraces and/or previous chest tube insertion. In order to free the lung, it is retracted away from the adhesions to provide adequate tension and facilitate the lysis performed with a hook cautery (**Figure 13.4**). The 30° thoracoscope, usually pointed toward the adhesions, allows their proper visualization and their relationships with surrounding structures. After the adhesions have been removed, the entire lung can be visualized. Sometimes, adhesions to the mediastinal pleura may be less obvious and more difficult to resect. Failure to recognize an adhesion may lead to tear visceral pleura and this may eventually become an unforeseen source of a prolonged postoperative air leak. Placement of forceps through the ports is useful for manipulation of the lung in order to plan the resection line. If possible, the stapler

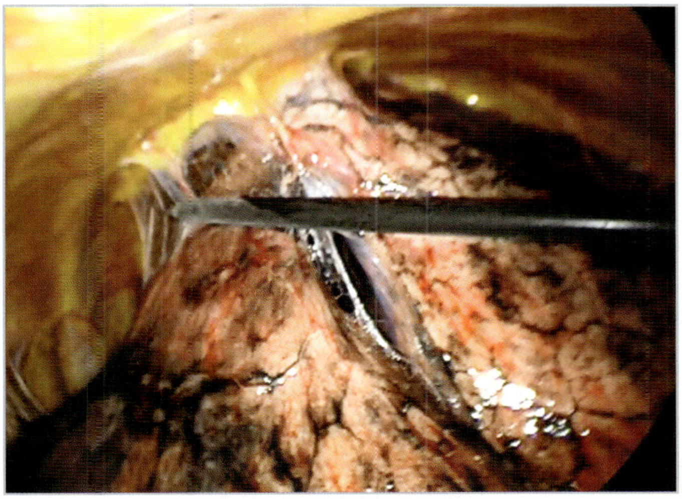

Figure 13.4 VATS for spontaneous pneumothorax. Adhesions due to previous pneumothoraces and/or previous chest tube insertion are lysed with a hook cautery.

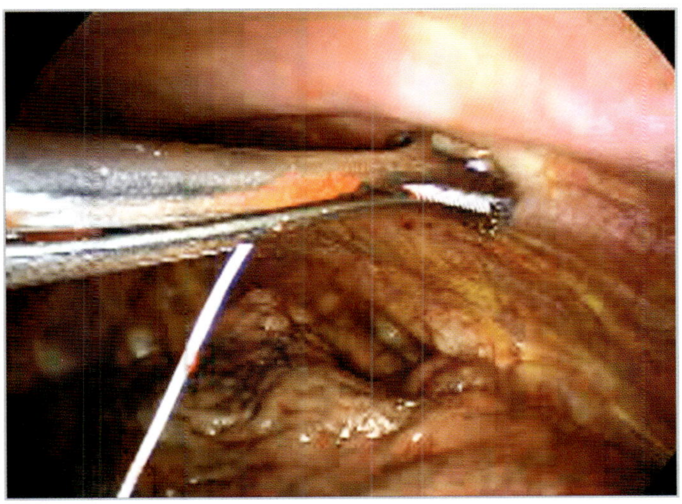

Figure 13.5 VATS for spontaneous pneumothorax. Pleurodesis is obtained by rubbing the parietal pleura with an abrasive mesh placed at the top of the ring forceps usually until the level of the 5th intercostal space.

should be placed through the anterior port because the rib spaces are wider anteriorly and, consequently, there is less postoperative pain. The check for any air leak and bleeding should be particularly careful along the staple line. We prefer to obtain pleurodesis by rubbing the parietal pleura with an abrasive mesh placed at the top of the ring forceps usually until the level of the 5th intercostals space (**Figure 13.5**). The procedure was concluded with the placing of a chest tube through the caudal port. The camera was placed in the posterior port to confirm good reinflation of the lung. Connection of the chest tube to suction is suggested.

Pneumothorax in cystic fibrosis

Cystic fibrosis is an autosomal genetic disease affecting a variety of organs, but especially involving respiratory tract and pancreas. The lungs undergo gradual destruction, as an effect of persistent microbial colonization, chronic inflammation, and recurrent infections caused by highly pathogenic bacteria, such as *Pseudomonas aeruginosa* and *Staphylococcus aureus*. The aim of treatment in cystic fibrosis patients is the safe and effective resolution of pneumothorax with prevention of recurrence. Historically, varieties of therapeutic interventions were employed, including sclerosant agents, pleural abrasion, intercostal drainage, pleurectomy and Heimlich flutter valve. Most of these methods were quite successful, but significant differences in the recurrence rates had been described, depending mostly by the employed procedure. Sclerosis and parietal pleurectomy appeared to be among the most effective methods of management. Pleural suction drainage was reported to have the lowest long-term success rate. These treatment suggestions were somewhat challenged by certain experts arguing the superiority of VATS. Their major arguments are focused on better safety, shorter postoperative period and less painkilling medications required, despite of the marginally higher recurrence rates observed with VATS.[11]

Catamenial pneumothorax

Catamenial pneumothorax is defined as spontaneous recurrent pneumothorax, occurring in women of reproductive age, in temporal relationship with menses. Catamenial pneumothorax is associated with thoracic and pelvic endometriosis, although endometriosis is not universally documented. Endometriosis is defined as the presence of ectopic endometrial tissue (stroma and glands) outside the uterine cavity. Thoracic endometriosis is not common but spontaneous pneumothorax is the most common clinical manifestation of thoracic endometriosis, occurring in 72–73% of patients, followed by catamenial hemoptysis, catamenial hemothorax, and endometriotic thoracic nodules. Pneumothoraces with catamenial character (with or without evidence of thoracic endometriosis) as well as pneumothoraces with evidence of thoracic endometriosis (with or without catamenial character) can be classified under the term catamenial and/or endometriosis related pneumothorax. Characteristic lesions of the disease spectrum described by the terms catamenial and/or thoracic endometriosis-related pneumothorax include single or multiple diaphragmatic lesions (fenestrations, diaphragmatic spots, and/or nodules), and/or visceral or parietal pleural lesions (spots and nodules). These lesions have not been revealed in all cases of catamenial pneumothorax, while they have been found in some cases without catamenial pneumothorax. Surgery is the treatment of choice of catamenial and/or thoracic endometriosis related pneumothorax, due to better results (regarding mainly less recurrences) in comparison to medical treatment only. VATS is considered the treatment of choice. Apart from routine lung inspection for bullae, blebs, and air leaks, a careful and meticulous inspection of the diaphragm as well as inspection of the parietal pleura, the lung, and the pericardium is of paramount importance. The procedure should be performed during menses, for better visualization of the endometriotic lesions. Magnification provided by VATS may facilitate identification of the lesions. Tissue sampling for histological documentation facilitates the diagnosis of thoracic endometriosis. Diaphragmatic plication and/or resection of the diseased area can be performed during VATS but sometimes through a utility thoracotomy. In order to avoid recurrences and provide samples for histology, diaphragmatic resection (along with removal of endometrial implants) is preferable to single diaphragmatic plication (that leaves endometrial implants untreated). Given the likelihood of occult defects and in order to avoid recurrences, systematic diaphragmatic coverage and reinforcement, usually by means of a mesh, is strongly suggested, including coverage of areas with normal appearance. Induction of pleurodesis is also encouraged.[12]

VATS LUNG BIOPSY FOR INTERSTITIAL LUNG DISEASES

Surgical lung biopsy for diffuse interstitial lung diseases is sometimes essential for accurate pathological diagnosis, treatment decision, and prediction of prognosis, and is recommended whenever there are no functional contraindications. Lung biopsy for diffuse interstitial lung diseases by thoracotomy, however, has been reported to be associated with substantial mortality because of postoperative acute respiratory distress syndrome, recognized as an acute exacerbation of interstitial lung disease. VATS has become the standard procedures for lung biopsy. Biopsy sites were determined through discussion with pulmonologists, diagnostic radiologists, and pathologists. In many cases, an early-phase lesion and a moderately advanced lesion as deemed from radiological findings were selected for biopsy.[13] The term interstitial lung disease encompasses a diverse group of diffuse parenchymal lung disorders that vary considerably in their clinical presentation, degree of lung function impairment, imaging characteristics, and histopathological changes.[14] These disorders are usually idiopathic, predominantly subacute, or chronic in their clinical course at initial diagnosis, and display a considerable range of inflammation and/or fibrosis on histopathological examination of lung tissue. Although the etiologies have been identified for some of these disorders, in the majority of cases, the ultimate cause remains unknown. The differentiation of a specific form of interstitial lung disease can present a formidable challenge to the clinician; therefore, an invasive approach may be often required to make a reliable diagnosis.[13]

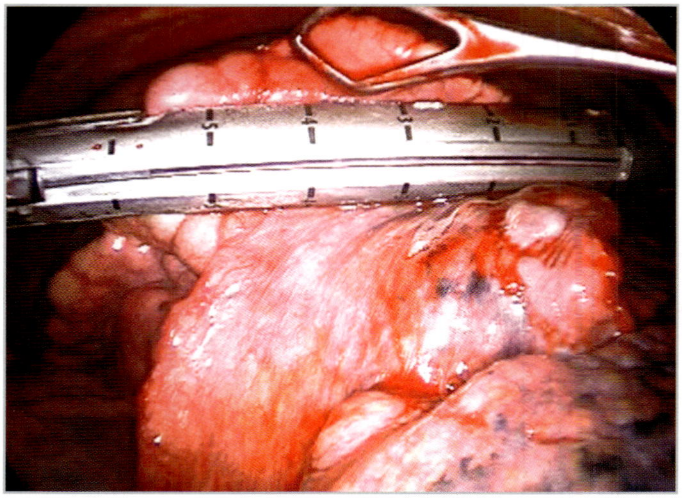

Figure 13.6 VATS for interstitial lung disease. Lung biopsy was obtained by performing a three-port VATS wedge resection with surgical stapling devices.

Technical notes

In the authors' experience, a three-port approach under one-lung ventilation was generally used. Lung biopsy was obtained by performing a wedge resection (non-anatomical lung resection) with surgical stapling devices. Selection of cartridge depended on the thickness and texture of the lung parenchyma as expected at the planned biopsy site. A border of at least 3 cm around the triangle-shaped has been included in order to sample a peribronchiolar area of lung parenchyma in the biopsy specimens (**Figure 13.6**). Since the disease condition had been deemed severe in several cases, steroids were administered immediately after resection of the biopsy specimen. One chest drainage tube was placed and connected to suction.

REFERENCES

1. Hansell DM, Bankier AA, MacMahon H, et al. Fleischner Society: glossary of terms for thoracic imaging. Radiology 2008; 246:697–722.
2. Thiessen NR, Bremner R. The solitary pulmonary nodule: Approach for a general surgeon. Surg Clin N Am 2010; 90:1003–1018.
3. Murrmann GB, van Vollenhoven FH, Moodley L. Approach to a solid solitary pulmonary nodule in two different settings – 'Common is common, rare is rare'. J Thorac Dis 2014; 6:237–248.
4. Bertolaccini L, Terzi A, Spada E, Acchiardi F, Ghirardo D. Not palpable? Role of radio-guided video-assisted thoracic surgery for nonpalpable solitary pulmonary nodules. Gen Thor Cardiovasc Surg 2012; 60:280–284.
5. Chen S, Zhou J, Zhang J, et al. Video-assisted thoracoscopic solitary pulmonary nodule resection after CT-guided hookwire localization: 43 cases report and literature review. Surg Endosc 2011; 25:1723–1729.
6. Bertolaccini L, Salgarello M, Terzi A. Radioguided video-assisted resection of non-palpable solitary pulmonary nodule/ground glass opacity: how to do it. J Vis Surg 2015.
7. Jiang L, Jiang G, Zhu Y, Hao W, Zhang L. Risk factors predisposing to prolonged air leak after video-assisted thoracoscopic surgery for spontaneous pneumothorax. Ann Thorac Surg 2014; 97:1008–1013.
8. Huang Y, Huang H, Li Q, et al. Approach of the treatment for pneumothorax. J Thorac Dis 2014; 6:S416–420.
9. Chou SH, Li HP, Lee YL, et al. Video-assisted thoracoscopic surgery for postoperative recurrent primary spontaneous pneumothorax. J Thorac Dis 2014; 6:52–55.
10. Goto T, Kadota Y, Mori T, et al. Video-assisted thoracic surgery for pneumothorax: republication of a systematic review and a proposal by the guideline committee of the Japanese Association for Chest Surgery 2014. Gen Thorac Cardiovasc Surg 2014; 63:8–13.
11. Kioumis IP, Zarogoulidis K, Huang H, et al. Pneumothorax in cystic fibrosis. J Thorac Dis 2014; 6:S480–487.
12. Visouli AN, Zarogoulidis K, Kougioumtzi I, et al. Catamenial pneumothorax. J Thorac Dis 2014; 6:S448–460.
13. Sonobe M, Handa T, Tanizawa K, et al. Videothoracoscopy-assisted surgical lung biopsy for interstitial lung diseases. Gen Thor Cardiovasc Surg 2014; 62:376–682.
14. Nguyen W, Meyer KC. Surgical lung biopsy for the diagnosis of interstitial lung disease : a review of the literature and recommendations for optimizing safety and efficacy. Sarcoidosis Vasc Diffuse Lung Dis 2013; 30:3–16.

Chapter 14 Emerging non-surgical techniques for volume reduction in emphysema

Joyce Chew, Tom Dymond, Donna Cummins, Jurgen Herre, Benedetta Bedetti, Marco Scarci, Ravi Mahadeva, Robert S George

INTRODUCTION

Chronic obstructive pulmonary disease (COPD) is an incurable disease of high prevalence and is predicted to be the 3rd leading cause of death worldwide by 2030 (WHO).[1] Pathologically, COPD encompasses diverse pathology including small airways narrowing, emphysema and large airway mucus hypersecretion that leads to clinical symptoms of breathlessness, sputum production and infective exacerbations. Specialist COPD phenotyping aids an understanding of the physiological and pathological relationships to the disease which facilitate targeted treatment. Emphysema is characterized by the destruction of alveolar tissue leading to the abnormal, permanent enlargement of airspaces distal to the terminal bronchioles. In addition to a loss of gas exchange surface area, this process also leads to the loss of lung elastic recoil, resulting in progressive hyperinflation and air trapping. Emphysema predominant COPD is characterized by progressive breathlessness, skeletal muscle deconditioning leading to loss of function, reduced quality of life (QoL), and increased mortality. The beneficial effects of treatments including smoking cessation, pulmonary rehabilitation and pharmacological treatment, such as inhaled bronchodilator therapy and corticosteroids, are modest at best particularly in severe emphysema.

The concept of lung volume reduction surgery (LVRS) for emphysema was initially described by Brantigan and Mueller in 1957 and later redefined and evaluated by Cooper et al. in a landmark study.[2] The aim of LVRS is to resect the most emphysematous part of the lung, allowing healthier, less compliant areas to function more effectively. Thus improving expiratory flow, diaphragmatic function, and respiratory muscle mechanics. In 2003, the most comprehensive trial of LVRS [National Emphysema Treatment Trial (NETT), $n = 1218$] demonstrated significant improvements in exercise capacity and QoL following bilateral LVRS.[3] Patients that had gained the maximum benefit and had increased survival were however confined to those with upper lobe predominant emphysema and low preoperative exercise capacity. The study also identified a high-risk group with excess surgical mortality; those with a forced expiratory volume in 1 second (FEV_1) of less than 20% of the predicted value, homogenous emphysema or carbon monoxide diffusing capacity (TLCO) of less than 20% of the predicted value. NETT further demonstrated that LVRS could be performed in non-high-risk patients with acceptable mortality of 5.5% within 90 days of LVRS, but with significant risk of complications 58.7% of the study participants developed at least one post-operative complication within 30 days of surgery. Major pulmonary and cardiovascular complications were recorded in 29.8% and 20% of patients, and included pneumonia, reintubation, tracheostomy insertion, failure to wean, cardiac arrhythmias, pulmonary embolus etc. Prolonged air leaks occurred in 28.1% of patients, resulting in prolonged postoperative hospital stay of over 28 days in many. Recent data however, has shown that with careful patient selection, discussion by an expert multidisciplinary team (MDT) and advances in surgery (e.g. unilateral video-assisted thoracoscopic LVRS), mortality and morbidity has significantly subsided.[4,5] Nevertheless, despite the published evidence, only 96 procedures were performed between 2009 and 2010 and 90 in 2010 to 2011 in the UK.[6,7] A survey conducted by the British Thoracic Society found that most respiratory physicians in the UK were unsure about the risk of death and associated prolonged hospital stay or significantly over-estimated them.[8] There was also a lack of access to a MDT to discuss management of patients with advanced COPD. The surgical lung volume reduction (LVR) data demonstrated that if patients are selected appropriately, reduction of pathological emphysematous hyperinflation has the potential for large improvements in symptoms and improvements in mortality in COPD unlike any other therapy for COPD other than long-term oxygen therapy.[9]

Thus surgical LVR is proven and effective in specific groups of patients. However the complexity of COPD disease and vulnerability of patients has contributed to the relatively high morbidity in some patient groups and benefit to only a restricted cohort of patients. This has prompted the search for ways to extend this potentially highly valuable treatment option to more patients. As mentioned previously, improved surgical techniques have resulted in improved outcomes. In addition, there has been a drive to develop less invasive modalities to achieve reduction of pathological hyperinflation, such as the use of endoscopic lung volume reduction (ELVR) technique, a rapidly expanding and promising field. A number of devices are now available either for clinical use or undergoing clinical trials. These include unidirectional airway valves, endobronchial coils, polymeric lung sealant, thermal vapor ablation and exhale airway stents. The main potential aim of these less invasive procedures is to achieve a reduction in post-procedural complications and a potential broadening of the eligibility criteria to include patients with significant co-morbidities or advanced/diffuse emphysema, which preclude surgical LVR.

ENDOBRONCHIAL VALVE THERAPY

Insertion of one-way endobronchial valves (EBV) is the most extensively investigated of these non-surgical techniques. There are currently two designs of valves available for use. The Zephyr valve (Pulmonx, Inc.) has a self-expanding, membrane-covered retainer that provides stability and prevents dislocation. The intrabronchial valve (IBV) (Spiration, Inc.) is an umbrella-shaped, one-way valve incorporating a nitinol skeleton consisting of five distal anchors holding the valve in place and six proximal struts covered by a polymer.[10] The majority of published data is with the Zephyr valve.

Endobronchial valve insertion can be performed with the patient under local anesthesia and sedation or general anesthesia. A delivery catheter is passed through a flexible bronchoscope and the valve is placed in the targeted segmental or sub-segmental bronchi that fixes to the bronchial wall. The valve obstructs the passage of air to the treated lobe during inspiration, while allowing air and secretions to escape during the expiratory phase. If effectively isolated, progressive expiration of air results in loss of volume in the target lobe. The initial randomized, multicenter Endobronchial Valve (Zephyr) for Emphysema Palliation Trial (Or VENT) in both the USA and in Europe that compared the Zephyr valve versus standard medical care showed small but statistically significant improvements in FEV$_1$, St George's Respiratory Questionnaire (SGRQ) score and 6-minute walk test (6MWT).[11] However, more detailed analysis identified a group of 'super-responders' characterized by correct valve placement with complete lobar exclusion, intact fissure of interest and heterogeneity between hyperinflated target and healthier non-target lobe. In these patients the FEV$_1$ demonstrated a sustained improvement at 6- and 12-monthly intervals (ΔFEV$_1$ 15–16%, $p = 0.02–0.04$). The EUROVENT study reported that at 12-month, the minimal clinically important difference (MCID) thresholds for FEV$_1$, cycle ergometry workload, 6-minute walk distance (6MWD) and SGRQ were met in 67%, 44%, 56% and 67% of this subgroup respectively.[11,12]

Two recent RCTs (STELVIO and BeLieVeR-HIFi) have confirmed the benefit of EBV in appropriately selected patients. STELVIO[13] investigated the efficacy and safety of placing endobronchial valves in patients with severe emphysema with intact fissures and absence of collateral ventilation as measured by Chartis system (balloon catheter occlusion of airway targeting target lobe). Patients were randomly assigned to EBV group (n=34) or standard medical care group (n=34). Changes from baseline to 6 months following intervention in FEV$_1$ (20.9 vs 3.1%, p=0.001), FVC (18.3 vs 4%, p=0.005) and 6MWT (19.6 vs. -3.6%, p< 0.001) were significantly greater in the EBV group compared with the standard medical care group. At the end of six months, patients who received standard medical care crossed over to receive EBV therapy and gained similar benefits to the original EBV-treated group. The main adverse events observed in the EBV group were pneumothorax (18%) of which half the patients required removal of a valve, COPD exacerbations (12%) and pneumonia (6%). Valve migration, dislocation and excessive coughing led to valve replacement in 15% of the cases. Other complications such as torsion of bronchus and excessive coughing have resulted to valve removal in 12% of the cases. One patient died due to end stage COPD with respiratory failure 58 days following treatment. It is important, therefore, to gain adequate experience in valve maintenance and how to manage complications in patients receiving EBV.

The BELIEVER HiFi study was a single centre, double blinded study comparing the use of endobronchial valves with a sham bronchoscopy procedure in patients with both heterogenous emphysema and fissure integrity of more than 90% on CT.[14,15] All patients underwent Chartis assessment before proceeding to the assigned intervention. 50 patients were randomly assigned equally to EBV insertion with standard medical (n=25) or sham procedure with standard medical care (n=25). The primary endpoint of the study was changes in FEV$_1$. By 3 months FEV$_1$ was improved by a mean of 24.8% in the intervention group as compared with 3.9% in the sham group. However, in the treatment group, 8 patients had indeterminate Chartis assessment or collateral ventilation present on Chartis assessment. The inclusion of sham bronchoscopy in the control group ensured a lower potential for a placebo effect. Valves were expectorated in 4 patients. Subsequent follow up open label trial was conducted. Patients who initially received sham bronchoscopy and standard medical care went on to have open label EBV treatment after completion of clinical trial (n=12). This data was combined with those in initial treatment group who did not have CV (n=19). 3-month follow up showed improvement in FEV$_1$ by 36.4% (SD36.4), reduction in residual volume (RV) by 0.49L (SD 0.76), and increase in the 6MWT distance increased by 32.6m (SD68.7).

The definition of homogenous emphysema is being debated. The feasibility of EBV treatment in patients with severe homogenous emphysema without collateral ventilation was assessed in the IMPACT RCT.16 Patients were assigned to either EBV group (n=43) or standard medical care group (n=50). Statistically and clinically significant improvement in lung function, exercise capacity, and quality of life associated with EBV therapy were sought. At 3 months FEV$_1$ has significantly improved in the EBV group as compared to standard medical care group (13.7% ± 28.2% vs -3.2 ± 13%;mean difference between groups of difference, 17%; p=0.0002). Both SGRQ and 6MWT have also improved (-8.63±11.25 vs. 1.01±9.36; and 22.63±66.63m vs. -17.34±52.8 m). The observed target lobe volume reduction at 3 months was -1195± 683 ml (p< 0.0001).

The magnitude of the functional improvements is significant though smaller compared to those seen in heterogenous patients. More work is needed to reproduce these results and assess benefits and duration of effect in this patient group.

Patient selection

Patient selection is critical to outcomes, particularly in determining risks and benefits of surgical and non-surgical volume reduction and pre- and post-procedure management. The UK's National Institute for Health and Care Excellence (NICE) guidelines recommends that patient selection should occur through a dedicated emphysema MDT.[17] The exact roles of core members of the MDT will vary with local expertise and practice – an example of a referral pathway is shown (**Figure 14.1**). There is a wide spectrum of clinical disease patterns encompassed within the spectrum of severe impairment of FEV$_1$ in severe COPD. Our practice is that the majority of patients have assessment by a COPD specialist team. Similarly, clinicians with specific training and expertise in interventional bronchoscopy, thoracic surgery and thoracic radiology are vital to the function of the MDT. Our own practice also includes a transplant physician, lung physiologist and specialist nurse as integral members of the team. In many MDTs patients are considered for either surgical or non-surgical LVR. The selection criteria should largely be based on clinical factors, degree of hyperinflation, motivation and goals of the patient collateral ventilation (CV) as well as emphysema pattern and physiological measures and risks (**Table 14.1**). For surgical LVR, quantitative perfusion scanning is a major tool to aid decision making with the computed tomography (CT) scan and assess benefit. However, in comparison lung perfusion scanning currently carries less weight for ELVR decision making than a CT scan where the degree of hyperinflation is critical. However, more work is needed in this area.

Clinical factors

It is important to understand the relative contribution of co-morbidities to symptoms and the relationship of emphysematous hyperinflation to clinical symptoms such as infective exacerbations and breathlessness; this is often the role of the COPD physician. The patient should be on maximum pharmacological treatment and have sustained benefits from pulmonary rehabilitation and must have achieved smoking cessation. All members of the MDT contribute to the appraisal of risks; the potential impact of procedures and predictable complications, e.g. optimizing fitness for bronchoscopy and surgery

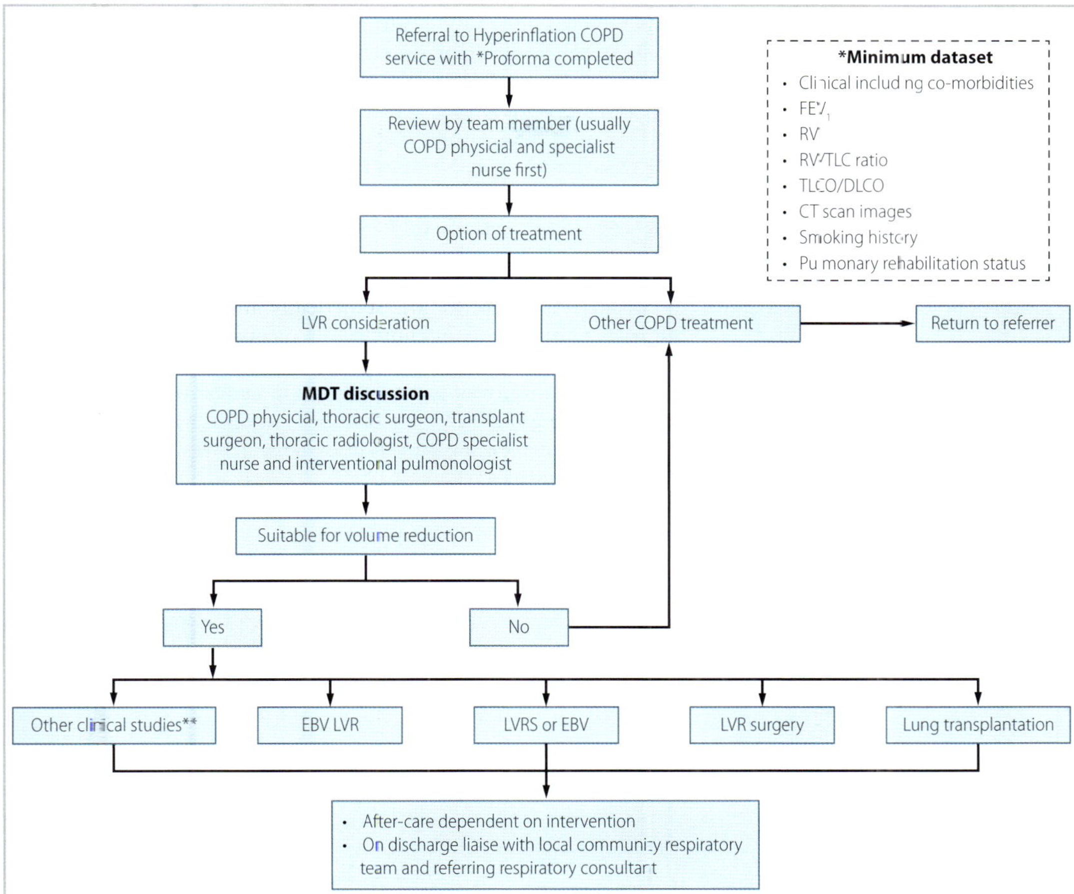

Figure 14.1 Our referral pathway for lung volume reduction in COPD. Local practice may vary. COPD, chronic obstructive pulmonary disease; LVR, lung volume reduction; MDT, multidisciplinary team; EBV, endobronchial valve; FEV_1, forced expiratory volume in 1 second; RV, residual volume; TLC, total lung capacity; TLCO/DLCO, carbon monoxide diffusion capacity; CT, computed tomography
**Other clinical studies refer to pharmacological or non-pharmacological related to volume reduction, some centers use endobronchial coil therapy.

Table 14.1 Patient selection criteria for endobronchial valve placement

Inclusion criteria	Exclusion criteria
Significant functional limitation from emphysema	Unfit for bronchoscopy
40–75 years of age	Clinically significant bronchiectasis
Non-smoking for 6 months prior	High sputum production as assessed at bronchoscopy
Heterogeneous emphysema on HRCT	High risk of pneumothorax and inability to tolerate
15% < FEV_1 < 45% predicted	TLCO< 20% predicted (relative contraindication)
TLC >100% predicted	Significant comorbidities limiting potential benefit
RV > 180% predicted	
Has shown benefit from pulmonary rehabilitation (no specific restrictions)	
Received maximal pharmacological treatment	

HRCT, high-resolution computed tomography; FEV_1, forced expiratory volume in 1 second; TLC, total lung capacity; RV, residual volume; TLCO, carbon monoxide diffusion capacity

and establishing the risk that co-morbidities pose in limiting the benefits or increase risks of procedures. Assessing pulmonary reserve is an important part of the discussion and should be case-specific to establish the potential and 'real' benefits to the patient.

Collateral ventilation

The 'super-responder' subgroup of patients identified in the VENT and EUROVENT study were generally observed to have developed complete lobar occlusion. There are several factors that can influence the development of complete lobar occlusion. The accurate placement of valve and correct selection of valve size is dependent on patient anatomy, operator's experience and technical skill. An important predictor of success of EBV therapy is the presence of CV between target and no-target lobe. Integrity of interlobar fissures on thin-slice CT is used as a surrogate that will help assess the presence or absence of CV. The sub-analysis of these trials revealed that patients who had complete interlobar fissure [(defined as > 90% completeness of the fissure between the target and adjacent lobes on at least one axis in the thin slice high-resolution computed tomography (HRCT)] experienced a marked improvement. Studies have shown that patients with greater heterogeneity in emphysema distribution achieved better outcomes, therefore in those where there is doubt over the degree of heterogeneity, formal emphysema quantification can be performed.[11,12]

Fissure integrity provides a useful surrogate for measurement of CV. More detailed assessment for CV can be performed using the Chartis Pulmonary Assessment System (Pulmonx Inc.) particularly in those with minor defects in fissure integrity. It consists of a single-use balloon catheter linked to flow and pressure sensors. The catheter balloon is inflated to obstruct the origin of the target lobe. The absence of CV manifests as a gradual reduction in the expiratory flow and rise in resistance. The main advantage of this system is the real time measurement of physiological changes. It is however invasive and can be complicated by difficult anatomy, coughing and mucous plugging of the catheter.[18]

As CV is believed to be secondary to anatomical or pathologically formed interlobular channels, HRCT fissure analysis is another avenue by which CV can be determined. This is performed visually by radiologists, but is prone to high inter-reader variability. Gompelmann et al. demonstrated in a retrospective analysis that fissure analysis correctly predicted the total LVR in 74% of patients as compared to the 77% predicted by the Chartis system.[19] As an alternative to manual fissure analysis, using the lung imaging software (Vida Diagnostics) has recently been utilized to assess CV through a model incorporating fissure integrity, low attenuation clusters and relative volume of small vessels. A retrospective comparison study (n = 146) reports comparable accuracy in selecting patients for LVR (Quantitative CT, 78.8% versus Chartis 75.8%).[20]

Given the lack of differences in diagnostic accuracy, the procedure selection for assessing CV is dependent on practical factors. Consideration should be given to logistics, patient tolerance, radiation risk, the availability of equipment/software and local expertise. There is the added benefit, when performing CHARTIS, of seeing the airways directly and assessing feasibility of valve insertion, secretions and the extent of tracheobronchomalacia.

Physiological measures

Accurate physiological assessment remains a key factor in determining which patients are suitable to undergo ELVR. A multimodal approach should include measuring different lung volumes, assessing exercise capacity, undertaking health-related questionnaires, and performing HRCT of the thorax. The primary aim of all LVR techniques is to improve lung volume by reducing hyperinflation and allowing greater airflow to perfused lung parenchyma. Data gained from the UPLIFT trial supported the concept of end-expiratory lung volume (EELV) being a determining factor of functional capacity and long term prognosis in stage II to IV COPD patients.[21] Assessment of static lung volumes via whole body plethysmography or helium-dilution techniques provide a multitude of measures, including the total lung capacity (TLC), residual volume (RV), inspiratory capacity (IC) and functional residual capacity (FRC). Changes in IC have been shown to correlate well with EELV.[21] Hyperinflation and gas trapping, which is a major driver of symptomatic limitations in COPD, can be measured using the ratio of RV/TLC.

It should be noted that all measurements throughout the LVR pathway should be gained through the same method, as helium-dilution has been shown to underestimate TLC compared to plethysmographic values. This is a source of current debate as both methods are open to inaccuracies in severely obstructed patients ($FEV_1 < 30\%$ predicted). One benefit of whole body plethysmography is that airways resistance can be measured during testing, often identifying grossly abnormal values in COPD patients. Those selected for the LVR pathway should also have their diffusing capacity measured to understand the level of parenchymal destruction and the severity of disease. As mentioned previously, the NETT trial identified patients with a low TLCO as those at most risk of mortality and morbidity following surgical LVR.

The most common forecaster of functional decline in patients with COPD is the serial change in predicted FEV_1, gained through spirometry. FEV_1 has been studied extensively in patients with COPD and has been a useful tool not only in assessing the severity of the disease but also its progress. Exercise capacity is routinely assessed using the 6MWT with the distance covered being the main outcome. Patients with advanced COPD can suffer skeletal muscle dysfunction, whereby cellular changes affect the muscle's force generating capacity and endurance capability. This state proves problematic when attempting to increase exercise capacity as it is usually linked to abnormal levels of dyspnea upon exercise. When selecting patients for LVR it is important to measure multiple potential areas that could improve with the intervention. QoL and the effect of respiratory symptoms are often assessed by standardized questionnaires such as the SGRQ, the shortened COPD specific version (SGRQ-C), modified Medical Research Council (mMRC) dyspnea scale and the five level version of the EuroQol 5D (EQ5D-5L).

Success from LVR is often measured by increases in FEV_1, but these changes can often occur in discordance to QoL and exercise capacity. In a European study, success from LVR was confirmed when the MCID in the walk distance, FEV_1 and RV post-ELVR was a 26-meter increase, ≥ 15% increase and >350 mL reduction respectively.[12]

Reduction in hyperinflation, measured during static lung volumes, also indicates the potential for improvements in QoL and exercise capacity but this is not always seen.[18] The current guidelines for the 6MWT do not include monitoring of peripheral capillary oxygen saturation (SpO_2) throughout the complete test or frequent dyspnea ratings.[22] This could mean that oxygen nadir may be missed especially if the patient stops during the test. Benefits gained post-procedure could include increased oxygenation or reduced breathlessness during exercise. Another area open for further investigation is the effect of ELVR on dynamic hyperinflation. Insertion of endobronchial valves is known to affect airflow into the target lobe at rest in successful cases but it is not yet known how this targeted atelectasis influences lung mechanics during exercise.

Safety and complications

The safety profile for EBV is considered more acceptable than surgical LVR as a whole. Death has been reported in three patients within the EBV trial literature. Causes were listed as tension pneumothorax, massive hemoptysis and the third was unspecified. These occurred across two RCTs and one case series. Other adverse complications are hemoptysis (EBV: 5–6%, Control: 0–2%), bronchospasm (5–9%), valve migration/expectoration/aspiration (5–7%), COPD exacerbation (EBV: 8–30%, Control: 1–22%), pneumothorax (EBV: 1–4%, Control: 0%), pneumonia distal to valve (1–7%) and respiratory failure (EBV: 1–4%, Control: 0–2%).[17]

Pneumothorax is an important complication directly related to the procedure. Post-EBV pneumothoraces are mainly thought to occur when shrinkage in the treated lobe facilitates expansion of the non-treated lobe with a subsequent risk of parenchymal tears ruptured bullae or blebs. Analysis of those patients who developed a post-procedure pneumothorax demonstrated a greater degree of volume reduction, and this was associated with greater improvement in FEV_1. Most pneumothoraces occur within 3 days of the procedure and can be managed conservatively. The impact could potentially be serious with respiratory failure and the risk of death in such already compromised individuals. Hence, these risks are discussed pre-procedure at the MDT and patients in most centers are monitored routinely for 3 days and issued with contact numbers for emergency use on discharge. Such pneumothoraces that are large or have significant compromise to the patient should be managed by the insertion of large bore intercostal chest drain with underwater seal. A persistent air leak or high flow leak with respiratory compromise may require the removal of at least one EBV or surgery.[23] Our routine referral practice is geographically large with some remote areas; hence we link directly with local respiratory nursing teams to provide monitoring of the patient's post-procedure.

Cost-effectiveness and prognosis

There has been a single study on the cost-effectiveness of EBV based on 5–10-year predictive modelling on a VENT subgroup. The model, based on the German statutory health insurance system, predicts an incremental cost-effectiveness ratio (ICER) of € 43,647 per quality adjusted life year (QALY) gained for EBV cohort at 5 years, and €21,920 at 10 years. The difference in ICER between the EBV and control cohorts was approximately € 10,000 at both time points (typical cost-effectiveness threshold of € 50,000 per QALY). Furthermore, this subgroup, all with complete fissures and high heterogeneity, showed substantial improvements in their GOLD staging even during the 12-month of VENT. 37.9% of patients in the EBV group have improved by one GOLD stage, with corresponding improvements in the SGRQ (51.44 to 42.79). In contrast, the control group either maintained or progressed to the next GOLD stage, and their SGRQ scores deteriorated (52.65 to 55.34). Taken together, this initial data would suggest that EBV is a cost-effective treatment in carefully selected patient groups (high heterogeneity and complete fissure) and can potentially lead to improved outcomes over conventional medical therapy.[24] It is established that surgical LVR improves long-term survival in those with upper lobe predominant emphysema and low preoperative exercise capacity. There is increasing patient years' data accumulating on EBV therapy and already a suggestion, albeit in small numbers of patients (n=19), that in those with atelectasis secondary to EBV therapy (n=5) may have a significant survival benefit as compared to those who do not develop atelectasis following the intervention (p=0.026).[25] It will not be long before we are in a position to evaluate this formally. What is clear is that in appropriately selected patients, physiological improvements can be sustained for several years (**Figure 14.2**).

EBV versus surgical LVR

This procedure is primarily a palliative one to improve patient symptoms. Surgical LVR or EBV therapy recommendation is influenced by several clinical factors and patient choice. In some cases, reimbursement and operational factors and local expertise are likely to play a role. It is important to have open discussions with the patients and relatives and the options tailored where possible. Starting with the individual with heterogeneous emphysema, in many cases the recommendation can be straightforward, e.g. young age, predominantly apical emphysema with CV between target and non-target lobe would favor surgical volume reduction. In those who are older, with co-morbidities in the absence of CV and/or high risk of surgery, EBV treatment is favored. A comparison of EBV LVR and surgical LVR in appropriately selected and risk-stratified patients would be helpful.

LUNG VOLUME REDUCTION COIL

Technique

Lung volume reduction coils (RePneu; PneumRx, Inc.) are made from pre-formed Nitinol wire that comes in variable sizes. The coil placement facilitates compression of the diseased parenchyma and redirects airflow to healthier parts of the lung, improving gas exchange and resulting in better lung function. Endobronchial nitinol coils can be inserted with the patient under general anesthesia or sedation. The airway to the diseased segment is identified bronchoscopically and a flexible guidewire is advanced under fluoroscopic guidance. A catheter is passed over the guidewire that is then removed and replaced with a straightened coil. This coil is held in place by a grasper. Upon catheter removal, the coil springs back into its pre-determined shape, which pulls on the surrounding diseased tissue causing a reduction in the lung volume.[10] Typically, 5–15 coils are inserted in each treated lobe and each lung is treated in separate procedures. (**Figure 14.3**) The coils are intended to remain in place indefinitely. Coil therapy is licensed in some countries, and available for use. However, in others such as the UK, NICE guidelines recommend that this procedure is used for research purposes only.[26]

Clinical efficacy and safety

The current evidence for clinical efficacy is based on two RCTs (RESET study, n = 47, and a RENEW study of 157 patients) and two case series (n = 60, n = 38). At 3-month follow-up, the RESET study demonstrated improvement in FEV_1 by 14.19%, reduction in the mean baseline SGRQ score by 8.11 points and the mean mMRC dyspnea score by 0.24 points. Similar results were found in the two case series, with mean increase in the 6MWD by 84.4m at 6-month follow-up. No deaths were reported, however the complications occurred were pneumothorax, exacerbation of COPD, chest pain and pulmonary infections.[26,27] A European multicenter trial also demonstrated acceptable safety profile and significant improvement in QoL, exercise capacity and pulmonary function with sustained results over 1 year. Further post hoc analysis of CT scan heterogeneity showed significant responses in both heterogeneous and homogenous emphysema, suggesting that LVR coil treatment may benefit patients with both heterogeneous and homogeneous emphysema.[28] Despite the low amount of published evidence, it is currently the only endoscopic procedure licensed for treatment in patients with CV.

The RENEW trial[29] was conducted to assess 1-year effectiveness and safety profile of endobronchial coils on exercise tolerance, quality of life and lung function in patients with either advance homogenous or heterogenous emphysema and severe lung hyperinflation.

Patients were randomly assigned to a coil treatment group (n=158) and to a standard medical care group (n=157). At 12-month follow up, the median change in the 6MWD was 10.3m with coil treatment vs -7.5m with usual medical care. The inter-group difference was only modest and the clinical importance was of uncertain significance. Similar modest improvement was obtained in the coil treatment group with a median increase in FEV_1 and a median reduction in the SGRQ by 7% and -8.9 points (p< 0.001), respectively. Major complications occurred in 34.8% of patients receiving coils vs 19.1% in the usual medical care group (p=0.002). These included pneumonia requiring hospitalization, COPD exacerbations, respiratory failure, hemoptysis, pneumothorax and death. Post hoc analysis of this trial showed that patients with residual volume of at least 225% with either heterogenous or homogenous distribution emphysema exhibited a superior treatment response.[29] From the evidence thus far, the coils are promising in selected patients with high RV (>225%), but our opinion is that further larger RCTs are needed before firm conclusions can be drawn. Further research is needed into their exact mechanism of action and target patient profile who are likely to benefit with a favorable risk/benefit profile.

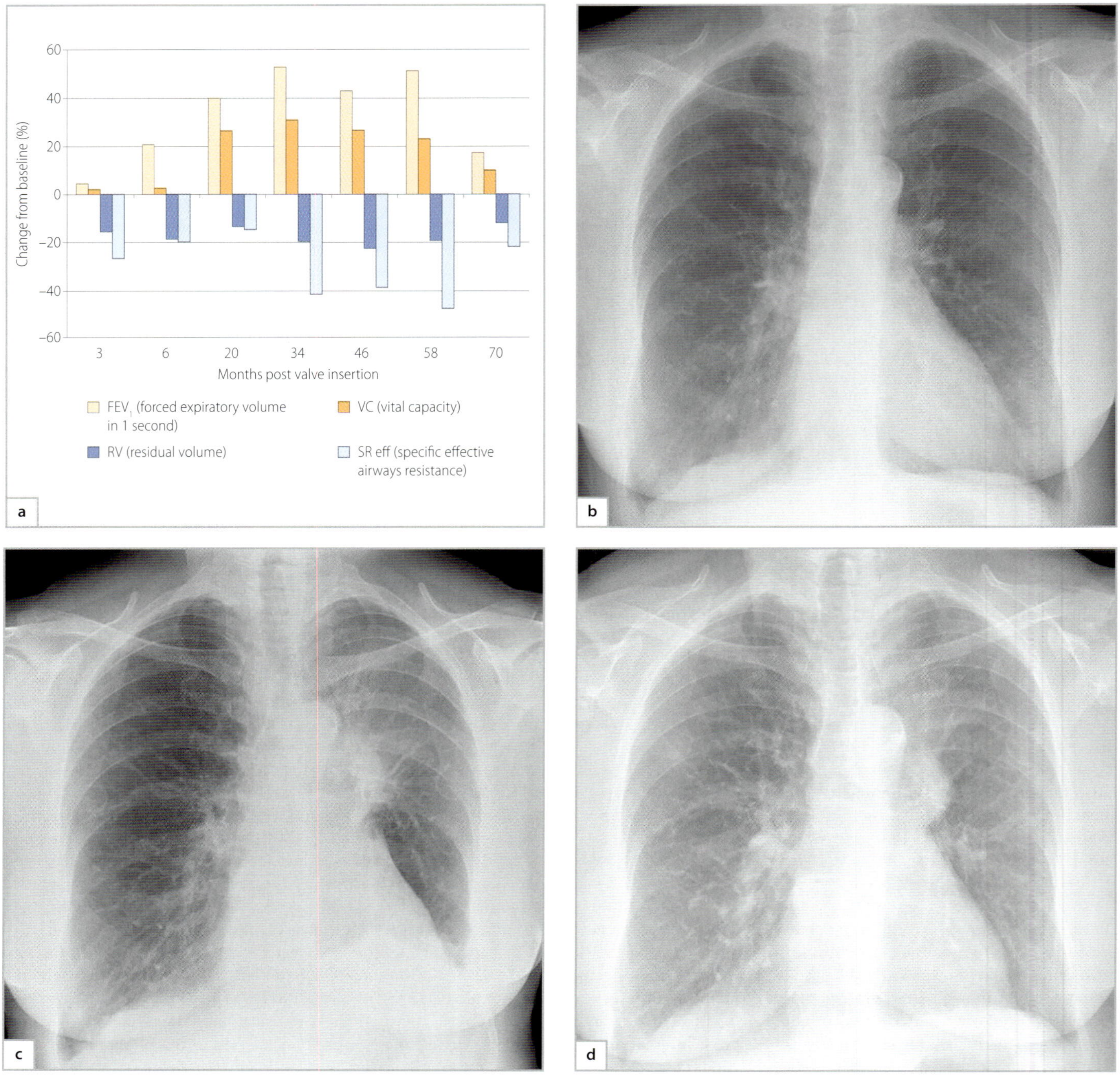

Figure 14.2 Patient treated with EBV therapy to the left upper lobe. They first gained a minimal clinically important difference (MCID) for FEV_1 6-month post-procedure, but continued to improve thereafter gaining a maximal improvement of > 50% of the baseline value. This MCID was still preserved at 70 months post-procedure and was associated with a significant and sustained improvement in breathlessness. The complex interactions between airflow dynamics, lung mechanics and cellular response post-procedure are not yet fully understood, so accurate follow-up is crucial in ensuring physiological benefits are being measured. (a) Long-term follow-up of a patient post-EBV LVR left upper lobe. SR eff gained during whole body plethysmography; FEV_1 improved by ≥ 15% at 6 months. RV MCID was reached by 3 months post-procedure and was maintained at 70 months (defined at the time of treatment as a reduction in RV of 350 mL, equivalent to an 11% drop in this patient). (b) Pre-procedure chest X-ray showing left upper lobe hyperinflation in keeping with severe emphysema (c) Post-procedure elevation of the hilum and loss of volume left upper lobe in keeping with successful volume reduction to the left upper lobe. (d) Five-year post-procedure chest X-ray demonstrating collapse of the left upper lobe with sustained efficacy of endobronchial valve volume reduction. Note: current recommended MCID values are reduction in RV by 430 mL, and improvement in FEV_1 by 100 mL.

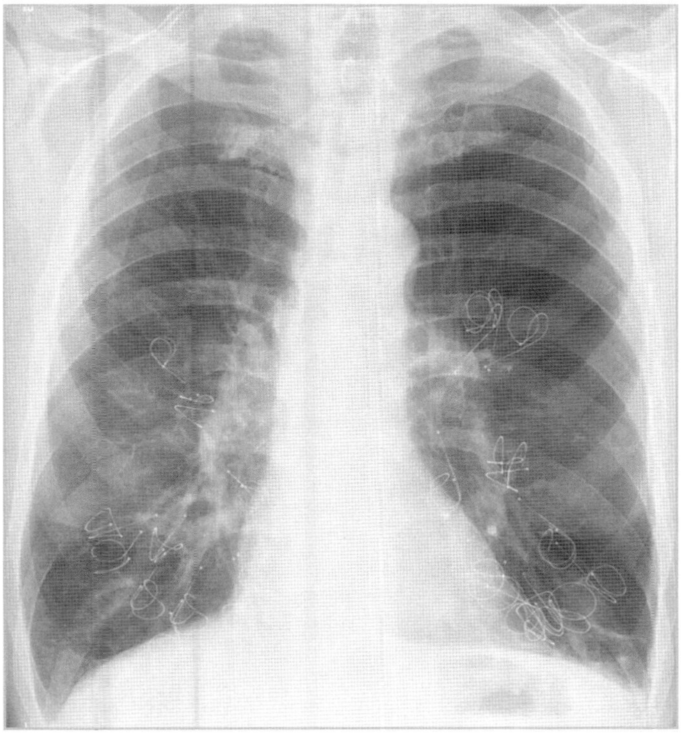

Figure 14.3 Chest radiograph showing endobronchial coils in a patient with severe homogenous severe emphysema.

POLYMERIC LUNG VOLUME REDUCTION

Also known as emphysematous lung sealant (ELS), this technique involves administering synthetic hydrogel foam sealant (AeriSeal; Aeris Therapeutics, Inc.) into the most emphysematous part of the lung. The sealant causes an inflammatory reaction that induces scarring and formation of fibrotic tissue, resulting in LVR. The process of remodelling takes several weeks; with the maximum effect achieved 8–12 weeks post-procedure. The procedure is performed under general anesthesia or sedation using flexible bronchoscope. The AeriSeal compound is delivered using a purpose-made catheter and injected into targeted sub-segments over a few seconds, followed by injection of 30 mL air, leading to a peripheral distribution of the hydrogel foam. By sealing the lung at alveolar level, the approach is independent of CV. In open-label pilot studies, ELS has been demonstrated to reduce lung volume, improving lung function and QoL with acceptable safety profile. However, an early terminated (due to business-related reasons) randomized trial (ASPIRE, $n = 57$) demonstrated that greater than 50% of patients in the treatment group experienced MCID in FEV_1, SGRQ, 6MWD, mMRC at 6 months.[30] 44% of the treated patients experienced adverse events requiring hospitalization (2.5-fold more than the control group, $p = 0.01$), with two deaths in the treated cohort. Treatment responders tended to be those experiencing respiratory adverse events. Despite the early termination, the authors concluded that minimally invasive ELS may be efficacious, yet significant risks (probably inflammatory) limit its current utility. A multicenter study by Herth et al. in 2011 demonstrated better efficacy in COPD GOLD stage III patients in terms of FEV_1, forced vital capacity and 6MWD.[31] This treatment is currently undergoing further evaluation prior to further clinical trials.

THERMAL VAPOR ABLATION

Bronchoscopic thermal vapor ablation (BTVA) uses heated water vapor to produce a thermal reaction leading to initial localized inflammatory response followed by permanent fibrosis and atelectasis. The remodelling results in reduction in tissue and lung volume within 8–12 weeks. Prior to the procedure, the dose of vapor is calculated according to the volume of lung to be treated. The water vapor is then heated to 75°C and is instilled via a balloon catheter that occludes the targeted proportion of the lung. This technique is irreversible but is independent of CV and employed in patients with predominantly upper lobe emphysema. A heterogeneous index of > 1.2 between upper and lower lobes was identified as a predictor to response. A non-controlled study ($n = 44$) on unilateral BTVA demonstrated a 48% reduction in lobar volume (717± 78.8 mL at 3 months and 715.5 ± 99.4 mL at 6-month, $p < 0.001$) with associated improvement in lung function parameters and QoL.[24] Common complications included a pronounced inflammatory reaction in the first few weeks after treatment, characterized by dyspnea, cough, fever and mild hemoptysis. It is recommended that all patients should receive prophylactic antibiotics and anti-inflammatory medication and be kept in hospital for observation following BTVA. The severity of the local inflammatory reaction correlates with the response to treatment. Moreover, there appears to be a correlation between the volume of the treated lobe of the lung and the scale of the inflammatory reaction. Patients with a treated lung volume of > 1700 mL frequently require readmission to hospital owing to pronounced local inflammation. However, by 6 months post-BTVA these patients experienced the greatest treatment benefit.[32] The STEP UP study[33] was a 2:1 randomized multi-center trial. Patients with upper lobe predominant heterogenous emphysema irrespective of CV were enrolled and staged therapy with vapor was delivered. Tissue-to-air ratio was calculated at a segmental level on HRCT to primarily identify the most damaged lung segment and secondly, to calculate the dose of the vapor energy needed to be delivered at the treatment site. Patients with very diseased lower lobes with tissue-to-air ratio of less than 11% were excluded. Only one segment was treated at the first treatment session and up to two segments were treated during the second treatment session 3 months later. 70 patients were randomly assigned to treatment group (n=46) and control group (n=24). The mean relative improvement in FEV_1 and SGRQ-C between the treatment group vs control group was 14.7% ($p < 0.0001$) and -9.7 points (p=0.0021), respectively. Serious adverse events were commonly due to acute COPD exacerbations (24%) and pneumonia/pneumonitis (18%). Pneumothorax rate were low. In their 12-month follow up study, most of the respiratory related serious adverse events (71%) occurred in the first 90 day after treatment. The rate of adverse events was similar in both groups after a 90-day period.

Vapor therapy potentially offers a treatment option in patients with heterogenous disease, irrespective of the presence of CV, with the advantage of targeting only the very diseased segments of the lung while preserving healthier segments. The treatment can also be delivered in stages over time in order to increase both magnitude and duration of benefit.[33] Additional trials are needed to confirm to evaluate the cost effectiveness and to reproduce the results of this treatment modality.

EXHALE AIRWAY STENTS

The airway bypass procedure, involves the placement of paclitaxel-coated stents into transbronchial passages to release trapped air. A Doppler catheter is used to identify safe locations remote from adjacent blood vessels where a transbronchial needle is used to pierce the airway wall followed by balloon dilation in the newly created passage. Following confirmation with the Doppler probe, the drug eluting stent is then deployed to support the newly created passageway.[10] This procedure was developed to target patients with diffuse homogenous emphysema. Unlike the other treatments described previously, these stents rely on the presence of CV to maintain their patency.

The exhale airway stents for emphysema trial (EASE, $n = 315$) showed only small and transient improvement in lung function. There were no significant difference in exercise capacity and symptom benefit. The mortality rate between the airway bypass group and the control group were not significantly different (6.7% versus 6.5%). The problems encountered were difficulty stenting some of the created passages, leading to eventual closure, stent expectoration and reduction in patency due to mucous plugging, granulation tissue and poor CV. Despite the lack of sustained results, the authors demonstrated that complex interventional bronchoscopy could be safely performed in this high-risk group of patients. Future developments in this treatment modality would aim to develop strategies to achieve sustainable results, perhaps through technique modification to overcome stent occlusion and expectoration.[34]

LUNG VOLUME REDUCTION SURGERY

Lung volume reduction surgery (LVRS) is not a new procedure, but, in spite of proven effectiveness in relieving symptoms of breathlessness in patients with severe emphysema, its adoption has been somehow slow. The cause is mainly due to the high mortality and morbidity reported in earlier series.

The introduction of endobronchial techniques together with the development of minimally invasive techniques, have determined a resurgence of interest for this operation.

Although this type of surgery is relatively easy to perform, the patients' limited functional reserve together with poor quality lung tissue make it a considerable technical challenge to avoid complications, especially prolonged air leak and respiratory failure.

Over the years, we developed a technique to reduce complications. Our current median length of stay for these categories of patients is 3 days.

Operative steps

1. We recommend a VATS three ports approach. We did experiment a non-intubated single-port approach to try to minimize the surgical insult, but we found that in this operation the potential slight reduction in morbidity is not justified by the potential complication. Often these patients have repeated episodes of pneumonia and COPD exacerbations which lead to complex adhesions. Lysis of adhesion via the single-port approach forces excessive retraction of the lung with potential for ongoing air leak. Whilst such technique is justified in case of lung resection for cancer, we feel that integrity of the visceral pleura and retraction of the lung above the intended staple line is paramount in minimizing troublesome air leakage.
2. It is recommended not to position the posterior port more lateral than the mid-axillary line. Such port is usually quite painful and patients do not have enough functional reserve to cope with that.
3. Pain control is essential. With standard VATS procedures (either single or multiport) we normally employ only intercostal nerve blockade. In LVRS patients, we insert a paravertebral catheter at the beginning of the operation to neutralize the latency period of all regional blocks. Such patients tend to retain CO_2, especially when excessive opioids are used to manage pain. Eventually, if not corrected, intubation is unavoidable with potentially negative effects on air leak. It is also important not to exert excessive pressure onto the ribs to avoid damaging intercostal nerves which will result in long lasting pain.
4. We perform a ' hockey stick' staple line starting from a couple of centimeters above the horizontal fissure and then remove most of the upper lobe. Pinching the upper lobe from top to bottom with an endoscopic lung grasper allows us to detect a 'line of transition' between the most disease part of the lung and the most preserved part. That is where we apply the stapler.
5. We strongly recommend the use of reinforced staplers. The use of dedicated reloads with tissue reinforcement is particularly useful in saving time and avoiding displacement of the reinforcement. Alternative buttress material is also acceptable.
6. Do not force the stapler insertion. Avoiding tearing the visceral pleura is essential in preventing air leak.
7. Once the lung resection is completed, we perform a pleural tenting. This is allowed to fall onto the lung and to cover the staple line. In case of air leak apposition of pleuras is key in stopping it. The pleural is removed from the apex of the chest up to a line 2 cm from the sternum and 3–4 cm from the spine. It is important to retain intact parietal pleura posteriorly to avoid leakage of local anesthetic from the paravertebral catheter.
8. We also believe that these patients have limited functional reserve and cannot cope with the potential pain caused by a bedside talc pleurodesis, therefore, we insufflate intraoperatively 8 g of talc between the lung and the newly created pleural tent.
9. Lastly we insert two drains in apical position (one anterior and one posterior) through the two most anterior ports.
10. Further intercostal nerve blocks are performed at the end together with local anesthetic infiltration of the ports.

Operative tips

1. Do not use open surgery instruments to retract the lung. Their straight configuration forces the surgeon to pull excessively onto the lung with potential for air leak.
2. Using powered staplers helps to position the staple line in the exact position without excessive tissue manipulation.
3. If the surgical view is impeded by air trapping, a small incision with scissors at the apex of the lung allows easy deflation.
4. If there are significant adhesions, the use of an energy device is beneficial in avoiding potential troublesome bleeding. Do not be tempted to detach the adhesions bluntly as the lung will tear.
5. Steroid therapy is one of the major determinants in postoperative air leak. Therefore, liaise with the referring chest physician in order to ensure that patients have stopped taking steroids at least 4–5 days before the surgery. Borderline high risk patients would benefit from hospital admission 4–5 days prior to surgery for pre-optimization therapy, which include intensive chest physiotherapy, intravenous antibiotics and a single dose of intravenous corticosteroids).
6. Inform your referring physicians that it is normal to potentially have a small apical pocket of fluid from the pleural tenting. In the absence of clinical signs of empyema, CT-guided drainage is prohibited.

CONCLUSION

Lung volume reduction for hyperinflation due to emphysema is an effective therapy to improve symptoms and QoL. The added benefit to date of surgical LVR is of an improvement in mortality. Patient selection is critical to good outcomes. The MDT, including a COPD physician, thoracic surgeon, interventional bronchoscopist and thoracic radiologist, provides a forum to discuss risks and benefits to individual patients and tailor risk management pre- and post-procedure to reduce morbidity. Minimally invasive surgical LVR has the most evidence base in selected patients with heterogenous emphysema, leading to improved QoL and an improvement in mortality. Of the non-surgical methods for LVR, EBV therapy using the Zephyr valve has the most convincing data to date in improving QoL in this devastating disease. Polymeric sealant, thermal vapor ablation and endobronchial coils offer the prospect of treatment for those which there are currently no treatment options to reduce hyperinflation: namely with more homogenous disease or those with heterogenous emphysema and a prohibitively high risk for surgery with CV. Coils are currently the most advanced in this respect. Further research is required to understand the relationship between COPD phenotype and symptoms, improvements in assessing patient symptoms outside of traditional anatomical and physiological measures of success and surgical and non-surgical techniques. The current progress in these areas offers the prospect of more meaningful benefits to more patients with COPD.

REFERENCES

1. WHO. COPD predicted to be third leading cause of death in 2030. Online. Geneva: WHO, 2008.
2. Brantigan OC, Mueller E. Surgical treatment of pulmonary emphysema. Am Surg 1957; 23:789–804.
3. Fishman A, Martinez F, Naunheim K, et al. A randomized trial comparing lung-volume-reduction surgery with medical therapy for severe emphysema. N Engl J Med 2013; 348:2059–2073.
4. Beckers F, Lange N, Koryllos A, et al. Unilateral lobe resection by video-assisted thoracoscopy leads to the most optimal functional improvement in severe emphysema. Thorac Cardiovasc Surg 2014; 64:336–342.
5. Rathinam S, Oey I, Steiner M, et al. The role of the emphysema multidisciplinary team in a successful lung volume reduction surgery programmet. Eur J Cardiothorac Surg 2014; 46:1021–1026.
6. Ciccone AM, Meyers BF, Guthrie TJ, et al. Long-term outcome of bilateral lung volume reduction in 250 consecutive patients with emphysema. J Thorac Cardiovasc Surg 2003; 125:513–525.
7. Cooper JD, Patterson GA, Sundaresan RS, et al. Results of 150 consecutive bilateral lung volume reduction procedures in patients with severe emphysema. J Thoracic Cardiovasc Surg 1996; 112:1319–1329.
8. McNulty W, Jordan S, Hopkinson NS. Attitudes and access to lung volume reduction surgery for COPD: a survey by the British Thoracic Society. BMJ Open Respir Res 2014; 1:e000023.
9. Criner GJ, Cordova F, Sternberg AL, Martinez FJ. The National Emphysema Treatment Trial (NETT) Part II: Lessons learned about lung volume reduction surgery. Am J Respir Crit Care Med 2011; 184:881–893.
10. Gompelmann D, Eberhardt R, Herth FJ. Endoscopic lung volume reduction. A European perspective. Ann Am Thorac Soc 2013; 10:657–666.
11. Sciurba FC, Ernst A, Herth FJ, et al. A randomized study of endobronchial valves for advanced emphysema. N Engl J Med 2010; 363:1233–1244.
12. Herth FJ, Noppen M, Valipour A, et al. Efficacy predictors of lung volume reduction with Zephyr valves in a European cohort. Eur Respir J 2012; 39:1334–1342.
13. Klooster K, ten Hacken NHT, Hartman JE, et al. Endobronchial Valves for Emphysema without Interlobar Collateral Ventilation. New England Journal of Medicine 2015 10;373:2325-2335.
14. Davey C, Zoumot Z, Jordan S, et al. Bronchoscopic lung volume reduction with endobronchial valves for patients with heterogeneous emphysema and intact interlobar fissures (the BeLieVeR-HIFi study): a randomised controlled trial. Lancet 2015 12;386:1066-1073.
15. Zoumot Z, Davey C, Jordan S, et al. Endobronchial valves for patients with heterogeneous emphysema and without interlobar collateral ventilation: open label treatment following the BeLieVeR-HIFi study. Thorax 2017;72:277-279.
16. Valipour A, Slebos D-J, Herth F, et al. Endobronchial valve therapy in patients with homogeneous emphysema. Results from the IMPACT Study. Am J Respir Crit Care Med 2016;194:1073-1082.
17. Insertion of endobronchial valves for lung volume reduction in emphysema. Interventional procedures guidance IPG465. Online. London: NICE, 2013
18. Herth F, Eberhardt R, Gompelmann D, et al. Radiological and clinical outcomes of using ChartisTM to plan endobronchial valve treatment. Eur Respir J 2013; 41:302–308.
19. Gompelmann D, Eberhardt R, Slebos DJ, et al. Diagnostic performance comparison of the Chartis System and high-resolution computerized tomography fissure analysis for planning endoscopic lung volume reduction. Respirology (Carlton, Vic.) 2014; 19:524–530.
20. Schuhmann M, Raffy P, Yin Y, et al. Computed tomography predictors of response to endobronchial valve lung reduction treatment. Comparison with chartis. Am J Respir Crit Care Med 2015; 191:767–774.
21. Celli BR, Decramer M, Lystig T, Kesten S, Tashkin DP. Longitudinal inspiratory capacity changes in chronic obstructive pulmonary disease. Respir Res 2012; 13:66.
22. ATS Committee on Proficiency Standards for Clinical Pulmonary Function Laboratories ATS statement: guidelines for the six-minute walk test. Am J Respir Crit Care Med 2002; 166:111–117.
23. Kemp SV, Zoumot Z, Mahadeva R, Shah PL. Pneumothorax after endobronchial valve treatment: no drain, no gain? Respiration 2014; 87:452–455.
24. Pietzsch JB, Garner A, Herth FJ. Cost-effectiveness of endobronchial valve therapy for severe emphysema: a model-based projection based on the VENT study. Respiration 2014; 88:389–398.
25. Hopkinson NS, Kemp SV, Toma TP, et al. Atelectasis and survival after bronchoscopic lung volume reduction for COPD. Eur Respir J 2011; 37:1346–1351.
26. Insertion of endobronchial nitinol coils to improve lung function in emphysema. Interventional procedures guidance IPG517. Online. London: NICE, 2015.
27. Shah PL, Zoumot Z, Singh S, et al. Endobronchial coils for the treatment of severe emphysema with hyperinflation (RESET): a randomised controlled trial. Lancet Respir Med 2013; 1:233–240.
28. Deslee, G, Klooster K, Hetzel M, et al. Lung volume reduction coil treatment for patients with severe emphysema: a European multicentre trial. Thorax 2014; 69:980–986.
29. Sciurba FC, Criner GJ, Strange C, et al. Effect of endobronchial coils vs usual care on exercise tolerance in patients With severe emphysema: The RENEW Randomized Clinical Trial. JAMA 2016;315:2178-89.
30. Come CE, Kramer MR, Dransfield MT, et al. A randomised trial of lung sealant versus medical therapy for advanced emphysema. Eur Respir J 2015; 46:651–662.
31. Herth FJ, Gompelmann D, Stanzel F, et al. Treatment of advanced emphysema with emphysematous lung sealant (AeriSeal®). Respiration 2011; 82:36–45.
32. Snell G, Herth FJ, Hopkins P, et al. Bronchoscopic thermal vapour ablation therapy in the management of heterogeneous emphysema. Eur Respir J 2012; 39:1326–1333.
33. Herth FJF, Valipour A, Shah PL, et al. Segmental volume reduction using thermal vapour ablation in patients with severe emphysema: 6-month results of the multicentre, parallel group, open-label, randomised controlled STEP-UP trial. Lancet Respir Med 2016;4:185–93.
34. Shah PL, Slebos DJ, Cardoso PF, et al. Bronchoscopic lung-volume reduction with Exhale airway stents for emphysema (EASE trial): randomised, sham-controlled, multicentre trial. Lancet 2011; 378:997–1005.

Chapter 15 VATS for empyema thoracis

John Kit Chung Tam, Harish Mithiran

When empyemata are opened by cautery or by knife; and the pus flows pure and white, the patient survives, but if it is mixed with blood; muddy and foul smelling, he will die.

Hippocrates 460–377 BC

INTRODUCTION

Parapneumonic effusions and empyema are one of the oldest diseases known to mankind. Empyema thoracis is defined as pus in the pleural cavity, and the precursor for empyema is mainly bacterial pneumonia and parapneumonic effusion.

Parapneumonic effusion occurs in 20–60% of patients with bacterial pneumonia; of these, 5–10% will progress to empyema. 30% of empyema are iatrogenic following intrathoracic procedures. Other causes include thoracic trauma, infected malignant effusion, and local extension of infection from the chest wall, mediastinum or subdiaphragmatic sources.

The mortality rate for patients with un-treated empyema thoracis is reported to be between 11–50%. Early recognition to its development is crucial to successful treatment. The surgical principle to treating empyema is to control the spread of infection and to evacuate all the infected material.

The main principles of empyema surgery are:

- Drainage of all loculated empyema fluid and evacuation of all empyema content
- Removal of the empyema cortex through complete decortication of the restrictive empyema peel on the pleura surfaces (visceral, parietal, diaphragmatic, and mediastinal)
- Sterilization of the pleural cavity through irrigation with water and antiseptics
- Complete lung re-expansion with restoration of normal pulmonary, diaphragmatic and chest wall mechanics

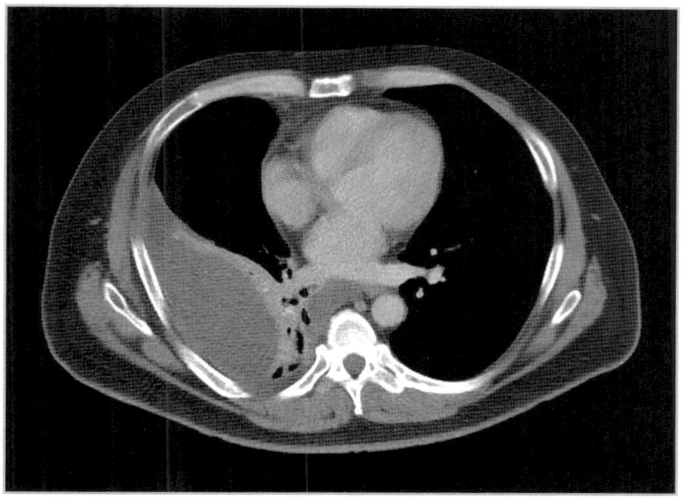

Figure 15.1 CT image of stage 1 empyema.

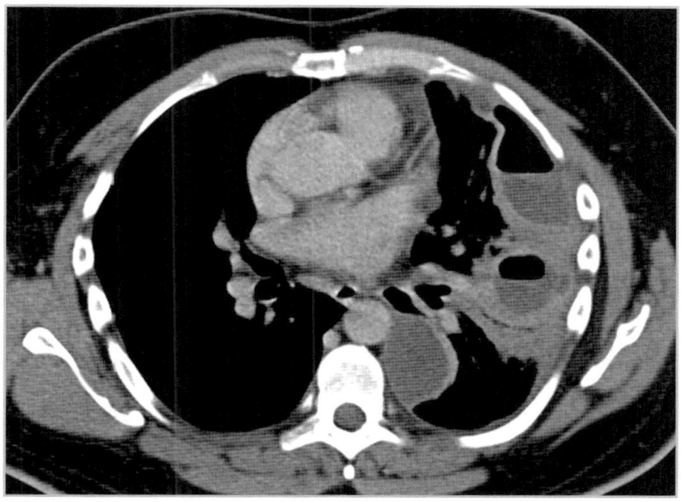

Figure 15.2 CT image of stage 2 empyema.

PARAPNEUMONIC EFFUSION

Parapneumonic effusions can be categorized into simple or complicated effusions. Simple uncomplicated effusions may be transudates or exudates with a negative gram stain and culture. These usually resolve with the appropriate antibiotics with or without simple drainage procedures through thoracentesis/thoracostomy. Complicated effusions are either loculated collections or early empyema that require further intervention. Light's criteria can be used to differentiate between uncomplicated versus complicated parapneumonic effusions.

STAGES OF EMPYEMA

The American Thoracic Society, in 1962, divided the progression of empyema in the pleural space into three stages. The exudative (stage I/acute phase), fibrinopurulent (stage II/transitional phase), and organizing (stage III/chronic phase). These three phases are evolving and can be arrested by appropriate intervention.

The exudative stage usually begins 2–5 days after the onset of pneumonia (**Figure 15.1**). The pleural membranes are inflamed and secrete a low density exudative fluid. There are thin fibrin deposits over the pleural surfaces. However, the pleura is not thickened, and the lung can fully re-expand once the fluid is evacuated. The pleural fluid has low LDH, normal glucose, and normal pH.

The fibrinopurulent stage usually starts 5–10 days after the onset of pneumonia (**Figure 15.2**). Thick fibrin is deposited over the parietal and visceral pleural surface, with resultant loculations within the pleural cavity. The pleural fluid cytology has raised polymorphonuclear leukocytes and positive gram stain. The pleural fluid chemistry will

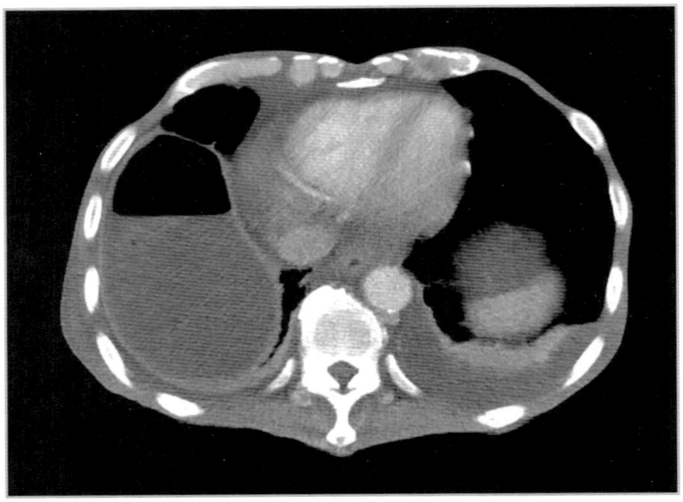

Figure 15.3 CT image of stage 3 empyema.

show pH <7.20, low glucose level (< 60 mg/dL), and elevated LDH. Antibiotic therapy and drainage must be performed without delay. At this stage, patients with multiple loculations, unsuccessful drainage by chest tube, or persistent sepsis will benefit from early VATS drainage and deloculation.

The organization stage sets in beyond 2–3 weeks (**Figure 15.3**). A thick inelastic pleural peel develops as fibroblasts infiltrates into the visceral and parietal pleural surfaces (**Figure 15.2**). This peel encases and restricts the lung. Decortication is required for the lung to regain its mobility and function.

DIAGNOSIS AND INVESTIGATIONS

Diagnosis of parapneumonic effusion and empyema are based on clinical history of pneumonia, raised white cell count, and an effusion on chest X-ray. Pleural fluid should be sampled and sent for pH, total protein, LDH, glucose, cell count with differential, and culture and sensitivity testing.

Large or complicated effusions should be further evaluated using computed tomography (CT) or ultrasound. These investigations will allow further characterization of the location and size of the loculations, pleural peel, and the condition of the underlying lung such as collapse consolidation, abscess cavity, or fistula. CT or ultrasound is also useful to localize, aspirate, or drain the effusion in order to obtain fluid samples for testing. A preoperative CT scan is essential for all patients who require surgical drainage and decortication.

MANAGEMENT

The three keystones to management of complicated parapneumonic effusion and empyema are drainage, decortication, and antibiotics. Large or complicated effusions should be evacuated early and completely. Decortication is necessary when lung expansion is restricted by empyema peel. A full course of appropriate antibiotic therapy is essential to completely treat the underlying pneumonia and to ensure pleural space sterilization.

TECHNIQUE

Patient is placed in standard lateral decubitus position with single-lung ventilation. VATS decortication can be performed through a conventional multi-portal approach using 3–5 incisions, double-port approach, or uniportal approach using a single small incision. Incision length ranges between 5 mm and 20 mm. Care must be taken when gaining entry into the pleural space, as dense scarring may result in inadvertent injury to the lung parenchyma. Digital dissection is performed before entry of the thoracoports and thoracoscope. Dense adhesions are taken down as the visceral pleura is separated from the parietal pleura. All loculations are opened up and all empyema fluid collections are completely drained and sent for microbiological testing. Loculations within the fissure and sulcus must also be completely drained.

After debridement and deloculation are performed to free up the entire pleural space, decortication is then performed on the visceral, diaphragmatic, parietal and mediastinal pleura. If the empyema is in stage 2 and the peel is not thick, the decortication can be done with a Yankauer suction, a peanut, a curved ring forceps or a curette. The aim is to completely remove all the empyema peel so as to expose the underlying pleural surface. If the empyema is in stage 3, the thickened organized pleural can be sharply incised to define a plane between the peel and the pleura. Once a plane is established, blunt dissection can be done with a Yankauer sucker or a peanut to avoid any lung parenchymal injury. During this process if there are any lacerations into the lung parenchyma, they should be repaired with Prolene sutures under thoracoscopic guidance. If there is a large raw surface of visceral pleural incontinuity that precludes suture repair, the area may be covered with hemostatic sealant or glue. During decortication care must be taken not to injure vital structures such as the subclavian or azygous vessels, aorta, vena cava, interlobar pulmonary artery, esophagus and phrenic nerve.

All empyema peel is dissected off the visceral pleural surfaces of the lung so that it can fully re-expanded. It is crucial to also dissect the peel off the diaphragm to restore normal physiologic mobility with respiration. Empyema cortex on the parietal pleura should also be decorticated to allow return of normal chest wall dynamics and to diminish the burden of infected content in the thorax.

Once decortication is completed and hemostasis achieved, the hemithorax is copiously irrigated with saline mixed with iodine or hydrogen peroxide. Two standard bore chest tubes are placed, one directed toward the apex and the other toward the costophrenic sulcus. The chest tubes are maintained on continuous suctioning, and are removed when drainage is less than 200 mL over 24 hours, no air leak, and patient is clinically aseptic and well.

Bronchoscopy is a useful adjunct immediately before or after the operation. Clearance of bronchial secretion facilitates successful single-lung ventilation intraoperatively, and ensures full lung re-expansion postoperatively.

CONCLUSION

In the beginning, VATS was only used as a diagnostic tool. Since the late 1990s, VATS was applied for drainage, debridement, and deloculation of early stage empyema. More recently, VATS is used for decortication of organized empyema. The efficacy of VATS in treating empyema has been evaluated in a number of retrospective studies. In summary, most studies showed that outcomes of VATS are superior or at least non-inferior compared to open surgery.[1-5] The reported success rates for complete decortication with the thoracoscopic approach have been reported to range between 68% to 100% for both stage II and stage III empyema.[6-9]

The success of performing VATS decortication is directly related to greater operative experience.[10] The main cited reason for conversion was delayed surgical intervention. The probability of thoracotomy increased from 28% to 81% if the operation was performed between 31-40 days instead of within 10 days after symptom onset.[11] Optimal timing of VATS drainage and decortication is found to be in patients with symptom duration of less than 4 weeks.[12]

Studies reported a reduction in operative time and intra-operative blood loss with VATS decortication compared to open surgery.[13-14] VATS decortication is also reported to result in less postoperative pain, postoperative air leak, chest drain duration, and length of hospital stay.[13-17] Importantly, VATS approach to decortication results in greater patient acceptance.[18]

A European expert consensus statement in 2015 supported the use of VATS as the initial treatment of choice for stage 2 or 3 empyema, and open thoracotomy when VATS is unsuccessful or when there is a long treatment delay of over 5 weeks.[19]

REFERENCES

1. Yamaguchi M, Takeo S, Suemitsu R, Matsuzawa H, Okazaki H. Video-assisted thoracic surgery for fibropurulent thoracic empyema: a bridge to open thoracic surgery. Ann Thorac Cardiovasc Surg 2009; 15:368–372.
2. Lackner RP, Hughes R, Anderson LA, Sammut PH, Thompson AB. Video-assisted evacuation of empyema is the preferred procedure for management of pleural space infections. Am J Surg 2000; 179:27–30.
3. Molnar TF. Current surgical treatment of thoracic empyema in adults. Eur J Cardiothorac Surg, 2007; 32:422–430.
4. Drain AJ, Ferguson JI, Sayeed R, Wilkinson S, Ritchie A. Definitive management of advanced empyema by two-window video-assisted surgery. Asian Cardiovasc Thorac Ann 2007; 15:238–239.
5. Olgac G, Fazlioglu M, Kutlu CA. VATS decortication in patients with stage 3 empyema. Thorac Cardiovasc Surg 2005; 53:318–320.
6. Luh SP, Chou MC, Wang LS, Chen JY, Tsai TP. Video-assisted thoracoscopic surgery in the treatment of complicated parapneumonic effusions or empyemas: outcome of 234 patients. Chest 2005; 127:1427–1432.
7. Petrakis IE, Kogerakis NE, Drositis IE, et al. Video-assisted thoracoscopic surgery for thoracic empyema: primarily, or after fibrinolytic therapy failure? Am J Surg 2004; 187:471–474.
8. Kim BY, Oh BS, Jang WC, et al. Video-assisted thoracoscopic decortication for management of postpneumonic pleural empyema. Am J Surg 2004; 188:321–324.
9. Lawrence DR, Ohri SK, Moxon RE, Townsend ER, Fountain SW. Thoracoscopic debridement of empyema thoracis. Ann Thorac Surg 1997; 64:1448–1450.
10. Waller DA, Rengarajan A. Thoracoscopic decortication: a role for video-assisted surgery in chronic postpneumonic pleural empyema. Ann Thorac Surg 2001; 71:1813–1816.
11. Stefani A, Aramini B, della Casa G, et al. Preoperative predictors of sucessful surgical treatment in the management of parapneumonic empyema. Ann Thorac Surg 2013; 96:1812–1819.
12. Chung JH, Lee SH2, Kim KT, et al. Optimal timing of thoracoscopic drainage and decortication for empyema. Ann Thorac Surg 2014; 97:224–229.
13. Chan DT, Sihoe AD, Chan S, et al. Surgical treatment for empyema thoracis: is video-assisted thoracic surgery "better" than thoracotomy? Ann Thorac Surg 2007; 84:225–231.
14. Vyas KS, Saha SP, Davenport DL, et al. Trends and practice patterns in the management of thoracic empyema. Asian Cardiovasc Thorac Ann 2014; 22:455–459.
15. Chung JH, Lee SH, Kim KT, et al. Optimal timing of thoracoscopic drainage and decortication for empyema. Ann Thorac Surg 2014; 97:224–229.
16. Bender MT, Ferraris VA, Saha SP. Modern management of thoracic empyema. South Med J 2015; 108:58–62.
17. Chambers A, Routledge T, Dunning J, Scarci M. Is video-assisted thoracoscopic surgical decortication superior to open surgery in the management of adults with primary empyema? Interact Cardiovasc Thorac Surg, 2010; 11:171–177.
18. Chan DTL, Sihoe AD, Chan S, et al. Surgical treatment for empyema thoracis: Is video-assisted thoracic surgery "better" than thoracotomy? Ann Thorac Surg 2007; 84:225–231.
19. Scarci M, Abah U, Solli P, et al. EACTS expert consensus statement for surgical management of pleural empyema. Eur J Cardiothorac Surg 2015; 48:642–653.

Chapter 16 VATS thymectomy

Thirugnanam Agasthian

INTRODUCTION

Common indications for thymectomy include myasthenia gravis and thymomas. Though there are many approaches to thymectomy there is no general consensus on the optimal approach – all seem to offer equal efficacy.[1-5] In recent years, the minimal invasive approach has gained popularity[2,5] and has rapidly become the preferred choice for small lesions.

INDICATIONS

Clinical indications for video-assisted thoracic surgery (VATS) thymectomy can be classified as follows:

- Non-thymomatous myasthenia gravis (unilateral right VATS approach)
- Well encapsulated thymomas (<5–6 cm) below level of innominate vein and invasive thymomas (unilateral approach, side of approach decided by location of tumor)
- Thymomas of 9–10 cm, large cystic thymomas especially on left side, tumors sitting on innominate vein (bilateral approach)

SURGICAL TECHNIQUE

VATS thymectomy is performed under general anesthesia. Lung isolation is obtained with a left-sided double lumen endotracheal tube. Further lung deflation is achieved with carbon dioxide insufflation (5–8 mmHg pressure at 4 L/min flow rate). The patient is positioned at 30° in a semi-supine position with a roll placed under the shoulder and with the ipsilateral arm held abducted over a padded L-screen for exposure of the axilla (**Figure 16.1a**). The semi-supine position gives better access to the opposite pleura, the thoracic inlet and the innominate vein. It also allows for quick conversion to a sternotomy if necessary. The surgeon and the camera assistant stands in front of the patient whilst the second assistant stands opposite the surgeon (**Figure 16.1b**).

The right side is the preferred approach for non-thymomatous myasthenia gravis especially in smaller women and children where there is more room for manipulation with the heart out of the way. It also gives better visualization of the innominate vein, and superior vena cava junction. The left-sided approach is used whenever a thymoma is located on that side.[6]

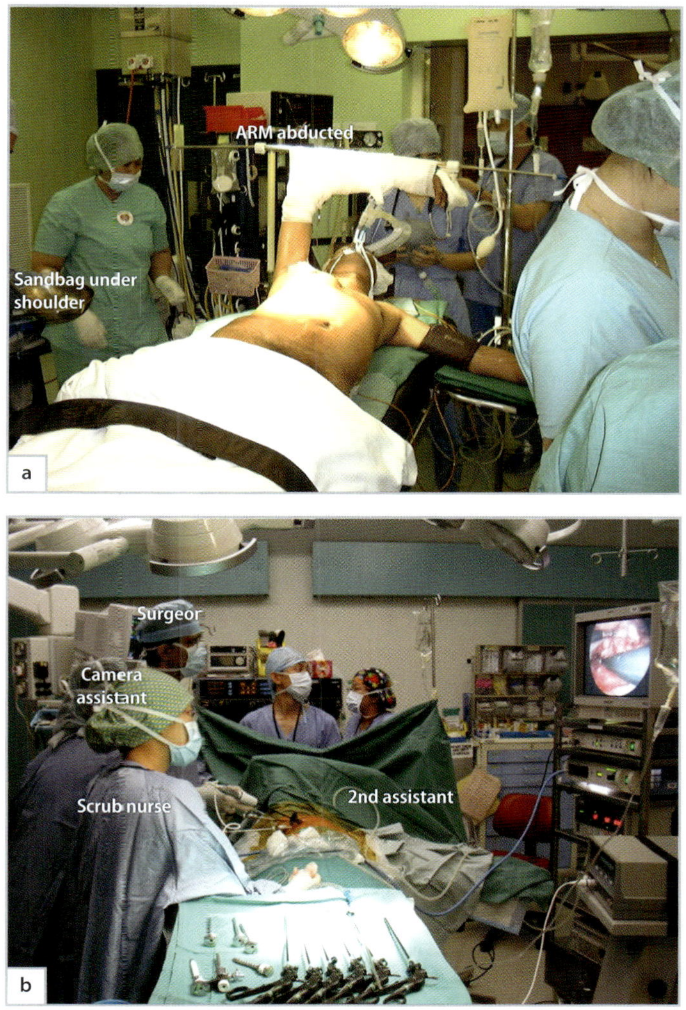

Figure 16.1 Patient positioning on OR set up for VATS thymectomy. (a) Patient position for right VATS thymectomy. (b) Operating room set up for right VATS thymectomy.

Three 5 mm and one 10 mm ports are inserted (**Figure 16.1a**). Although in my initial experience three ports (2 × 5 mm and 1 × 10 mm) were used, the additional 4th medial 5 mm working/retraction port enhances exposure and quickens the surgery, especially in large hyperplastic glands with abundant perithymic fat and thymomas. A 30° angled camera was placed in the lateral 5 mm port at the anterior axillary line, the other ports being working ports (**Figure 16.2b**). The right mediastinal pleura is opened first and the right phrenic nerve is then identified and preserved. The thymus and its perithymic fat are mobilized from neck to diaphragm and phrenic nerve to phrenic nerve. Superior horns are dissected from the innominate vein first before the body and inferior horns of the thymus are mobilized. This is to prevent the weight of the gland from obstructing the surgical field of vision which makes subsequent dissection of the gland from the innominate vein difficult. All horns are dissected right up into the neck and delivered into the chest. This is achieved by directing the 30° camera up into the chest inlet with the assistant's finger pressing on the suprasternal notch. Accessory horns usually under the innominate vein should be searched for routinely.[5]

Identification and prevention of injury to both phrenic nerves are mandatory to ensure a safe complete thymectomy. In the unilateral approach the thymus is dissected right up to the opposite phrenic nerve which is identified by opening the contralateral pleura and shifting the camera medially to the 10 mm port with retraction of the

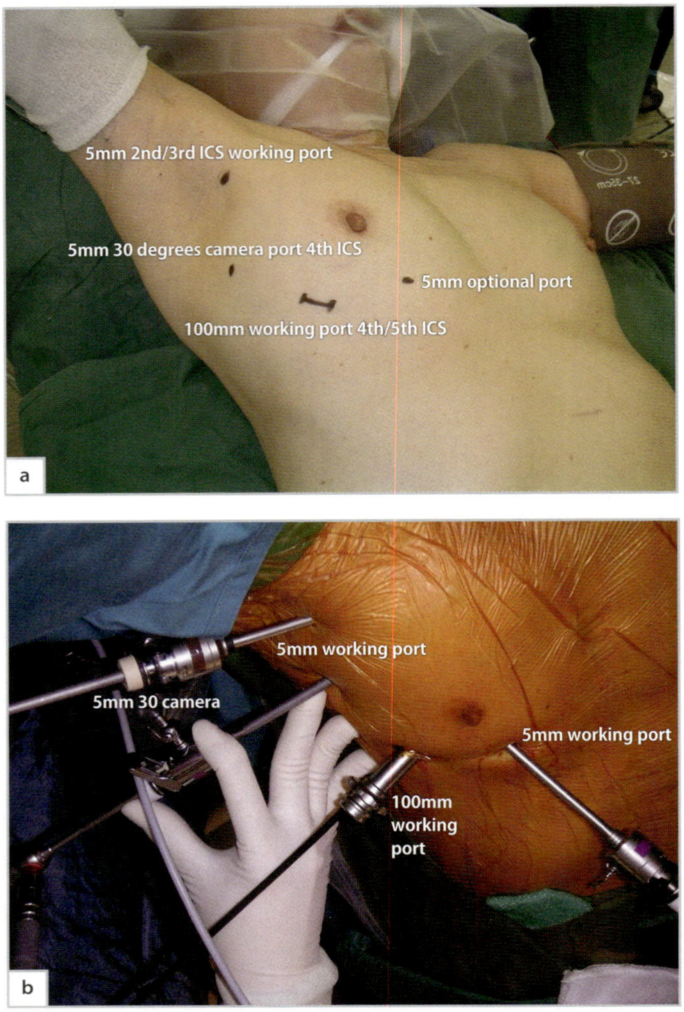

Figure 16.2 Port and instrument placements for right VATS thymectomy. (a) Port placements for Right VATS thymectomy. (b) Instrument placements for right VATS thymectomy.

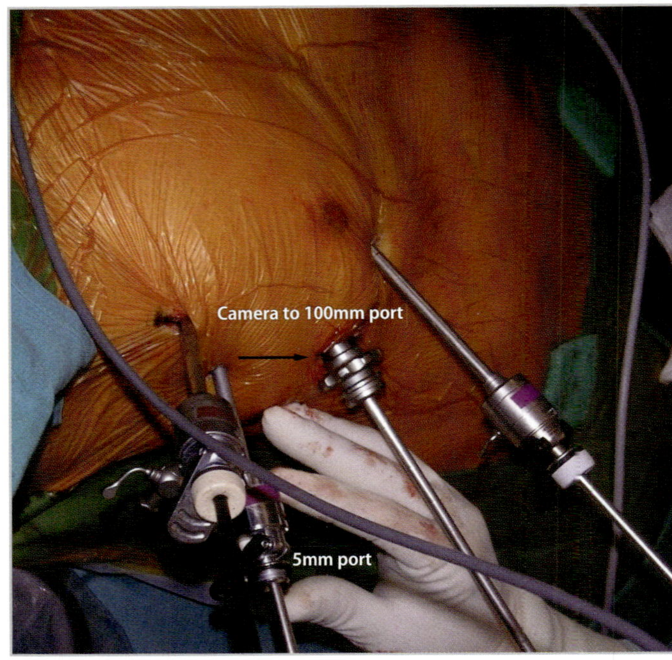

Figure 16.3 Camera and instrument placements for visualization of contralateral phrenic nerve in unilateral VATS approach.

opposite lung by the second assistant through the medial most 5 mm port (**Figure 16.3**). Sometimes to further improve visualization of the opposite phrenic nerve, perithymic and aortopulmonary window fats, intermittent stoppage of ventilation of the opposite lung is done.[5] Thermal injury to the nerves can be minimized by using an energy source like the bipolar dissector or ultrasonic harmonic scalpel.[7] The routine use of energy source also allows for quick dissection and safe coagulation of the feeding thymic vessels.[7]

The specimen is removed by appropriate enlargement of the 10 mm port, through which a chest tube is placed. As both pleural cavities are opened one chest tube suffices as both pleural spaces function as one compartment.

VATS THYMECTOMY FOR NON-THYMOMATOUS MYASTHENIA GRAVIS

Radical complete thymectomy is paramount in myasthenia gravis as long term neurological outcomes can be adversely affected by an incomplete thymectomy.[7] In a unilateral VATS approach for myasthenia gravis complete radical anatomical thymectomy is feasible as the 30-degree lens and small instruments offer superior magnified panoramic visualization and exposure to all aspects of the chest from neck to diaphragm and phrenic nerve to phrenic nerve. This allows en-bloc removal of the thymus, perithymic and aortopulmonary fats and tissue from the thoracic inlet to the diaphragm and phrenic nerve to phrenic nerve. All horns are dissected up into the neck and delivered into the chest. The contralateral phrenic nerve, perithymic and aortopulmonary window fats are easily visualized by changing the camera port more medially and opening the opposite pleura (**Figure 16.3**). Radicality and completeness is further ensured at time of surgery by anatomical inspection of the resected gland for completeness, and also to inspect and remove residual fat and ectopic thymic tissue from the thymic bed and possible ectopic sites.[8]

Clinical improvement in myasthenia gravis in my series was seen in 94.7% of patients who improved one or more Osserman grades. 69.3% (64) improved two or more grades. Using the MGFA post intervention status classification, 80% (74) of patients remain asymptomatic, 21% were in complete remission without medication, 42.9% with reduced therapy, 18.6% were in remission with medication unchanged, 14.7% required more medication, and 5.3% had not improved with surgery.[5] Though five patients had a myasthenia crisis early in our series, no patients have reported postoperative problems since 2001. This is due to improved preoperative pharmacological control especially with liberal use of intravenous immunoglobulins and high dose steroids, without the fear of possible sternotomy-related complications. Though many published series appear to have better outcomes in patients with variables such as age, gender, duration of preoperative symptoms and histology, in our series we found there was no significance to any of these variables.[5] The additional benefits for VATS in myasthenia gravis are:[2,5,10]

- A significant number of myasthenia gravis patients are young females where superior cosmesis through VATS would increase patient acceptability and earlier patient referral

- As many of these myasthenia patients are on high dose steroids and multiple immunosuppressants, VATS helps to minimize wound and sternotomy-related complications
- Less chest wall trauma and pain with better preservation of postoperative pulmonary function in VATS, allows for less pulmonary-related complications and early extubation, especially in those with severe myasthenia gravis combined with respiratory involvement[6]
- Decrease immunological surgical stress responses in VATS may decrease severity and frequency of postoperative myasthenic issues[7]

VATS THYMECTOMY FOR THYMOMAS

Vats thymectomy for thymomas has initially been confined to small (< 2 cm) well-encapsulated intrathymic thymomas. Larger tumors were not subjected to VATS due to the risks of a breach of tumor capsule with tumor seedling, port-site implantation and possible iatrogenic capsular injury during extraction of larger specimens making subsequent histological analysis inaccurate.[9]

With increased experience in VATS thymectomy larger well-encapsulated tumors can be resected by modifying the VATS technique used for standard non-thymomatous myasthenia gravis. My first experience with large thymomas involved a 73-year-old man who was severely emaciated from recurrent infections from hypogammaglobulinemia, secondary to a 9-cm thymoma.[5] It was successfully removed by VATS as he was deemed not fit for major open surgery. This case demonstrated that even larger thymomas can be removed successfully by VATS. Therefore, over the years with increasing experience in VATS thymectomy, indications were extended to larger thymomas by modifying the VATS technique to incorporate oncologically sound principles which was coined the 'no touch tumor last' technique. The principles of this technique are:

- Unlike in VATS thymectomy for non-thymomatous myasthenia gravis where the right side is the preferred side of approach, for thymomas the side of the approach is determined by site of tumor location. This is to ensure safe dissection of the tumor under direct vision (**Figure 16.4b**).
- The non-tumorous part of the thymus and perithymic fat is always dissected first so it can be used for grasping and traction when dissecting the tumor at the end of the process
- The tumor is always dissected last. This is to minimize tumor handling and manipulation. Also, when the tumor is dissected first, it's weight under gravity will obstruct the surgical field of vision and make subsequent dissection of the gland difficult and oncologically hazardous. When the tumor is dissected last, the non-tumorous horns and thymic fat can be used for traction and grasping and not the tumor thus minimizing risk of capsular damage
- All specimens are removed via an endobag by appropriate enlargement of the 10 mm port incision to prevent capsular damage. Through this incision, a size 28F chest tube is placed at the end of the surgery (**Figure 16.4b** and **c**).

Between 1998 and 2011, 158 patients underwent VATS thymectomy of which 80 were for thymomas which were resected using this technique. 41(51.3%) were associated with myasthenia gravis. The right-sided approach was used in 79.3% of patients. 44.8% were males. Mean age was 52.3 years (range, 22–83 years). Mean duration of surgery was 149.8 minutes (range, 60–289 minutes). Mean length of stay was 5 days (range, 2–15 days). Mean size of thymomas was 50 mm (range, 10–90 mm). Thirty-three were in Masoaka stage I, 34 in stage II, 12 in stage III and 1 in stage IV. All patients had clear surgical resection margins on pathological analysis. There were no operative deaths and operative morbidity was 6.9%. Morbidity included superficial wound infection in four patients, myasthenic crisis in one and phrenic nerve injury in one.

Mean follow up was 5.5 years (range, 1–11 years). Of the 67 patients with stage 1 and 2 thymomas, one had a local relapse. This was a patient in stage 1 with a 5-cm tumor who was treated before the adoption of the modified 'no touch, tumor last technique'. In this case, the mistake was to dissect the tumor first followed by the rest of the non-tumorous thymus gland as this was easier to do. However, once the tumor was dissected, the weight of the tumor under gravity made subsequent visualization and dissection of the gland difficult. Also, with dissecting the tumor first there was less normal surrounding tissue to grasp when dissecting the tumor from its bed which increased the risk of breaching the tumor capsule. It is likely that this is what happened to this patient who recurred locally 4 years later and underwent median sternotomy to resect the local recurrence followed by radiotherapy.[5]

As 51.3% of the thymomas were associated with myasthenia gravis, the surgery has to be both oncologically sound and radical to ensure good long-term neurological outcomes. Principles of radical thymectomy as for non-thymomatous myasthenia gravis should be followed to ensure good neurological outcomes.[5]

93.8% of thymoma patients associated with myasthenia gravis improved by one or more Osserman grade after surgery. Mean Osserman grade improvement post-surgery was 2.88 (range, 1–5). 84% remain asymptomatic and 25% in complete stable remission without medications for more than 6 months. Using Cox multivariate regression analysis, the presence of thymoma had no adverse impact on neurological outcomes after surgery.[5]

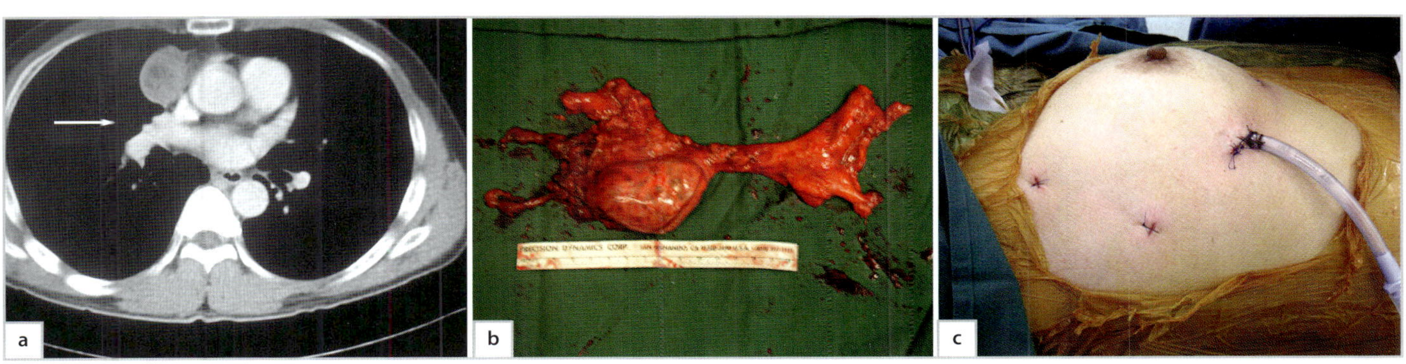

Figure 16.4 VATS thymectomy for thymomas. (a) Unilateral VATS approach for well encapsulated thymoma (b) 5 cm well encapsulated stage 1 thymoma. (c) Incisions for right VATS thymectomy.

Table 16.2 Tumor characteristics for bilateral VATS approach

Age(years)	Size(CM)	Histology	Indication for surgery
14	10	Type A, stage 1 cystic thymoma	Large left cystic tumor
16	8	Mature teratoma	Large left-sided tumor with small chest cavity
19	9	Seminoma	Large right tumor abutting innominate vein
22	4.5	Post-chemotherapy non-seminomatous germ cell tumor	Sitting on innominate vein
35	7.5	Type AB, stage 1 thymoma	Large right tumor abutting innominate vein
44	8	Type A, stage 1 thymoma	Large left tumor
44	8	Type AB, stage 1 thymoma	Large left tumor
48	4.8	Type B2, stage 3 thymoma	Sitting on innominate vein
56	8	Type B, stage 1 thymoma	Large left tumor
74	9.5	Type AB, stage 1 thymoma	Large left tumor
64	10	Type A, stage 1 thymoma	Large tumor sitting on innominate vein
62	9	Stage 3 thymoma	Large cystic thymoma invading pericardium, phrenic nerve and abutting on innominate vein

REFERENCES

1. Kattach H, Anastassiadis K, Cleuziou J, et al. Trans-sternal thymectomy for myasthenia gravis: surgical outcome. Ann Thorac Surg 2006; 81:305–308.
2. Yim,Manlulu A, Tak Wai L, Wan I, et al. Video-assisted thoracic surgery thymectomy for non thymomatous myasthenia gravis. Chest 2005; 128:3454–3460.
3. Sonnett JR, Jaretzki A IIIrd. Thymectomy for non-thymomatous myasthenia gravis: A critical analysis. Ann NY Acad Sci 2008; 1132:315–318.
4. Shrager JB, Deeb, ME, Mick R, et al. Transcervical thymectomy for myasthenia gravis achieves results comparable to thymectomy by sternotomy. Ann Thoracic Surg 2002:74:320–326.
5. Agasthian T, Lin SJ. Clinical outcomes of video-assisted thymectomy or myasthenia gravis and thymoma. Asian Cardiovasc Thorac Ann 2010; 18:234–239.
6. Yim APC, Mineo TC, Pompeo E, Ambrogi V. Thoracoscopic thymectomy "Which side to approach?" Ann Thorac Surg 1997; 64:584–585.
7. Soon JL, Agasthian T. Harmonic scalpel in video-assisted thoracoscopic thymic resections. Asian Cardiovasc Thorac Ann 2008; 16:366–369.
8. Ruckert JC, Czyzewski D, Pest S, Muller JM. Radicality of thoracoscopic thymectomy- anatomical study. Eur J Cardiothorac Surg 2000; 18:735–736.
9. Ashour M. Prevalence of ectopic thymic tissue in myasthenia gravis and its clinical significance. J Thorac Cardiovasc Surg 1995; 109:632–635.
10. Agasthian T, Soon JL. Clinical outcomes of VATS for thymomas. Interact Cardio Vasc Thorac Surgery 2008:7.
11. Ruckert JC, Walter M, Muller JM. Pulmonary function after thoracoscopic thymectomy vs median sternotomy for myasthenia gravis. Annals of Thoracic Surgery 2000:70:1656–1661.
12. Agasthian T. Can invasive thymomas be resected by video-assisted thoracoscopic surgery? Asian Cardiovasc Thorac Ann 2011; 19:225–227.

Chapter 17 Pericardial window

Simon CY Chow, Calvin SH Ng

INTRODUCTION

Pericardial effusion (PE) is a commonly encountered clinical scenario. It may be due to local pericardial disease or secondary to systemic illnesses. Causes can range from thyroid dysfunction, infection, inflammatory disease, uremia to disseminated malignancies. Around half of patients with pericardial effusion develop cardiac tamponade requiring urgent drainage. Hence pericardial effusion itself contributes to significant morbidity and carries a risk of mortality. The prognosis of pericardial effusion depends on the underlying cause, and the ideal intervention for PE should not only achieve palliation of symptoms and prevention of recurrence, but also serves to obtain adequate samples for diagnosis. Options of pericardial drainage vary from non-surgical to surgical and include needle pericardiocentesis, pericardial drains, balloon pericardiotomy, pericardial window and pericardiectomy. Surgical pericardial drainage is preferred for patients with recurrent effusion, while needle pericardiocentesis may be a better immediate option for patents with cardiac tamponade and hemodynamic instability. Subxiphoid and open transthoracic pericardial window have been well established as safe and effective options for pericardial drainage, however with the recent surge of interest in minimally invasive surgery and the rapid development of thoracoscopy, video-assisted thoracoscopic (VATS) pericardial window is increasingly practised by surgeons. In this chapter, we will introduce and explore the different methods of pericardial drainage, with particular focus on VATS pericardial window and recent advances in minimally invasive approaches.

INDICATIONS AND APPROACHES

Cardiac tamponade is a life-threatening condition, and urgent image-guided percutaneous needle pericardiocentesis for patients with unstable hemodynamics and features of tamponade on echocardiogram is usually the best initial approach. However, needle pericardiocentesis is mostly a temporizing measure and over 50–60% of pericardial effusion tends to re-accumulate. Hence surgical means of drainage for patients with recurrent pericardial effusion is recommended. Different surgical approaches exist for pericardial drainage and the most commonly performed procedure is pericardial window. Other alternatives include pericardiectomy and pericardio-peritoneal shunt.

Different surgical approaches to achieve pericardial fenestration and the creation of a window in the pericardium have been described in literature. The most well described approach is the subxiphoid pericardial window (SXP) followed by the transthoracic open pericardial window via anterior thoracotomy. Since the 1990s surgeons have been performing pericardial window with the VATS approach. Until recently, uniportal and needlescopic VATS thoracic surgery have been described.[1] A number of studies have found the VATS approach to be safe and feasible for a wide variety of thoracic and mediastinal conditions and it has been associated with less wound pain, as well as a better and speedier recovery in patients postoperatively.[2] In addition, innovative techniques such as natural orifice transluminal endoscopic surgery (NOTES) have been explored and are currently under investigation in animal studies.

PATIENT SELECTION AND PREOPERATIVE PLANNING

Patients with recurrent pericardial effusion should be considered for surgery. All patients should have a formal transthoracic echocardiogram to document the thickness of the pericardium and effusion, as well as to look for features of tamponade. Echocardiogram may in some cases provide evidence for an unsuspecting diagnosis for the pericardial effusion, such as aortic dissection, myocardial infarction or even an infiltrating cardiac tumor. Computed tomography (CT) of the thorax can reveal the extent of pericardial effusion, including the presence of loculations and masses both within and surrounding the pericardium, as well as pleural diseases such as pleural effusion that can be managed concomitantly during surgery. Hence, a CT scan has an important role in providing information for deciding the type of approach, as well as the laterality of the approach.

Anesthetic concerns differ for different surgical approaches. The subxiphoid and transthoracic open approach can be performed under local anesthesia with sedation in the supine position. These approaches are recommended in patients who are marginal candidates for surgery or during emergencies as urgent subxiphoid pericardiocentesis can be performed if the patient deteriorates on the surgical table before the operation. In addition, these approaches do not require one-lung ventilation and decubitus positioning. For the VATS approach, patients can be positioned in the lateral decubitus position, or supine with 30° tilt, with double lumen endobronchial tube intubation and one-lung ventilation. The VATS approach is not recommended in patients who are hemodynamically unstable or intolerant of one-lung ventilation.

SUBXIPHOID PERICARDIAL WINDOW

The SXP is arguably not a true window procedure, as it does not involve the creation of a passage of drainage of pericardial fluid into another body cavity. SXP can be done under local or general anesthesia with the patient positioned in the supine position. A 3–4 cm vertical incision is made over the xiphoid process. The xiphoid process is either retracted or excised. The retrosternal plane is entered with direct visualization of the diaphragmatic aspect of the pericardium. An incision is made over the pericardium and the effusion is released. Finger palpation of the pericardium is performed to determine the presence of and, in appropriate circumstances, breakdown of adhesions or loculations. A biopsy of the pericardium is sent for further investigations and the pericardial fluid should also be collected for biochemical, microbiological and histological studies. Subsequently, a large bore thoracostomy tube is inserted into the pericardial space and kept for 72–96 hours. Apart from the immediate release of pericardial fluid, an additional mechanism of SXP in treating pericardial effusion is the symphysis of the pericardium and epicardium induced by sclerotic inflammatory reaction stimulated by the presence of the thoracostomy tube. The SXP is the most commonly described method of pericardial drainage. In a latest systemic review including 10 studies on SXP and malignant pericardial effusion, overall 93.2% of the patients did not require repeated pericardial intervention, with symptomatic recurrence rates at 5.5% and complication rates at 3.9%.[3-5] The SXP is a relatively simple procedure and is the preferred approach in patients with unstable hemodynamics and multiple comorbidities as it can be performed in supine position under local anesthesia, with the option of emergent percutaneous pericardiocentesis intraoperatively.

TRANSTHORACIC AND VATS PERICARDIAL WINDOW

The transthoracic or VATS pericardial window is a true window in the sense that it creates a communication between the pericardial and pleural cavity, allowing effusion to flow into the pleural space. This prevents the pericardial effusion from causing hemodynamically significant tamponade. Traditionally, pericardial windows are done via the open approach with an anterior thoracotomy in the 5th intercostal space. One-lung ventilation is not a pre-requisite and the procedure can be done under local anesthesia. With swab sticks retracting the lung, a pericardial window is created with electrocautery or scissors, and the pericardial and pleural fluid is drained. To conclude the procedure, a thoracostomy tube is inserted into the ipsilateral pleural cavity.

The VATS approach, on the other hand, involves the creation of small instrument port incisions over the thoracic cavity, and under thoracoscopic guidance provides excellent visualization of the thoracic cavity enabling access to the pericardial region without the need for long incisions. Pericardial window via the VATS approach has been reported to be feasible and safe for treatment of effusions and can offer concomitant treatment of other thoracic conditions involving the pleura as it allows simultaneous access into the pleural cavity.[6-8]

The conventional three-port VATS approach is performed under general anesthesia with the patient in the lateral decubitus position and the table flexed at 30° to open up the intercostal spaces. This procedure requires double lumen endobronchial tube intubation with one-lung ventilation. Traditionally the three ports include a 10-mm camera port and two additional instrument ports positioned in a triangulating manner. A common configuration of the three-port strategy includes placement of the camera port in the region of 6th to 8th intercostal space over the mid axillary line, and two working ports around the 4th to 6th intercostal space in the mid and anterior axillary. The exact port site positions may be adjusted according to preoperative imaging, surgeon preference and the anatomy of the pathological process. In most circumstances, 0 degree thoracoscope is sufficient, and conventional instruments familiar to the surgeon, such as sponge forceps and Roberts clamps can be used. Upon entrance into the cavity, a systematic exploration of the pleural cavity, in particular the mediastinum over the pericardium is performed and any pleural fluid is drained. It is important to identify and avoid injuring the phrenic nerve before making the incision into the pericardial space, which is usually anterior to the phrenic nerve. Pericardial fluid is aspirated and sent for appropriate investigations. A 3 cm by 3 cm pericardial window is then created with electrocautery. Some surgeons attempt deloculation of intrapericardial adhesions of the pericardial cavity, although that should be done with caution as bleeding may be difficult to control, and there is no data to suggest it is necessary. Meticulous hemostasis of the pericardial fat and pericardium edge should be performed. Routinely, a large bore thoracostomy tube is inserted into the ipsilateral pleural cavity and kept until the drain output is acceptable. For patients with concomitant malignant pleural effusion, talc pouldrage may be instilled into the pleural cavity postoperatively if drain output remains high.

In a recent systematic review including three studies (70 patients) on VATS pericardial window and malignant pericardial effusion, around 90% of patients did not require further pericardial intervention during follow-up, with 9% overall symptomatic recurrence and complication rates at 4.8%.[5] Reported complications included arrhythmias, pulmonary embolism and respiratory failure. Among the earliest studies on VATS pericardial window, Geissbuhler et al. performed VATS pericardial window for 24 patients with recurrent and loculated effusions. In that series, 72% of the patients had septations and loculations intrapericardially. 87% of patients had double lumen intubation and 13% underwent VATS window creation under local anesthesia and intravenous sedation. Additional talc pleurodesis was performed in 25% of patients suffering from malignant pleural effusion. The mean operating time was 45 minutes (40–60 minutes), with 1 requiring conversion due to fibrosed pericardium. The mean postoperative chest drainage duration was 3.3 days and mean hospitalization duration was 10.4 days (range 4–33 days). The postoperative complication rate was 12% (3 patients) and included pulmonary embolism, supraventricular arrhythmia and minor cerebrovascular events. There was no treatment-related 30-day mortality. One (4%) patient amongst the surviving patients had asymptomatic recurrence of pericardial effusion 1 month postoperatively.[6] Similar VATS approaches have been described in various studies thereafter (**Table 17.1**). Comparisons have been made between the VATS approach and SXP. O'Brien et al. found VATS to be associated with higher postoperative morbidities, and with a higher incidence of pneumothorax and air leak than SXP. Unsurprisingly, the same study also found a longer duration of anesthesia for the VATS group compared to SXP (117.1 minutes versus 81.1 minutes) owing to the need for double lumen endobronchial intubation.[13]

NEEDLESCOPIC VATS

The introduction of needlescopic instruments allows for even smaller incisions, to further reduce access trauma and hasten recovery. Needlescopic VATS (nVATS) have been performed in thoracic surgeries such as bullectomy, pleurodesis and sympathectomy with promising results in terms of reduction of morbidity and earlier recovery. Technical details of the two-port or three-port nVATS approach vary with patient anatomy and surgeon preference. One such approach for the three-port nVATS involves the use of two 3 mm working ports at the 6th intercostal space on the mid-clavicular and mid-axillary line, and a 10-mm thoracoscopic port at the 8th intercostal space forming a triangle (**Figure 17.1**). After the creation of the pericardial window with 2 mm endograspers and the diathermy, the pericardium can be retrieved via the 10 mm port with the 3 mm endograspers under direct vision, sharing the port with the 5 mm thoracoscope. Extra care should be taken when manipulating needlescopic instruments within the thoracic cavity due to the very sharp tip which can easily injury visceral organs (**Figure 17.2**). The 3-mm stab wounds are closed with single nylon sutures and a 24-Fr chest drain is inserted in the camera port (**Figure 17.3**). From our own experience, total operative time was around 25–30 minutes and the patients were drain free and discharged 2 days postoperatively.[15] Trials comparing nVATs and traditional three-port VATS for sympathectomy and pleurodesis have found nVATS to be a safe procedure with less access trauma and better cosmesis. So far no trials have been performed specifically describing case series of pericardial window with nVATS, but it is not inconceivable that with smaller wounds, the recovery from surgery for patients especially with malignancies may be more favorable.

Table 17.1 VATS pericardial window case series: efficacy and complications

References	No. of patients	Technique	Mean operation time	Hospital stay and drain time (mean days)	Recurrence	Complications
Geissbuhler et al.[6]	24	3 ports 13% under local anesthesia and IV sedation	45 minutes	Drain duration: 3.3 days Hospital stay: 10.4 days	1/22 recurrence in 3 months	12% (3 patients): • peripheral pulmonary embolism • minor cerebrovascular event • supraventricular arrhythmia no treatment related mortality
Muhammed et al.[11]	15	GA, DLT 2–3 ports	111.3 minutes	Drain: 3.4 days Hospital: 10.2 days	0 recurrence in 3 months	0% complications and mortality
Nataf et al[10]	22	GA, DLT 2–3 ports	N/A	Drain: 48 hours	1 /22 recurrence	No complication 3 deaths < 3 months due to underlying cancer progression
Palma et al.[9]	26	GA, DLT 3 ports	52 minutes	N/A	1/26 recurrence	1% conversion for bleeding 3/26 complications: • ventricular tachycardia • acute pulmonary edema • prolonged intubation
Neragi Miandoab et al.[8]	62	GA, DLT 2–3 ports	N/A	Hospital stay: 8.7 days	5/62 recurrence	1/62 postoperative ventilator support No procedural-related deaths
Katlic et al[12]	13/353	GA , DLT , 2 ports	28 minutes for all procedures	N/A	N/A	3% complications in general including CVA, airleak, empyema, respiratory and renal failure No procedural related deaths
Georghiou et al.[7]	18	GA, DLT 2–3 ports	46 minutes	Drain time: 2.3 days Hospitalization: 6.4 days	0/18 recurrence in 3 months	1/18 supraventricular arrhythmia No procedural related deaths
Ohtsuka et al.[14]	10	GA, DLT 3 ports	27 minutes	N/A	N/A	One non-procedural death at 6 days postoperatively due to low cardiac output
O'Brien et al.[13]	15/71	GA, DLT 2–3 ports	Anesthesia time: 117.1 minutes	Drain time: 3.3 days Hospitalization: 12.4 days	1/15 recurrence in mean 22 months follow up	4/15 complications: • Pneumothorax after drain removal • Prolonged airleak

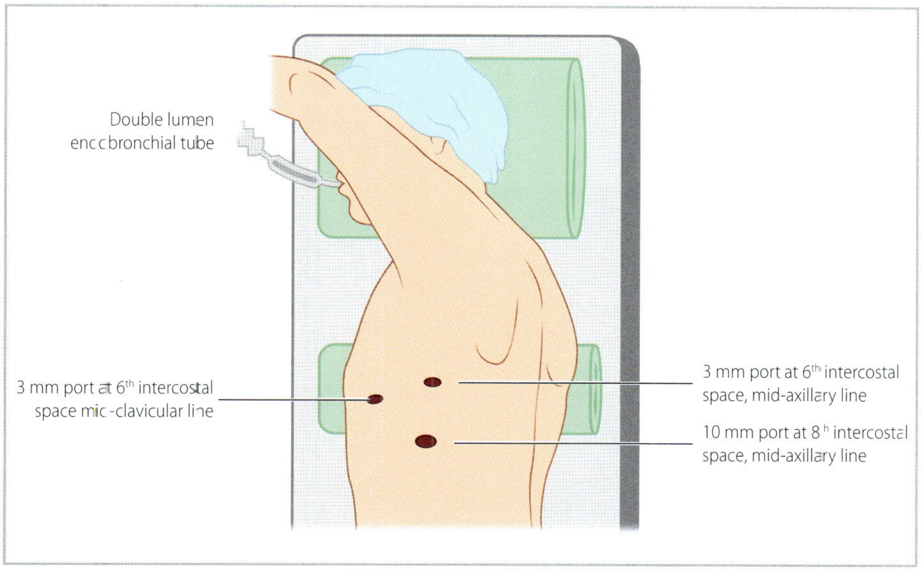

Figure 17.1 Lateral decubitus operating position and incision sites for needlescopic three-port VATS pericardial window.

UNIPORTAL VATS

The development of uniportal VATS has gained momentum and popularity amongst thoracic surgeons worldwide. Uniportal VATS approach has displayed great versatility and is being reported in major lung resections including lobectomies and pneumonectomies, as well as complex lung resections requiring reconstruction of major pulmonary vessels. Numerous studies have shown that uniportal VATS is as safe and equally effective as conventional three ports VATS for various thoracic conditions.[16-18] Uniportal VATS pericardial window

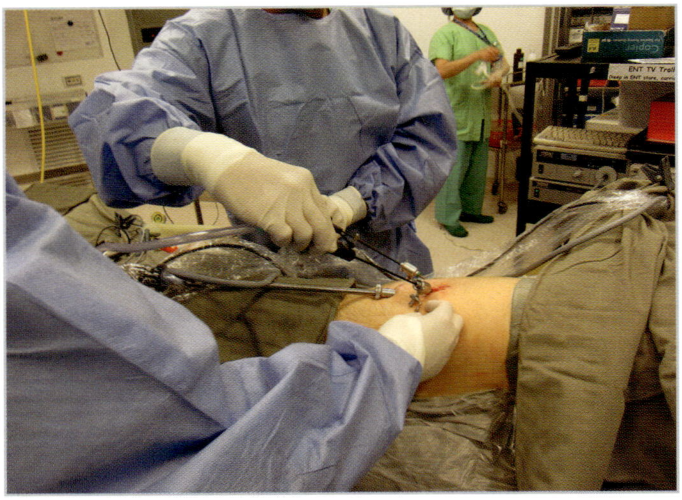

Figure 17.2 Intraoperative needlescopic VATS pericardial window with 3 mm endo-instruments and 10 mm thoracoscope.

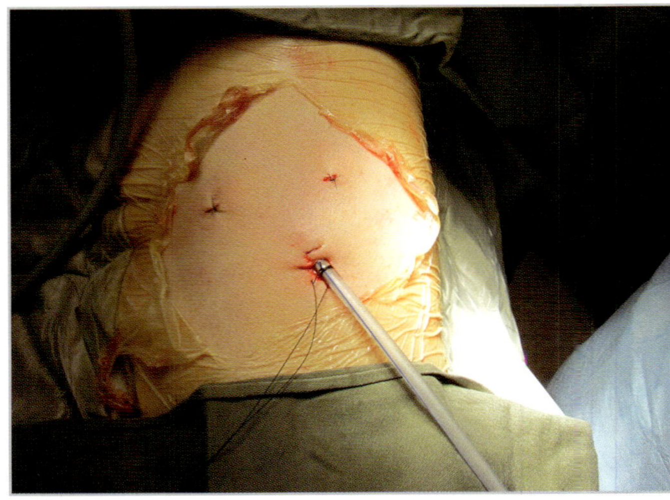

Figure 17.3 At completion of needlescopic VATS pericardial window, the drain is placed in the camera port and the needlescopic 3 mm wounds sutured with interrupted 4-0 Dermalon.

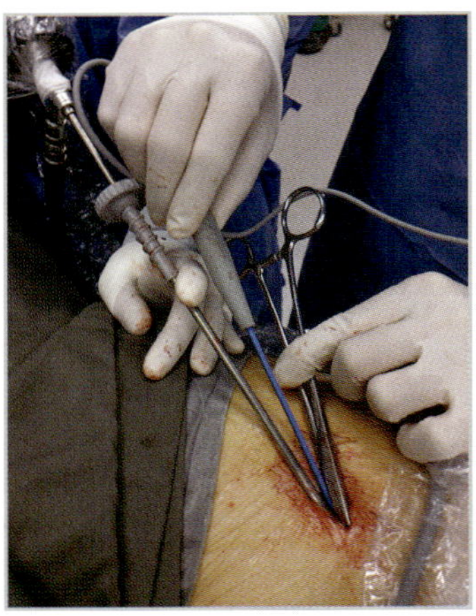

Figure 17.4 Uniportal incision of 2.5 cm with 5 mm instruments and thoracoscope inserted through the same incision.

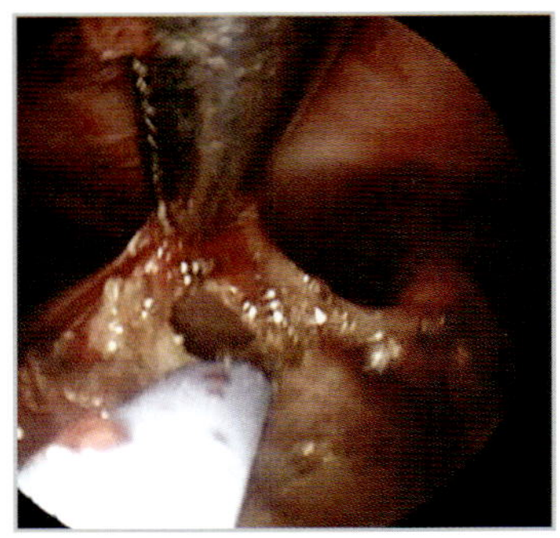

Figure 17.5 Thoracoscopic view of pericardial window creation via uniportal access with diathermy, and variable angulated Snowden-Pencer endograsper.

was first described by Rocco and colleagues in 2006.[19] In that report, 4 patients with malignant pleuro-pericardial effusions had a uniportal pericardial window performed under general anesthesia via single-lung ventilation. Patients were placed in supine positon or with hemithorax elevated 45° with a roll, and then a 2.5 cm incision was created in the 5th intercostal space along the mid-axillary line (**Figure 17.4**). The pleural cavity was inspected using a 5 mm videothoracoscope. The pericardium was opened under direct vision anterior to the phrenic nerve (**Figure 17.5**), and circumferentially enlarged with endoscissors inserted parallel to the thoracoscope. A thoracostomy tube was inserted through the same incision and removed postoperatively (**Figure 17.6**). To date, cases of uniportal VATS pericardial window have been reported as part of larger studies looking into the feasibility and versatility of single-port surgery. Song et al. reported their own series of uniportal VATS in a heterogeneous group of patients with mediastinal and thoracic pathologies.[20] Of the 264 cases in the series, 3 cases of single-port pericardial window were reported. The pleural cavity was accessed via a 2.5–3.0 cm long incision in the 6th to 7th intercostal space. All 3 cases of pericardial window formation did not require conversion or further incisions, but there was limited

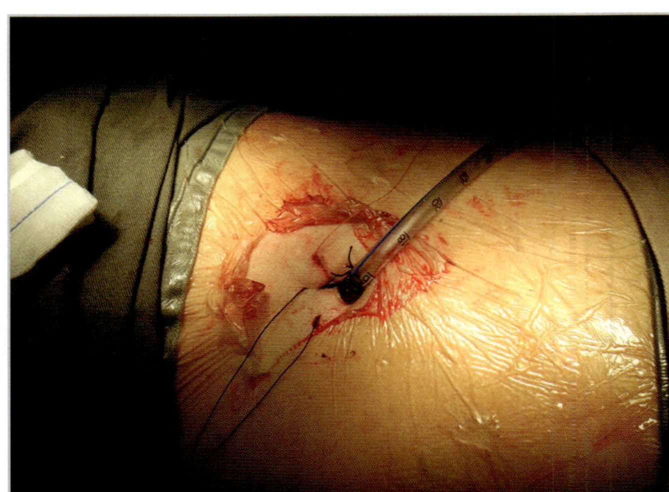

Figure 17.6 At completion of uniportal pericardial window, a drain is placed at the single incision site.

data on patients' follow-up. In a recent larger case series of 644 cases of uniportal VATS thoracic surgery spanning 10 years, Rocco et al. further demonstrated the versatility of uniportal VATS. In his cohort, 17.8% of the 644 patients operated under uniportal VATS had pathologies other than lung nodules or pleural effusion. 95.6% of the patients had the surgery performed under general anesthesia with reported conversion rates at 3.7%.[21] Although no specific data concerning the number of cases, overall success and any complications of the pericardial window is available from the paper, the study has further reinforced the increasing consensus that uniportal VATS is feasible and safe in a wide variety of thoracic and mediastinal conditions.

A possible concern regarding uniportal VATS is the limited working space, resulting in instrument fencing and frequent soiling of the videothoracoscope. Hence meticulous preoperative planning is important, as application of endoscopic instruments may be hindered by suboptimal positioning of the incision necessitating a second-port for better intrathoracic manipulation. As a result, flexible, long curved or angled instruments have been developed to facilitate uniportal VATS, and special considerations and techniques are described to minimize fencing.[22] The proposed advantages of uniportal VATS over three port VATS are less pain and paresthesia as well as better patient satisfaction postoperatively. Although conclusive large scaled studies are lacking to prove the superiority of uniportal VATS over traditional three port approach, multiple studies have shown it is an equally effective and safe alternative to two- or three-port VATS in a wide variety of thoracic and mediastinal conditions.[16-18]

NOTES

Natural orifice transluminal endoscopic surgery is based on the concept of accessing the operative field via natural orifices such as the mouth, vagina, rectum or urethra. The first NOTES was performed by Ott et al. in 1901. NOTES for thoracic surgery has lagged behind in comparison to the development in abdominal surgery, due to greater reluctance in accessing the thoracic cavity through the trachea or oesophagus, which is associated with devastating complications such as pericarditis or mediastinitis. Nevertheless, animal models have shown that access for thoracic surgical procedures is possible via esophagotomies and tracheotomies. The transluminal esophagotomy approach was first described by Sumiyama which involves creating a submucosal plane in the esophagus by the injection of saline or gas. Subsequently, a viscerotomy is made at a different level of the esophagotomy and is sealed with endoclips after the procedure. Fritscher-Ravens and Sumiyama reported their experiences with a transesophageal pericardial window in animal models.[23-24] In one series, 3 cm pericardial windows were successfully created in 5 pigs. One pig sustained aortic injury while the remaining showed patent pericardial windows in necropsy 1 week later. However, the risk of mediastinitis is still considerable and warrants significant attention. Two animals from the study of Fritscher-Ravens developed severe mediastinitis and mediastinal abscess due to spillage of refluxed gastric contents into the mediastinum. In that series, the infectious morbidity was 34%. Liu et al. explored the feasibility of transtracheal and transoral pericardial window in porcine and canine models. For the transtracheal approach, 58.3% of the studied animals developed tension pneumothorax secondary to carbon dioxide insufflation during scope entry, with intraoperative mortality of 25%. In the transoral approach, the videoscope was inserted via a 12 mm incision over the vestibulum oris down to the periosteum of the mandible. The pretracheal plane was entered and continued into the substernal space with subsequent entrance into the mediastinal pleura in the upper part of the thoracic cavity. A flexible endoscope was used to explore the thoracic cavity and the pericardial window was created using a needle knife. The procedure was successful in 10 canines with 2 developing hemorrhage and significant bradycardia intraoperative.[25] Overall it appears the success of NOTES in thoracic surgery can eliminate the need for skin incisions altogether but its safety remains a concern and further modifications and well-thought out steps in the development of NOTES is required prior to its applicability to humans.

CONCLUSION

The pericardial window is an effective option of pericardial drainage for patients with pericardial effusion. VATS pericardial window has been shown to be as effective and safe as traditional procedures such as the subxiphoid and open transthoracic approach. With the aid of a thoracoscope, VATS pericardial window offers a wider and more comprehensive visualization of the thoracic cavity and an added benefit of concomitant pleural drainage. Shorter incisions and uniportal VATS minimize access trauma and further reduce postoperative wound discomfort and pain. The interest in NOTES offers promise for thoracic surgeries without scars, but its safety and feasibility remain to be substantiated in human studies.

REFERENCES

1. Ng CS, Lau KK. Gonzalez-Rivas D, Rocco G. Evolution in surgical approach and techniques for lung cancer. Thorax 2013; 68:681.
2. Li WW, Lee TW, Lam SS, et al. Quality of life following lung cancer resection: video-assisted thoracic surgery vs thoracotomy. Chest 2002; 122:584–589.
3. Becit N, Unlu Y, Ceviz M, et al. Subxiphoid pericardiostomy in the management of pericardial effusions: case series analysis of 368 patients. Heart 2005; 91:785–790.
4. Moores DWO, Allen KB, Faber LP, et al. Subxiphoid pericardial drainage for pericardial tamponade. J Thorac Cardiovasc Surg 1995; 109:546–552.
5. Jama GM, Scarci M, Bowden J, Marciniak SJ. Palliative treatment for symptomatic malignant pericardial effusion. Interact Cardiovasc Thorac Surg 2014; 19:1019–1026.
6. Geissbuhler K, Leiser A, Fuhrer J. Video-assisted thoracoscopic pericardial fenestration for loculated or recurrent effusions. Eur J Cardiothorac Surg 1998; 14:403–408.
7. Georghiou GP, Stamler A, Sharoni E, et al. Video-assisted thoracoscopic pericardial window for diagnosis and management of pericardial effusions. Ann Thorac Surg 2005; 80:607–610.
8. Neragi-Miandoab S, Linden PA, Ducko CT, et al. VATS pericardiotomy for patients with known malignancy and pericardial effusion: survival and prognosis of positive cytology and metastatic involvement of the pericardium: a case control study. Int J Surg 2008; 6:110–114.
9. Palma JH, Gaia DF, Guilhen JC, Branco JN, Buffolo E. Video-thoracoscopic pericardial drainage in the treatment of pericardial effusions. Rev Bras Cir Cardiovasc [online] 2009; 24:44–49.
10. Nataf P, Cacoub P, Regan M, et al. Video-thoracoscopic pericardial window in the diagnosis and treatment of pericardial effusions. Am J Cardiol 1998; 82:124–126.
11. Muhammad MI. The pericardial window: is a video-assisted thoracoscopy approach better than a surgical approach? Interact. Cardiovasc Thorac Surg 2011; 12:174–178.
12. Katlic MR, Facktor MA. Video-assisted thoracic surgery utilizing local anesthesia and sedation: 384 consecutive cases. Ann Thorac Surg 2010; 90:240–245.
13. O'Brien PK, Kucharczuk JC, Marshall MB. Comparative study of subxiphoid versus video-thoracoscopic pericardial window. Ann Thorac Surg 2005; 80:2013–2019.

14. Ohtsuka T, Wolf RK, Wiring P, Park SE. Thoracoscopic limited pericardial resection with an ultrasonic scalpel. Ann Thorac Surg 1998; 65:855–856.
15. Ng CSH, Wong RHL, Yeung ECL, et al. Needlescopic video-assisted thoracoscopic pericardial window. Surgical Practice 2012; 16:84–85.
16. Ng CSH. Uniportal VATS in Asia. J Thorac Dis 2013; 5:S221–225.
17. Lau RW, Ng CS, Kwok MW, et al. Early outcomes following uniportal video-assisted thoracic surgery lung resection. Chest 2014; 145:50A.
18. Gonzalez-Rivas D, Paradela M, Fernandez R, et al. Uniportal video-assisted thoracoscopic lobectomy: two years of experience. Ann Thorac Surg 2013; 95:426–432.
19. Rocco G, La Rocca A, La Manna C, et al. Uniportal video-assisted thoracoscopic surgery pericardial window. J Thorac Cardiovasc Surg 2006; 131:921–922.
20. Song IH, Yum SW, Choi WS, et al. Clinical application of single incision thoracoscopic surgery: early experience of 264 cases. J Cardiothor Surg 2014; 9:44.
21. Rocco G, Martucci N, La Manna C, et al. Ten-year experience on 644 patients undergoing single-port (uniportal) video-assisted thoracoscopic surgery. Ann Thorac Surg 2013; 96:434–438.
22. Ng CSH, Wong RHL, Lau RWH, Yim APC. Minimizing chest wall trauma in single port video-assisted thoracic surgery. J Thorac Cardiovasc Surg 2014; 147:1095–1056.
23. Sumiyama K, Gostout CJ, Rajan E, et al. Pilot study of transesophageal endoscopic epicardial coagulation by submucosal endoscopy with the mucosal flap safety valve technique. Gastrointest Endosc 2008; 67:497–501.
24. Fritscher-Ravens A, Patel K, Ghanbari A, et al. Natural orifice transluminal endoscopic surgery (NOTES) in the mediastinum: Long-term survival animal experiments in transesophageal access, including minor surgical procedures. Endoscopy 2007; 39:870–875.
25. Ko PJ, Chu Y, Wu YC, et al. Feasibility of endoscopic transoral thoracic surgical lung biopsy and pericardial window creation. J Surg Res 2012; 175:207–214.

Chapter 18 First rib and thoracic outlet

Miguel Congregado

INTRODUCTION

Thoracic outlet syndrome (TOS) is caused by compression of neurovascular elements that traverse the superior thoracic outlet from the chest to the upper extremities. Although it is difficult to know the true incidence, this disease is estimated to affect 0.3–2% of the general population and is three times more common in women than in men. Previously, TOS had several names depending on the etiologic factor that caused the compression, such as scalene, costoclavicular, hyperabduction, cervical rib, or first rib syndrome. Peet unified these conditions in 1956 by coining the term 'TOS,' which referred to all pathological processes that cause compression of the neurological and vascular bundle at this level.[1]

It is very important to understand that, regardless of the cause of compression, the common location against which pressure is exerted is always the first costal arch. **Figure 18.1** outlines possible causes of TOS such as the presence of a posterior scalene muscle or hypertrophy of the medial and anterior scalenes, a costoclavicular ligament, a bifid first rib or traumatic or congenital malformations of this bone, or the presence of a cervical rib or a vertebral transverse mega-apophysis. Therefore, surgical treatment must always consist of the removal of the first rib because this achieves, on the one hand, an increase in the size of the gap and, on the other hand, its removal necessarily entails sectioning of the scalene muscles, costoclavicular ligament, and other accessories or abnormalities such as those extending from the cervical rib to the upper face of the first costal arch.

HISTORICAL PERSPECTIVE

Galeno and Vesalio previously described the presence of a cervical rib centuries ago, and until 1927, it was thought that this was the root cause of TOS.[2] In addition, Coote published the results of the first successful extirpation of the cervical rib in 1861.[3] Shortly thereafter, Sir James Paget, in 1875, and von Schroetter, in 1884, described thrombosis syndrome in the subclavian-axillary vein.[4,5] Other authors have studied various causes and consequences of compression of the superior thoracic outlet such as adventitious ligaments, scalene muscles, costoclavicular ligaments, hyperabduction, and the pectoralis minor muscle.[6-9] The important role of the first rib in this syndrome was proposed by Bramwell and Brinckner, among others.[10,19]

Regarding surgical treatment, Murphy was the first surgeon to resect the first rib in 1910.[11] Clagett emphasized the usefulness of first rib resection using an incision similar to that used in a posterior thoracoplasty, while Falconer and Li proposed an anterior approach for this extirpation.[12,13] In 1966, Roos presented and described the transaxillary approach for resection of the first rib.[14] Finally, Urschel, after treating more than 5,102 surgical patients, created a number of clinical guidelines and steps to follow, suggesting the axillary approach as the best method, the supraclavicular approach when aneurysms of the subclavian artery are present, and the posterior approach in cases of recurrence.[15]

Currently, in the age of minimally invasive surgery, there is growing interest in a new extirpation technique for the first rib using videothoracoscopy, which has shown very good results.[16]

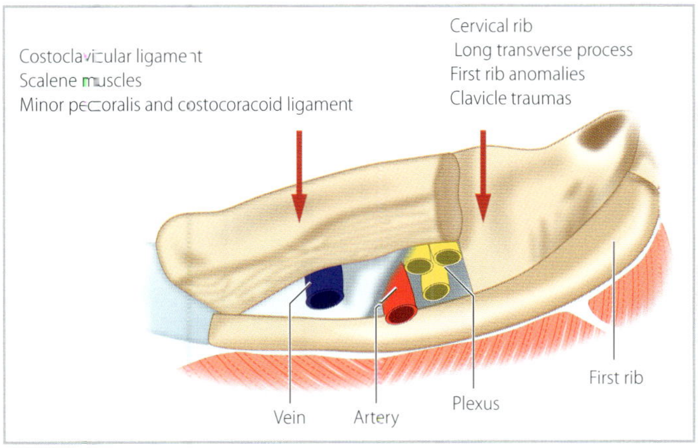

Figure 18.1 Causes of thoracic outlet syndrome. Compression of the neurovascular bundle can occur for all of these causes with different origin.

CLINICAL ASPECTS

The clinical aspects of this process depend on the compressed structure(s) and potentially exhibit neurological and/or vascular symptomatology. The most common symptom is nerve compression, and when there is involvement of the brachial plexus, the patient presents pain and paraesthesia in 95% of cases; only 10% of patients complain of muscle weakness. Pain and paraesthesia are segmental in 75% of cases and occur in 90% of cases that involve the distribution of the ulnar nerve. The pain is usually insidious and typically affects the neck, shoulder, arm, and hand. Other clinical signs that may present in relation to neurological compression, but in this case are related to the sympathetic chain, are changes in the color and temperature of the upper limb and Raynaud's syndrome.

The symptoms that appear when compression of the subclavian artery is present are those related to ischemia with trophic changes, loss of pulse, and claudication of the affected arm. Additionally, when compression of the space above the outlet predominates, i.e. the subclavian vein (the least common in TOS), edema, venous distension of the peripheral wall when attempting to drain the upper limb, or thrombosis of the vein in Paget–Schroetter syndrome can be observed.

DIAGNOSIS

The diagnosis of TOS begins with a good clinical history and physical examination. A series of Maneuvers s can be performed that force compression in the thoracic outlet and reveal the syndrome, such as the Adson test (which decreases the interscalene space and magnifies a persistent compression of the brachial plexus or subclavian artery), the costoclavicular test or military position, the hyperabduction test, and the Roos test or arm claudication.

Upon clinical suspicion, the best complementary tests to confirm this difficult diagnosis include angiography and CT angiography in different positions of the arm, where vascular compression can be visualized, and neurological conduction velocity studies to determine if compression of the brachial plexus is present. The latter type of compression is the most difficult to prove, and the best test to date consists of measuring the motor conduction velocity of the ulnar nerve. Normal measurements are 85 m/s in the thoracic outlet, 55 m/s at the elbow, 59 m/s in the forearm, and 2.5–3.5 m/s in the wrist. In patients with TOS, the conduction velocity of the ulnar nerve in the thoracic outlet drops to an average of 53 m/s, but it is considered a positive test if the velocity is less than 85 m/s, and it is a surgical indication if the velocity is less than 60 m/s.[17] However, affected TOS patients have been observed in which the tests cannot confirm this decrease in motor conduction, but the clinical presentation includes very disabling pain, and therefore, the final diagnosis is mainly clinical and symptomatic.

ANATOMICAL CONSIDERATIONS

From the upper opening of the chest, the subclavian vessels and brachial plexus cross the cervicoaxillary canal to reach the upper extremities. This cervicoaxillary canal is divided by the first rib into two sections: a proximal section composed of the scalene triangle and costoclavicular space and a distal section that consists of the armpit (axilla). In proximal TOS, more compressions are produced, and this disease is of the most interest. This space is limited above by the clavicle, below by the first rib, anteromedially by the costoclavicular ligament, and posterolaterally by the medial scalene muscle and the long thoracic nerve. The anterior scalene muscle, which is inserted in the scalene tubercle in half of the first costal arch, divides the costoclavicular space into two compartments. The subclavian vein runs through the anteromedial and the subclavian artery, and the brachial plexus pass through the posterior or scalene triangle, as shown in **Figure 18.2**.

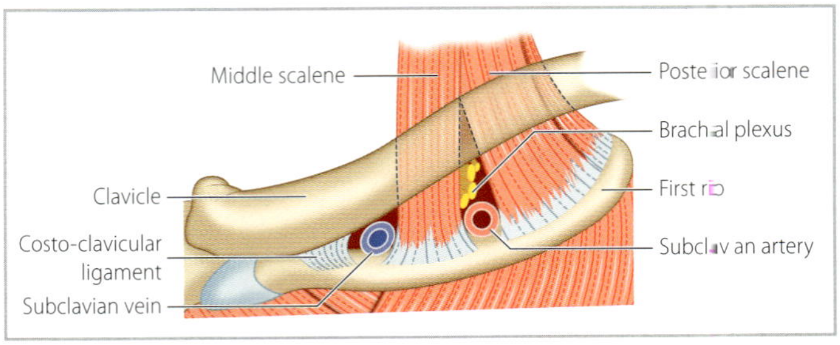

Figure 18.2 Anatomy of the costoclavicular space and scalene triangle.

Table 18.1 Surgical indications in thoracic outlet syndrome

Indications for resection of the first rib
1. Failure of conservative treatment
2. Ulnar motor conduction velocity < 60 m/s
3. Subclavian vein thrombosis (Paget–Schroetter syndrome)
4. Subclavian artery aneurysm
5. Clinical intense and acute arterial compression
m/s: meters per second

TREATMENT

Treatment of patients suffering from TOS, in principle, consists of physiotherapy and reserving surgery if that method fails. Physiotherapy in these patients should include heat massages, active exercises of the neck, and stretches of the anterior scalene, trapezius, and shoulder girdle muscles, as well as teaching them to maintain proper posture, which frees the space in the thoracic outlet. Removal of the first costal arch is indicated in situations that are listed in **Table 18.1**.

SURGICAL TECHNIQUES

Since Murphy, in 1910, resected the first rib for TOS, different techniques and approaches have been developed that include the supraclavicular, infraclavicular, transaxillary, thoracotomy, and posterior approaches and very recently, videothoracoscopy. The most commonly used methods are discussed below.

Supraclavicular approach

The supraclavicular approach presents the highest incidence of injuries to the brachial plexus, as it has the disadvantage that to gain access to the first costal arch, the surgeon must reposition the brachial plexus and subclavian vessels, which may cause possible injury to the phrenic and long thoracic nerves.

In addition, it should be noted that most patients are women, and the wound is very unsightly. However, this approach is used in hospitals with little experience with TOS, possibly due to a false sense of security from having vessels exposed before a possible hemorrhage during rib resection. It is also an approach chosen in cases where there is clear arterial failure and aneurysm of the subclavian artery that requires bypass therapy or vascular resection and anastomosis.

Posterior approach

The posterior thoracotomy technique provides a very poor visual field and also requires sectioning of very powerful back muscles such as the trapezius and rhomboids. This technique is reserved almost exclusively for cases of recurrent TOS after previous intervention for extirpation of bone remnants and brachial plexus neurolysis.

Transaxillary approach

The preferred approach in experienced hospitals is the transaxillary or the Roos technique, which has the following advantages no major muscle is sectioned, the first rib or cervical rib can be extirpated without repositioning the brachial plexus or the vessels, and the wound remains hidden in the armpit, which produces better esthetic results. In contrast, the disadvantages of this technique include that the wound is very deep, and visualization of the rib and neurovascular bundle is negligible (it is felt rather than seen, as shown in **Figure 18.3**), which requires more skill and experience than other approaches.

Videothoracoscopic approach

Finally, at the beginning of the 21st century, the possibility of removing the first rib by videothoracoscopy was described. Wolf was the first surgeon to perform this procedure at the end of the 20th century,[18] but the procedure included a very limited series, and the description of the procedure was not complete; therefore, reproducibility was not possible. In 2011, we published the resection technique of the first costal arch by videothoracoscopy. This report has aroused great interest in this technique, which has the same advantages as the transaxillary

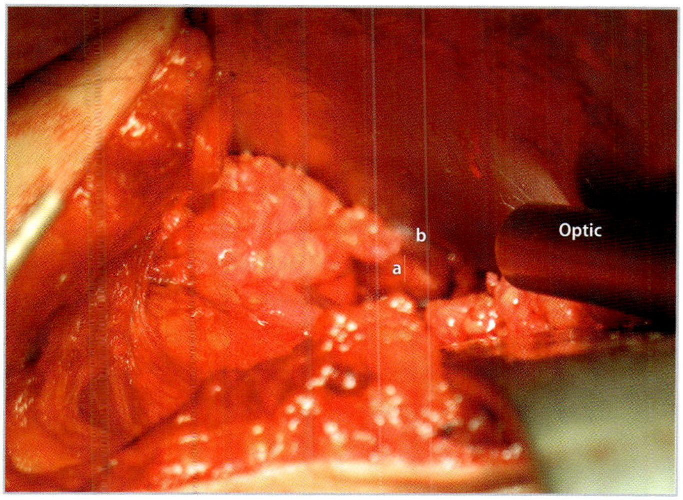

Figure 18.3 Transaxillary approach. Vision of the depth of the wound is possible with this technique using optic lighting. The edge of the rib (a) and subclavian vein (b) can be hardly located.

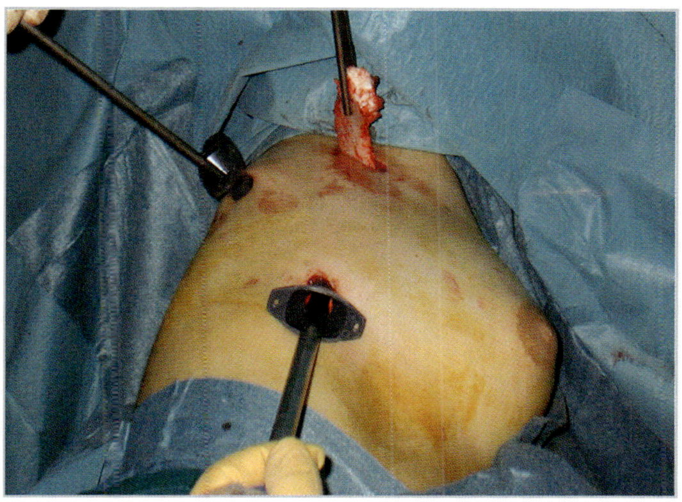

Figure 18.4 Removal of the first rib by videothoracoscopy.

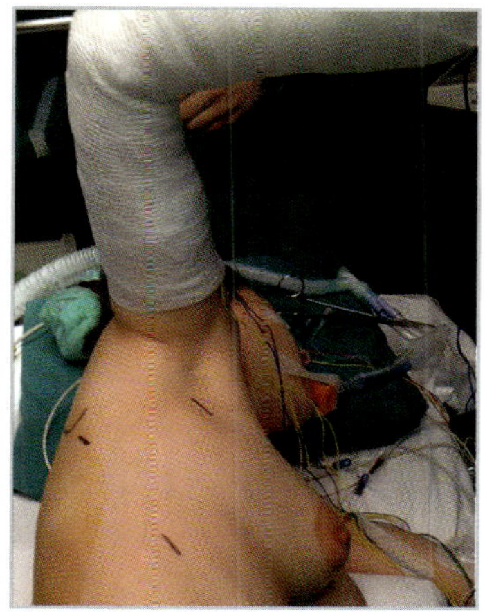

Figure 18.5 Position of the patient on the operating table for the videothoracoscopic technique.

approach (removal of the rib if traction or dissection of the vascular or neurological elements is needed) but without its disadvantages, and it produces a perfect visual field without the problem of axillary wounds (**Figure 18.4**). To date, this technique has been performed in other hospitals in the world, in some cases with the support of the da Vinci surgical robot, but there are still no studies that compare its results with other techniques.

Technique description

The patient is placed in the lateral decubitus position with their arm in fixed abduction to the arc of the operating table. The brachial plexus is monitored using interoperative neurophysiological monitoring throughout the procedure (**Figure 18.5**). We practiced three entrances: one measuring 12 mm in the 7th intercostal space in the midaxillary line for the entrance optics, another measuring 12 mm or 5 mm in the 6th intercostal space and posterior axillary line, and the last one in the 2nd or 3rd intercostal space on the border of the underarm hair. The latter entrance is extended approximately 3 cm because dissection and extraction of the first rib is performed at this location. The procedure begins with identification of the first rib, which in its anterior segment is easy, but its rear edge is hidden. The parietal pleura is opened with scissors, and electrocoagulation is performed over the first rib from front to back, starting from the internal mammary artery and continuing throughout the costal plane (**Figure 18.6a**). For the posterior segment, an ultrasonic scalpel can be used to prevent injury to structures, such as the sympathetic chain or the stellate ganglion, by electrocoagulation. Once the internal face of the rib has been exposed, dissection of the lower or external edge of the rib begins with Maurer and Semb curettes. Because the first costal arch is very flat, its external face can be seen immediately, and by pulling inwards, dissection of this plane can begin with the periosteum, taking care to not damage the subclavian vessels and the plexus. At this point, the rib mobility allows a perfect view of the neurovascular bundle above and below the costal arch, and a dissector can be passed by the upper or inner edge of the rib separating it from the subclavian artery and vein (**Figure 18.6b**). This is one of the key points of the intervention and is performed with perfect visualization, unlike the axillary approach. The next step is sectioning the anterior margin of the rib, which we carry out with the costal cartilage because it is easier to section than bone. For this step, we use Kerrison forceps, an endoscopic gouge or a discectomy (**Figure 18.6c**). After sectioning the first costal cartilage, and to completely free the front part of the rib, the strong costoclavicular ligament is sectioned, which is one of the most difficult steps of the intervention; its consistency causes it not yield to the periosteum, and it cannot be sectioned with the Kerrison forceps. Therefore, the most common approach is sectioning it with scissors or an ultrasonic scalpel with strict visual control of the subclavian vein. Once this ligament is released, the rib easily descends to traction and is only anchored by the scalene muscles that can be easily sectioned with a perfect visual field of the veins, arteries, and brachial plexus (**Figure 18.6d**). The anterior scalene muscle is sectioned near the scalene tubercle of the first rib with an ultrasonic scalpel to prevent injuries to the phrenic nerve, and the medial scalene muscle can be deinserted along with the periosteum from the first costal arch without damaging the long thoracic nerve.

Finally, rib dissection is continued dorsally while disinsertion of its vertebral articulations is performed to extract the rib in one piece (**Figure 18.7**). In other cases, there is no choice but to section the rib as dorsally as possible with a costotome, and the bone remnants are removed with rongeurs; injuries of the C8 and T1 roots of the brachial

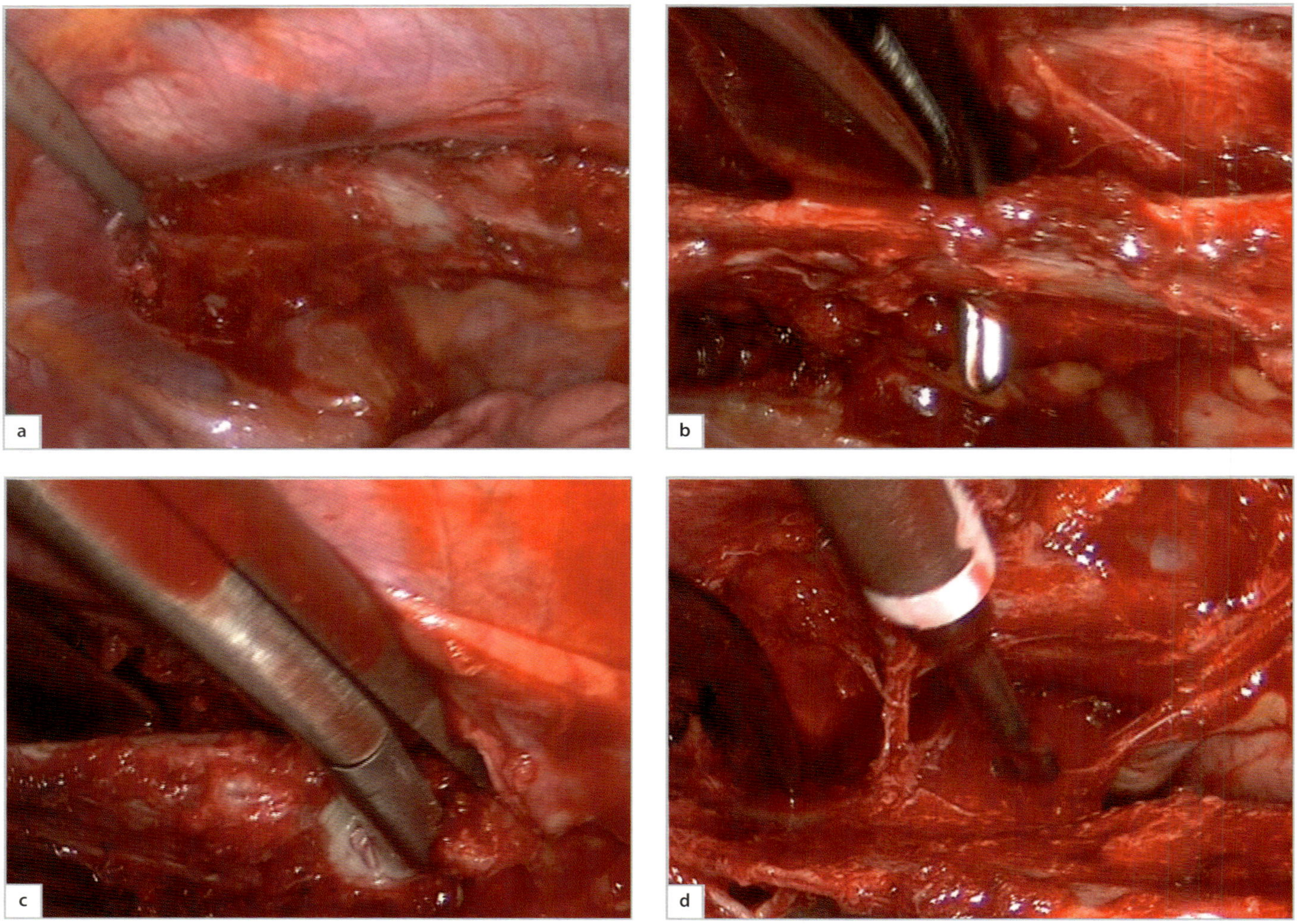

Figure 18.6 (a) Endoscopic view of the first costal arch. (b) Dissection of the first rib. (c) Sectioning of the costal cartilage. (d) Dividing of the anterior scalene muscle.

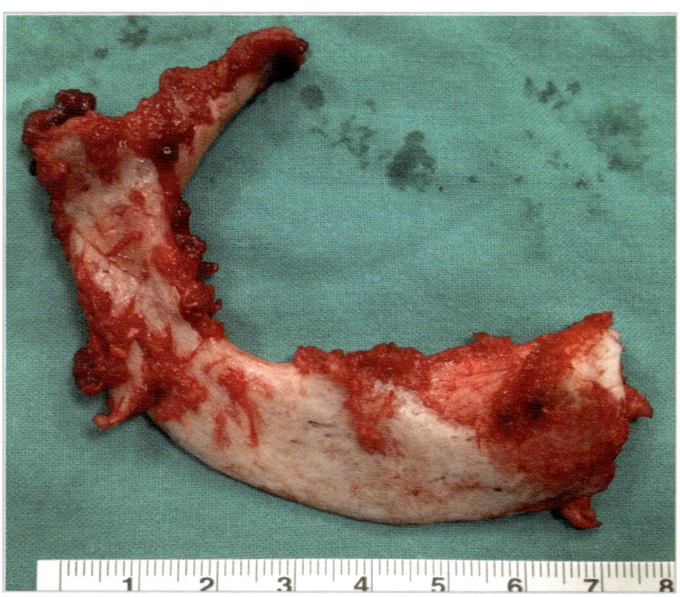

Figure 18.7 The first rib is completely removed by videothoracoscopy.

plexus are avoided. The rib is removed through the upper entrance. Hemostasis is thoroughly reviewed, and a 19F pleural drainage tube is placed. At the time of wound closure, it is only necessary to suture the skin.

In recent years, in our institution, we have operated on 20 cases of TOS by removing the first costal arch by videothoracoscopy, which has shown very good results, similar to those published to date in the literature.[19,20] With regard to the literature and a comparative study of other techniques that we are conducting, we propose that removal of the first rib for surgical treatment of TOS by videothoracoscopy is a feasible, safe, and reproducible procedure, and very good results have been obtained with very low morbidity. Moreover, compared to the technique of resecting the first costal arch by the transaxillary approach, videothoracoscopy appears to result in shorter hospitalization time.

In our experience, videothoracoscopy is an especially useful technique in obese patients or patients with Paget–Schroetter syndrome because it obviates dissection of the wall (with many newly formed or dilated vessels), and in this type of subject the transaxillary route is very difficult, technically complex, and produces high morbidity.

Nevertheless, studies with a larger number of cases are needed to obtain consistent evidence regarding which is the best approach for costal resection in TOS.

REFERENCES

1. Peet RM, Hendriksen JD, Anderson TP, Martin GM. Thoracic outlet syndrome: evaluation of the therapeutic exercise program. Proc Mayo Clin 1956; 31:281–287.
2. Adson AW, Coffey JR. Cervical rib: a method of anterior approach for relief of symptoms by division of the scalenus anticus. Ann Surg 1927; 85:839–857.
3. Coote H. Pressure on the axillary vessels and nerves by an exostosis from a cervical rib; interference with the circulation of the arm; removal of the rib and exostosis, recovery. Med Times Gaz 1861; 2:108.
4. Paget J. Clinical Lectures and Essays. London: Longmans Green, 1875.
5. Von Schroetter L. Erkrankungen der Gefasse. In: Nothnagel CWH, (Ed). Handbuch der Pathologie und Therapie. Vienna: Holder, 1884.
6. Law AA. Adventitious ligaments simulating cervical ribs. Ann Surg 1920; 72:497–499.
7. Ochsner A, Gage M, DeBakey M. Scalenus anticus (Naffziger) syndrome. Am J Surg 1935; 28:699.
8. Brintnall ES, Hyndman OR, Van Alien WM. Costoclavicular compression associated with cervical rib. Ann Surg 1956; 144:921.
9. Wright IS. The neurovascular syndrome produced by hyperabduction of the arm. Am Heart J 1945; 29:1–19.
10. Bramwell E. Lesion of the first dorsal nerve root. Rev Neurol Psychiatr 1903; 1:236.
11. Murphy T. Brachial neuritis caused by pressure of first rib. Aust Med J 1910; 15:582–585.
12. Brickner WM. Brachial plexus pressure by the normal first rib. Ann Surg 1927; 85:858.
13. Clagett OT. Presidential address: Research and prosearch. J Urol Nephrol (Paris) 1962; 44:153–166.
14. Falconer MA, Li FWP. Resection of the first rib in costoclavicular compression of the brachial plexus. Lancet 1962; 1:59–63.
15. Roos DB. Transaxillary approach for first rib resection to relieve thoracic outlet syndrome. Ann Surg 1966; 163:354–358.
16. Urschel HC Jr. Anatomy of the thoracic outlet. Thorac Surg Clin 2007; 17:511–520.
17. Loscertales J, Congregado M, Merchan RJ. First rib resection using videothoracocopy for the treatment of thoracic outlet syndrome. Arch Bronconeumol 2011; 47:204–207.
18. Urschel HC Jr, Razzuk MA, Wood RE, et al. Objective diagnosis (ulnar nerve conduction velocity) and current therapy of the thoracic outlet syndrome. Ann Thorac Surg 1971; 12:608–620.
19. Ohtsuka T, Wolf RK, Dunsker SB. Port-access first-rib resection. Surg Endosc 1999; 13:940–942.
20. Ghefter MC, Yoshida WB, Cataneo DC, et al. Thoracic outlet syndrome – cervical rib resection by video-assisted thoracoscopic surgery. J Vasc Bras 2012; 11:219–225.

Chapter 19 Management of chylothorax

Benjamin Wei, Robert Cerfolio

INTRODUCTION

The development of chylothorax may occur de novo or as a postoperative complication. An undrained chylothorax may lead to respiratory difficulty due to compression of the lung. Even after drainage proper management of chylothorax is critical because of the negative immunologic and nutritional effects of prolonged loss of lymphatic fluid from the body. The mortality rate of untreated chylothorax may reach 50%.[1] Minimally invasive techniques for drainage, pleurodesis, and thoracic duct ligation have decreased the surgical impact of intervention for chylothorax.

INITIAL EVALUATION

Generally, the etiology of the chylothorax may be surmised by the patient's history. Iatrogenic chylothorax may occur after lung resection, esophageal resection, or congenital cardiac surgery. Procedures involving cannulation of the subclavian vein, such as pacemaker implantation and central line insertion, and operations in the neck more rarely result in chylothorax. Excluding cases resulting from iatrogenic injury, malignancy is the most common cause of chylothorax. Hematologic malignancies such as lymphoma and chronic lymphocytic leukemia, and primary and metastatic cancers infiltrating the lung and/or lymphatic channels of the chest are the usual culprits. Obstruction of the thoracic ducts due to congenital malformations, radiation, tuberculosis, and fibrosing processes may result in the development of chylothorax due to increased hydrostatic pressure. Lymphangioleiomyomatosis (LAM) is a rare but notable cause of chylothorax. Finally, chylothorax may be idiopathic, although many of these patients are eventually found to harbor a malignancy of some kind.

Lymphatic fluid can leak from the thoracic duct anywhere along its course from the diaphragmatic hiatus to the junction with the subclavian vein, or from its tributaries in the mediastinum. Uncommonly, chylous fluid from the abdomen can traverse the diaphragm resulting in chylothorax.

The presentation of the patient with chylothorax depends on whether the patient already has a chest tube in place. In patients without a chest tube, chylothorax manifests as a pleural effusion; in patients with a pre-existing chest tube, it may be suspected if there is a 'milky' consistency to the drainage or drainage is excessive or occurs for an unusually prolonged length of time. One difficult to diagnosis scenario is a chylothorax after pneumonectomy. Since the hemithoracic fills with fluid it is only suspected when a patient has a larger than expected mediastinal shift and severe shortness of breath and a tap of the pleural effusion shows a milky effluent and chyle.

Pleural fluid testing to confirm the presence of chylothorax is warranted. A triglyceride level of > 110 mg/dL is diagnostic of chylothorax.[2] Occasionally, the level will be < 110 mg/dL in the presence of chylothorax, especially in a patient who is fasting. If suspicion remains high for chylothorax, the pleural fluid should be examined for chylomicrons by lipoprotein electrophoresis.

If the chest radiograph shows that the pleural space is well drained, further imaging may not be necessary. If undrained fluid is suspected, a computed tomography (CT) scan is warranted to evaluate the characteristics of the effusion and to differentiate it from a parenchymal process. Laboratory values such as prealbumin, transferrin, and albumin may be useful for monitoring the patient's nutritional status, but are not essential for planning the management of chylothorax.

NONOPERATIVE MANAGEMENT

The first consideration in management of chylothorax is often whether or not it is well-drained. If a moderate to large effusion exists, the patient will often have dyspnea warranting drainage. This may be accomplished by thoracentesis, small-bore catheter placement, or tube thoracostomy. Once the effusion is drained, medical intervention is initiated. Octreotide injections (200 mg every 8 hours subcutaneously) are started. Gastrointestinal side effects (nausea, vomiting, diarrhea) can occur and blood sugar should be monitored, especially in diabetic patients. Oral intake is stopped, and the patient started on a medium-chain triglyceride (MCT) diet, which typically consists of 1 tablespoon of supplementation 3–4 times per day. If chylous output continues to be significant, either manifesting as reaccumulation or via chest tube output, total parenteral nutrition (TPN) and NPO status may be necessary. In patients with a malignant or autoimmune etiology, treatment of the underlying disease often leads to resolution of the chylothorax.

Operative intervention for chylothorax should be considered when continued output/reaccumulation occurs in spite of nonoperative interventions. For patients with either high-output (> 1 L/day) or postesophagectomy chylothoraces, surgery should be considered earlier. Our recently published algorithm and management strategy for post-lung resection chylothoraces is shown in **Figure 19.1**.[3]

Thoracic duct embolization/disruption

Embolization of the thoracic duct may be considered if surgical therapy for chylothorax is not desired or fails. Pedal lymphangiography is performed, and once the cisterna chyli is opacified, percutaneous access to it via a transabdominal approach is achieved. After the leak is identified, embolization of the thoracic duct below the leak can be done with coils or glue. If catheterization of the cisterna chyli is unsuccessful, needle interruption/disruption of the thoracic duct can be accomplished. The efficacy of thoracic duct embolization/disruption has been ~70% in resolving chylothorax in the largest reported series.[4-6] The expertise needed for pedal lymphangiography and thoracic duct embolization can limit the application of this method to larger centers experience in the technique.

OPERATIVE MANAGEMENT

The choice of operation depends on the radiographic appearance of the chest in terms of side and presence/absence of loculations. Pleurodesis alone can be very successful, although generally we perform thoracic duct ligation as well if a chylothorax is located predominantly on the right side. If bilateral effusions are present, we recommend that the side with the more significant effusion be operated on. The effusion on the opposite side may respond to thoracentesis or catheter drainage alone. If the chylothorax is after esophagectomy and the patient

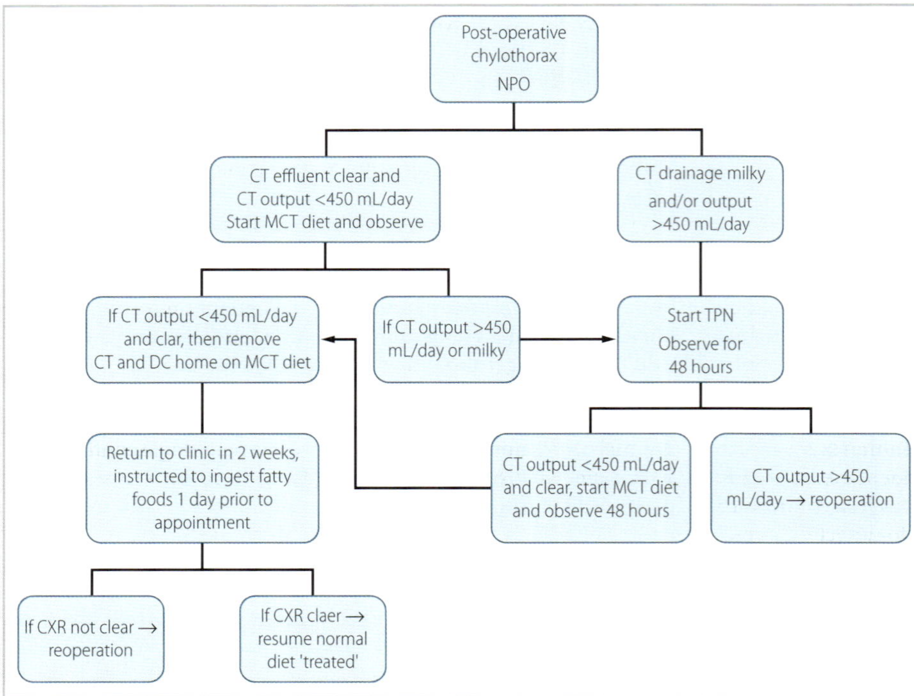

Figure 19.1 Management approach for patients with chylothorax occurring after lung resection.

had a right-sided dissection, we prefer to go back in the right chest robotically or laparoscopically to clip it at the diaphragmatic hiatus.

VATS drainage of effusion/ decortication

Patients with a loculated effusion generally benefit from operative drainage and decortication rather than simple chest tube drainage. VATS has been shown to be a very effective technique for decortication, resulting in decreased operative time and length of stay and fewer postoperative complications compared to decortication via thoracotomy.[6] Decortication may be accomplished with a variety of 2-port and 3-port techniques. We have found the use of a camera port in the 8th intercostal space and a ~3-cm utility port in either the 5th or 6th intercostal space anteriorly to be effective in nearly all cases. The use of the extra-small Alexis wound retractor (Applied Medical; Rancho Santa Margarita, CA) for the utility port is helpful in allowing greater ease of insertion of VATS instruments as well as avoiding the loss of maneuverable space around the lung during suctioning. The use of a 10-mm suction instrument (Scanlan International; Saint Paul, MN) is useful when dealing with semi-solid or gelatinous fluid. Principles of surgery include:

- Complete release of the lower lobe from the diaphragmatic surface
- Removing peel from trapped lung
- Avoidance of injuries to structures such as the azygos vein, mammary vessels, and phrenic nerve
- Complete drainage of significant pockets of fluid

For patients with minimal adhesions and no peel, uniportal VATS drainage of effusion can be accomplished through a single-port in the 8th intercostal space. Other authors have reported the utility of uniportal VATS for pleural effusions.[8]

VATS pleurodesis

Pleurodesis should be considered in patients with refractory chylothorax or patients who are going to the operating room anyway for VATS to deal with a loculated effusion caused by chyle. Pleurodesis is generally warranted also in patients going to the operating room for thoracic duct ligation, as it adds little time or risk to the procedure. In addition, patients with a left-sided chylothorax may first be approached with VATS drainage accompanied by pleurodesis alone, as the thoracic duct is more difficult to access from the left chest.

Pleurodesis can be achieved by either chemical or mechanical means. Chemical agents used include talc and doxycycline. The efficacy of chemical pleurodesis is better studied in the treatment of malignant effusions. Most studies of patients with pleural effusions treated with pleurodesis (not limited to those with chylothorax) have demonstrated an increased efficacy of talc (80–90%) compared to doxycycline (50–70%). Studies of pleurodesis specifically in chylothorax patients are summarized in **Table 19.1**. Disadvantages of talc include the risk of developing acute respiratory distress syndrome, which can be decreased by limiting the dose to <5 g, and possible carcinogenic risk, although this may not be applicable to purified forms of pharmaceutical-grade talc used typically in the operating room.[9]

No head-to-head comparison of the different chemical agents or chemical versus mechanical pleurodesis exists for patients specifically with chylothorax. Our general preference is to use talc for older patients, patients with known malignancy, and patients

Table 19.1 Studies of patients with chylothorax undergoing pleurodesis

Author	Number of patients	Etiology	Agent used	Success rate (%)
Mares et al.[18]	19	Lymphoma	Talc, poudrage	100
Paul et al.[19]	6	Multiple	Talc	83
Cho et al.[20]	27	Pulmonary resection	Talc, minocycline	100
Akin et al.[21]	26	Pulmonary resection	Talc	73
Peillon et al.[22]	4	Spontaneous	Talc	100

Table 19.2 Commonly used dosages for chemical pleurodesis

Agent	Dosage
Talc	5 g powder (poudrage)
	5 g in 50 mL normal saline (slurry)
Doxycycline	500 mg
Iodine	20 mL of 10% solution

with chylothorax refractory to thoracic duct ligation and/or other mechanical/chemical pleurodesis. Mechanical and/or doxycycline pleurodesis is reasonable in younger patients without malignancy undergoing VATS pleurodesis for the first time. The use of iodine has also been shown to be safe and effective in other settings, such as pneumothorax and malignant pleural effusion, and could be considered for chylothorax as well.[10,11] The standard dose for commonly used agents for pleurodesis is shown in **Table 19.2**.

In terms of method of delivery, no definitive evidence exists for the superiority of bedside instillation versus VATS pleurodesis; the former may be preferred in patients with a very limited life expectancy and/or prohibitive medical or pulmonary comorbidities.

Minimally invasive (VATS or robotic) thoracic duct ligation

Ligation of the thoracic duct is can be performed either in the right or left chest. The thoracic duct traverses the diaphragm in the left hemithorax via the aortic hiatus, and then ascends in the right chest running parallel between the aorta and azygos vein (**Figure 19.2**). The duct can be interrupted anywhere along this part of its course through the thorax, although we have found it most easily accessed through the right chest near the level of the inferior pulmonary vein. At this location, the thoracic duct is found running parallel between the azygos vein and the aorta. The esophagus may need to be partially mobilized to identify the duct. The duct then crosses to the left side at the level of the 5th thoracic vertebra, exist the chest and enters the neck where it rises above the clavicle and generally drains near where the left internal jugular vein meets the left subclavian vein. Injuries to the duct can therefore occur during surgery in the lower neck.

Zoetmulder et al. were the first to report thoracoscopic ligation of the thoracic duct in 1994.[12] Ingestion of heavy cream the night before duct ligation can assist in the identification of the duct, although is not strictly necessary. We recommend performing duct ligation prior to pleurodesis if both procedures are to be done in the same sitting, so that visibility is not compromised during identification of the thoracic duct. Any number of ports can be used; it is helpful to have the working port(s) placed anteriorly as the target area is located in the posterior portion of the hemithorax. Our standard port positioning is shown in **Figure 19.3**.

First, the inferior pulmonary ligament is divided and the esophagus is mobilized anteriorly. The lung can be retracted anteriorly; alternatively, a nearly prone position can assist in visualization. The thoracic duct is identified between the azygos vein and the aorta. Either direct ligation of the duct may be performed, which is our preferred technique, or mass ligature of the tissue between the azygos vein and the aorta may be done. If direct ligation is chosen, the thoracic duct may be interrupted with clips or a ligature. The duct is generally divided, although this is not required. Frozen section pathologic confirmation of thoracic duct tissue can be obtained if the surgeon is unsure about

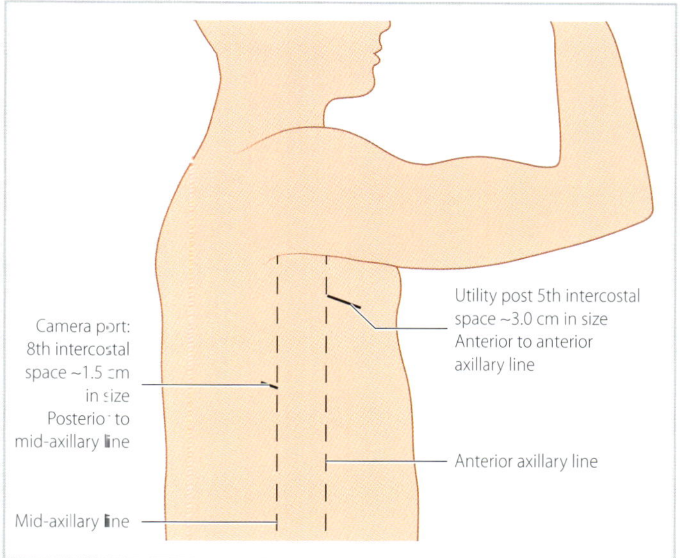

Figure 19.3 VATS port positioning for thoracic duct ligation.

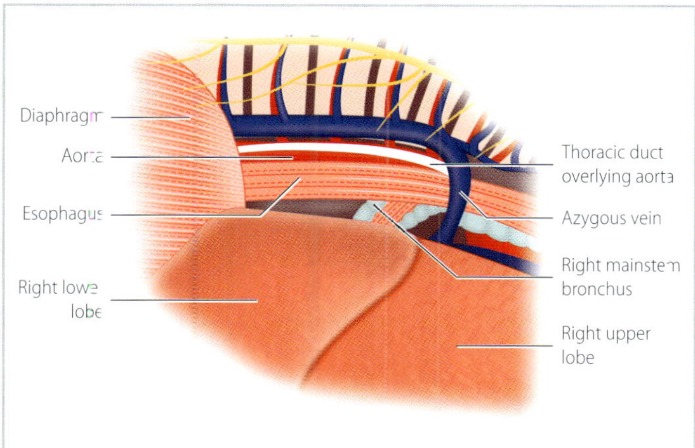

Figure 19.2 Location of thoracic duct in the right hemithorax during VATS.

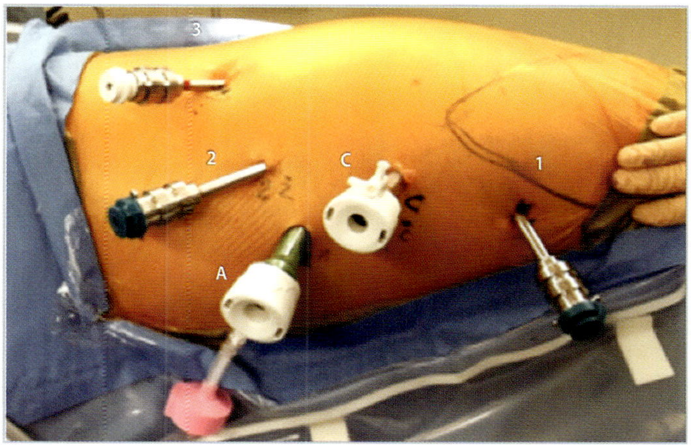

Figure 19.4 Robotic port positioning for thoracic duct ligation: (C) camera port (1) robotic arm 1 (2) robotic arm 2 (3) robotic arm 3 (A) assistant port.

whether or not the structure divided is the thoracic duct. Mass ligation is a good choice when the duct cannot be definitively identified. Multiple sutures are placed surrounding the tissue between the azygos vein and aorta overlying the vertebral body.[13]

Pleurodesis is done if indicated, and a single chest tube can be left in the chest. There is no clear advantage of suction or water seal in this situation, although we generally prefer suction for 24–48 hours if pleurodesis is added. We advance the diet over the next 24–48 hours from clears to a low-fat diet. The chest tube may be removed when the output is < 200 mL/day and the quality of the output is serous rather than milky. Large scale studies of the efficacy of VATS thoracic duct ligation comparing it open ligation have not been done, but most case series report excellent results with an 80–100% success rate12.[14]

A single case of robotic thoracic duct ligation for chylothorax has been reported in the literature, although some routinely perform the procedure prophylactically during robotic esophagectomy.[15] Patient and port positioning is similar to esophagectomy, and shown in **Figure 11.4**. Robotic arm no. 3 may not be necessary for this procedure. The thoracic duct is identified and ligated as described in the above section. The advantages and disadvantages of robotic as opposed to VATS for thoracic duct ligation mirror those of robotic versus VATS in general. Namely, robotic technology generally permits for a better view and better dexterity, while being more expensive and requiring specialized training.

Laparoscopic thoracic duct ligation

Uncommonly, a laparoscopic approach to ligating the thoracic duct may be favored over VATS. Patients with a hostile chest, contraindications to single-lung ventilation, or who have failed VATS thoracic duct ligation may be better candidates for the procedure. Patient and port positioning resembles that for laparoscopic Nissen fundoplication or gastric mobilization during esophagectomy. A liver retractor is used to expose the diaphragmatic hiatus after the patient is placed in reverse Trendelenburg position. The gastrohepatic ligament is divided and the right crus of the diaphragm identified. The esophagus is mobilized and retracted to the patient's left. The thoracic duct is identified to the right of the aorta on top of the vertebral body and ligated. Successful resolution of chylothorax with laparoscopic thoracic duct ligation has been reported in a few case reports.[16,17]

REFERENCES

1. Cerfolio RJ. Chylothorax after esophagogastrectom. Thorac Surg Clin 2006; 16:49–52.
2. Maldonado F, Hawkins FJ, Daniels CE, et al. Pleural fluid characteristics of chylothorax. Mayo Clin Proc 2009; 84:129.
3. Bryant AS, Minnich DJ, Wei B, Cerfolio RJ. The incidence and management of postoperative chylothorax after pulmonary resection and thoracic mediastinal lymph node dissection. Ann Thorac Surg 2014; 98:232–237.
4. Marcon F, Irani K, Aquino T, et al. Percutaneous treatment of thoracic duct injuries. Surg Endosc 2011; 25:2844–2848.
5. Itkin M, Kucharczuk JC, Kwak A, et al. Nonoperative thoracic duct embolization for traumatic thoracic duct leak: experience in 109 patients. J Thorac Cardiovasc Surg 2010; 139:584–589.
6. Boffa DJ, Sands MJ, Rice TW, et al. A critical evaluation of a percutaneous diagnostic and treatment strategy for chylothorac after thoracic surgery. Eur J Cardiothorac Surg 2008; 33:435–439.
7. Tong BC, Hanna J, Toloza EM, et al. Outcomes of video-assisted thoracoscopic decortication. Ann Thorac Surg 2010; 89:220–225.
8. Alar T, Ozcelik C. Single-incision thoracoscopic surgery of pleural effusions for diagnosis and treatment. Surg Endosc 2013; 27:4333–4336.
9. Wehner AP. Cosmetic talc should not be listed as a carcinogen: comments on NTP's deliberations to list talc as a carcinogen. Regul Toxicol Pharmacol 2002; 36:40–50.
10. Mohsen TA, Zeid AA, Meshref M, et al. Local iodine pleurodesis versus thoracoscopic talc insufflation in recurrent malignant pleural effusion: a prospective randomized control trial. Eur J Cardiothorac Surg 2011; 40:282–286.
11. Agarwal R, Paul AS, Aggarwal AN et al. A randomized controlled trial of the efficacy of cosmetic talc compared with iodopovidone for chemical pleurodesis. Respirology 2011; 16:1064–1069.
12. Zoetmulder Frans, Rutgers E, Baas P. Thoracoscopic ligation of a thoracic duct leakage. Chest 1994; 106:1233–1234.
13. Christodoulou M, Ris H, Pezzetta E. Video-assisted right supradiaphragmatic thoracic duct ligation for non-traumatic recurrent chylothorax. Eur J Cardiothorac Surg 2006; 29:810–814.
14. Wurnig PN, Hollaus PH, Ohtsuka T, et al. Thoracoscopic direct clipping of the thoracic duct for chylopericardium and chylothorax. Ann Thorac Surg 2000; 70:1662–1665.
15. Thompson KJ, Kernstine KH, Grannis FW, et al. Treament of chylothorax by robotic thoracic duct ligation. Ann Thorac Surg 2008; 85:334–336.
16. Vassallo BC, Cavadas D, Beveraggi E, Sivori E. Treatment of postoperative chylothorax through laparoscopic thoracic duct ligation. Eur J Cardiothorac Surg 2002; 21:556–557.
17. Tsubokawa N, Hamai Y, Hihara J, et al. Laparoscopic thoracic duct clipping for persistent chylothorax after extrapleural pneumonectomy. Ann Thorac Surg 2012; 93:e131–132.
18. 18. Mares DC, Mathur PN. Medical thoracoscopic talc pleurodesis for chylothorax due to lymphoma: a case series. Chest 198; 114: 731-5.
19. 19. Paul S, Altorki NK Port JL, Stiles BM, Lee PC. Surgical management of chylothorax. Thorac Cardiovasc Surg 2009; 57: 226-8.
20. 20. Cho HJ, Kim DK, Lee GD et al. Chylothorax complicating pulmonary resection for lung cancer: effective management and pleurodesis. Ann Thorac Surg 2014; 97: 408-13.
21. 21. Akin H, Olcmen A, Isgorucu O et al. Appraoch to patients with chylothorax complicating pulmonary resection. Thorac Cardiovasc Surg 2012; 60: 135-9.
22. 22. Peillon C, D'Hont C, Melki J et al. Usefulness of video thoracoscopy in the management of spontaneous and postoperation chylothorax. Surg Endosc 1999; 13: 1106-9.

Chapter 20 VATS plication of the diaphragm

Nur Ismail, Joel Dunning, Pankaj Mishra

INTRODUCTION

Eventration of the diaphragm is an umbrella term describing a rare condition in which the right or left hemidiaphragm, or both have ascended abnormally high into the chest. The muscle retains its continuity without any defect, the insertions are normal and there is no interruption in the pleural or peritoneal layers.[1-5] In congenital cases, the elevated hemidiaphragm may appear normal or show degeneration of varying degree – thin membranes without muscular fibers. Even in extensive cases, this thinning is noted to be limited to the central portion of the diaphragm.[1] In acquired cases, there is a loss of contractility of the diaphragm that leads to progressive muscular atrophy, thinning and distension of the dome. Diaphragmatic paralysis is often described in conjunction with diaphragmatic eventration in literature. Although they are technically different, they give rise to the same physiological disturbance and radiological findings. The goal of treatment is also the same, which is to reduce dysfunctional caudal excursion of the diaphragm during inspiration by plication.

The physiological consequences of diaphragmatic dysfunction include atelectasis and ventilation – perfusion mismatch, preferential redistribution of pulmonary blood flow to the contralateral lung, paradoxical movement of the affected hemidiaphragm, and shift of the mediastinum to the contralateral side. Furthermore, the positive intra-abdominal pressure pushes the diaphragm upwards, creating a vicious cycle and worsening pulmonary function.

Etiology

Diaphragmatic dysfunction may be congenital or acquired. Acquired causes could be due to trauma, iatrogenic, e.g. damage to phrenic nerve during harvest of internal mammary artery for coronary artery bypass grafting; neoplastic disease, e.g. lung cancer invading the phrenic nerve; Infection such as herpes zoster, diptheria or influenza. Neuromuscular disorders on the other hand typically give bilateral diaphragmatic paralysis, which includes multiple sclerosis, myopathies, muscular dystrophy, Guillain–Barré syndrome, and Parsonage–Turner syndrome (**Table 20.1**).

Table 20.1 Causes of diaphragmatic dysfunction

Causes
Congenital
Idiopathic
Phrenic nerve injury: • Iatrogenic • Malignancy • Trauma
Phrenic mononeuritis: • Diabetes • Vasculitis • Infection
Neuromuscular disorders: • Multiple sclerosis • Poliomyelitis • Myopathies • Muscular dystrophies • Parsonage–Turner syndrome

Presentation

Most adult patients remain asymptomatic and the diagnosis is made incidentally after chest radiography.

Respiratory symptoms include dyspnea, cough, chest pain and recurrent chest infection due to the associated atelectasis from the compression of the basal part of the lung.

Abdominal symptoms such as dyspepsia, nausea, vomiting and belching have also been described. These symptoms are probably due to the displacement of abdominal contents upward.

Cardiac symptoms are rare but include palpitations and arrhythmia, probably owing to the displacement of the mediastinum.

Complications such as diaphragmatic rupture, gastric rupture and gastric or splenic flexure volvulus have been described in literature.[6-10]

INVESTIGATIONS

Imaging

A high-riding hemidiaphragm is almost always picked up on the chest radiograph (**Figure 20.1**). On a lateral film, the difference of level between the normal and the elevated leaf may be more appreciated than it appears from the AP film. Fluoroscopy and sniff test is useful in confirming the diagnosis of unilateral diaphragmatic dysfunction. Sniffing during a fluoroscopy may reveal paradoxical movements of a diaphragm; however it is not as useful in diagnosing bilateral diaphragmatic paralysis.[11] Ultrasound scan has a benefit of being more accessible, portable and less radiation than fluoroscopy. Lack of thickening of diaphragm in inspiration is consistent with diaphragmatic paralysis.[12] CT scan is not routinely performed to evaluate diaphragmatic function, however it is useful in excluding diaphragmatic hernia and in cases of trauma or suspected underlying malignancy, which helps in preoperative planning. MRI scan although costly, could also be used to exclude diaphragmatic rupture (**Figure 20.2**). It has the advantage of obtaining sequential images that can reveal dynamic changes in the diaphragm during inspiration that may be more useful than still MRI.[13]

LUNG FUNCTION TEST

Patients with diaphragmatic weakness or paralysis will have a marked fall in the FVC in supine position compared to standing or sitting. This is due to the gravitational effect on the abdominal content in erect posture. The lying FVC in a normal diaphragm is 5–10% less than

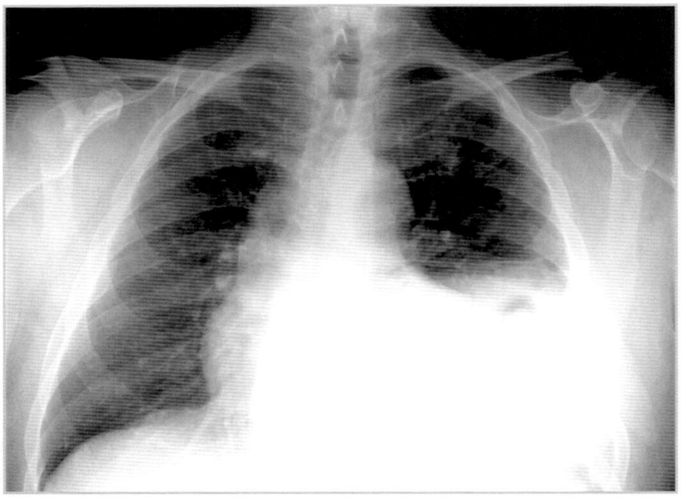

Figure 20.1 Chest radiograph showing high riding left hemidiaphragm.

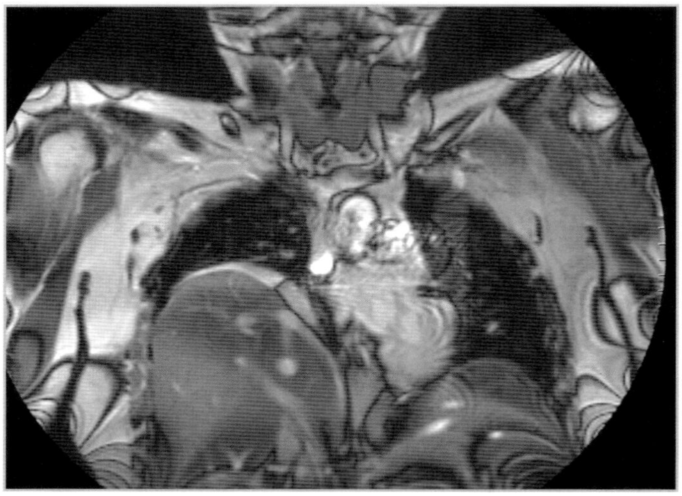

Figure 20.2 MRI showing paralytic/high-riding right hemidiaphragm.

when upright, in weakened or paralysed diaphragm the lying FVC is 30% less than in erect posture.[14]

MANAGEMENT

Although diaphragmatic eventration/paralysis is a benign condition, it has a progressive course. Surgery is indicated in symptomatic patients. The aim of surgery is to reduce the abundant diaphragmatic surface and to lower the diaphragmatic dome. This returns the abdominal contents back to their normal position, prevents the displacement of mediastinum, and allows for greater lung expansion. Diaphragmatic plication could be approached via thoracotomy, VATS or robotics.

OPERATIVE TECHNIQUES (VATS PLICATION OF DIAPHRAGM)

The first report of a surgical repair was published by Morrison in 1923. Since then various techniques and approaches have been employed.

Plication of diaphragm by VATS was first described in 1995 by Gharagozloo.[15] A year later, Mouroux reported a more technically applicable VATS procedure – performed through two ports and a 4-cm mini thoracotomy, diaphragm is pushed down to create a transverse fold, using two superposed back and forth continuous sutures. The first suture starts from periphery and proceeds to cardiophrenic angle, invaginating the abundant diaphragm and maintaining its excess inside the abdomen. The second suture stretches the dome at the desired tension.[16]

One of the challenges of plicating the diaphragm through minimally invasive approach is the estimation of tension and feel of the diaphragm during the procedure. The advantages of minimally invasive approach are less postoperative pain, earlier hospital discharge and better cosmesis.

Various techniques have been described for VATS plication of the diaphragm: number of ports, plication techniques (sutures versus staplers, interrupted versus continuous, pledged versus non-pledgeted, direction of plication).

Visouli et al. described a three-port VATS technique with oblique plication line starting from cardiophrenic recess to costophrenic recess using nylon sutures, U-stitches and Teflon pledgets. The diaphragm is incised if there is suspicion of adhesion to abdominal viscera. The abundant diaphragmatic dome in between the pleats is inverted and invaginated underneath the approximated pleats (**Figure 20.3**).[17]

A four-port VATS technique was described by Hwang et al., using an oblique diaphragmatic plication. Continuous running non-absorbable suture was used, starting at the anterolateral and proceeding to posteromedial costophrenic recess, invaginating the abundant diaphragm and progressively inverting it caudally.[18]

Dunning described a three 5 mm ports technique using CO_2 insufflations to push the diaphragm down. 8–15 interrupted, pledgeted U-stitches were used, with the aid of endo-stitch. The diaphragm is invaginated so there is a layer of diaphragm under the suture line to avoid inadvertent suturing of intra-abdominal viscera.[19]

Moon et al. have described the use of endostaplers instead of stitches. The abundant diaphragm was pulled, rolled and plicated without being resected. This is repeated five times until desired tension of diaphragm achieved.[20] Reports have described rupture of staple line, torn diaphragm and herniation of intestine into the thorax following plication of diaphragm using endostaplers.[21,22] Reinforcement of staple line with sutures or patch may be of advantage when using endostaplers.

A uniportal VATS technique for plication of diaphragm has been described by Wu et al., using interrupted sutures from medial portion to the lateral, pleat is created by pushing the flaccid part downward.[23]

As thoracic surgery evolves to more minimally invasive surgery, diaphragmatic plication has followed similar approach. Robotic VATS plication has recently come to light. Several of the limitations of VATS surgery such as instrument fencing, and instrument manipulation between the ribs have been addressed and improved with the robotics approach as it allows no or minimal movement at the level of the ribs and maximal articulation and manipulation in the thoracic cavity instead. Thus, in our experience it leads to enhanced recovery with minimal postoperative discomfort.

POSTOPERATIVE CARE

Chest drain is usually removed 2–3 days after surgery when drainage is minimal. Immediate complications such as intra-abdominal viscera injury should be looked out for. Following discharge, patients are followed up in outpatient clinic with chest radiograph to ensure no recurrence or complications such as ruptured diaphragm, hernia and repair failure have occurred. Lying/supine lung function test is a useful tool to assess quality of repair and improvement in lung function test.

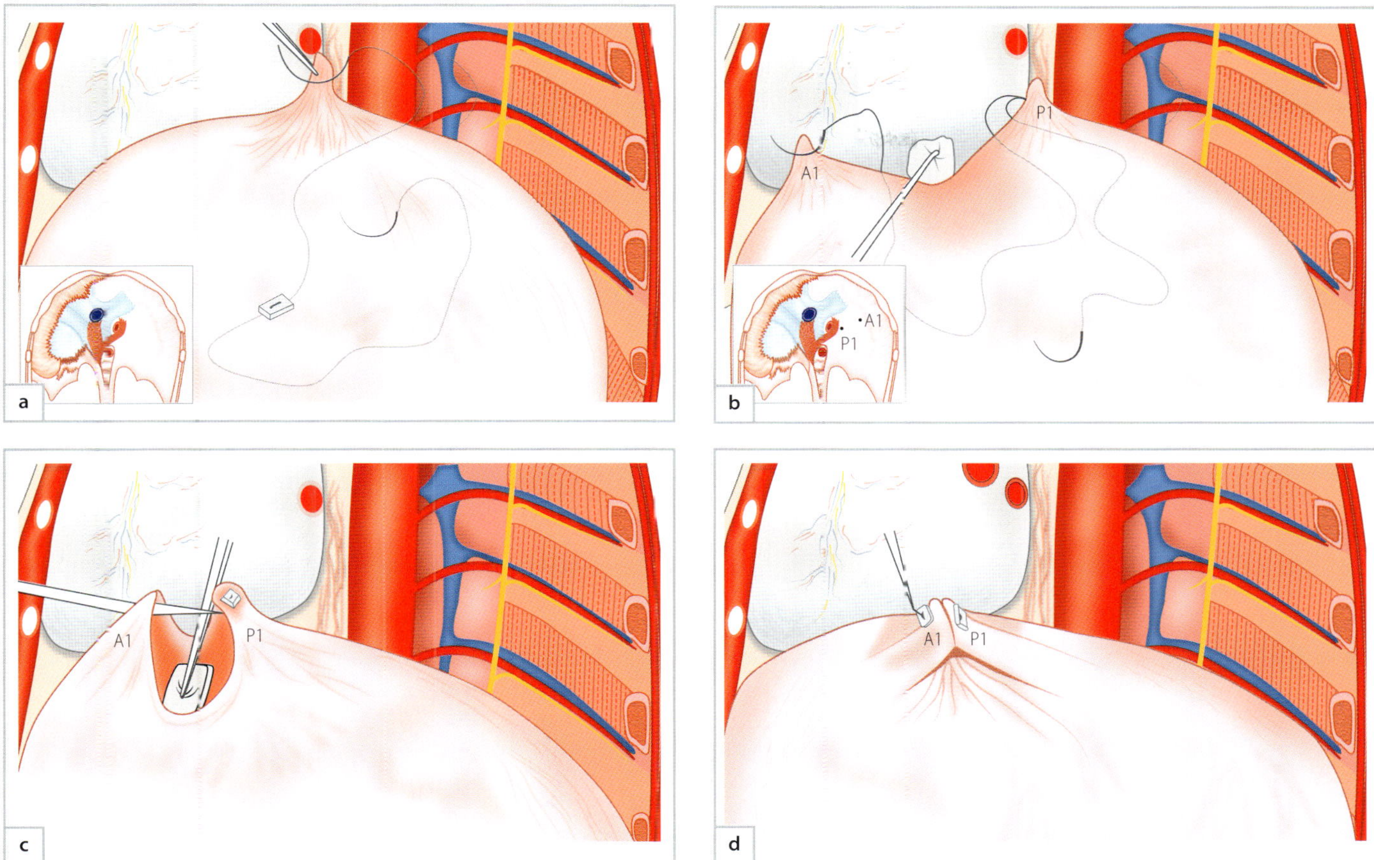

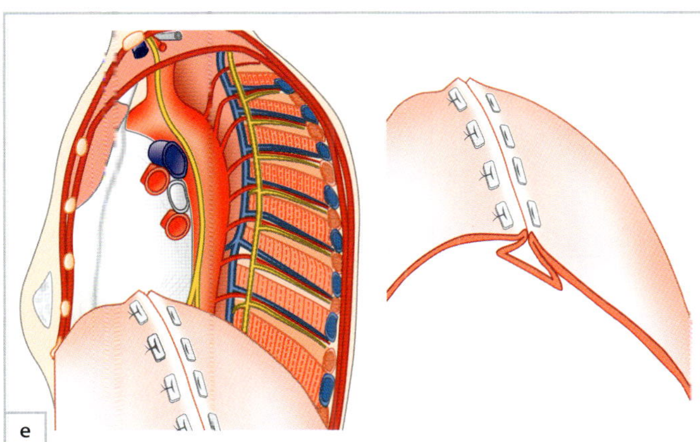

Figure 20.3 (a) Thin redundant diaphragm is lifted easily when grasped between forceps at its dome. (b) A non-absorbable, pledgetted suture is used to take generous bites on the loose redundant diaphragm and a posterior and anterior pleats are created (P1 and A1). (c) The P1 and A1 (posterior and anterior pleats) points which are reinforced with pledgetts on both sides are gently approximated; the redundant fold of diaphragm is gently pushed downward which aids in invagination of excessive diaphragm between the two pleats. (d) Approximated anterior and posterior pleats (A1 and P1). (e) By repeating the same, a line of approximation is created bringing together the anterior and posterior pleats. An oblique plication line is created starting anteromedially toward the cardiophrenic angle and progressing posterolaterally toward the costophrenic recess. Usually 8–10 such sutures are required (techniques described by Visouli et al. J Thorac Dis, with permission[17]).

REFERENCES

1. Christensen P. Eventration of the diaphragm. Thorax 1959; 14:311–318.
2. Mouroux J, Venissac N, Leo F, Alifano M, Guillot F. Surgical treatment of diaphragmatic eventration using video-assisted thoracic surgery: a prospective study. Ann Thorac Surg 2005; 79:308–312.
3. Mantoo SK, Mak K. Congenital diaphragmatic eventration in an adult: a diagnostic dilemma. Singapore Med J 2007; 48:e136–137.
4. Gatzinsky P, Lepore V. Surgical treatment of a large eventration of the left diaphragm. Eur J Cardiothorac Surg 1993; 7:271–274.
5. Nathan N, Iles PB. Acute respiratory failure with an abnormal chest radiograph. Respiration 2005; 72:205–209.
6. Morcillo-López I, Hidalgo-Mora JJ, Baamonde A, et al. Gastric and diaphragmatic rupture in early pregnancy. Interact Cardiovasc Thorac Surg 2010; 11:713–714.
7. Kanojia RP, Shanker R, Menon P, et al. Eventration with diaphragm perforation leading to secondary diaphragmatic hernia and intestinal strangulation. Hernia 2010; 14:531–533.
8. Oh A, Gulati G, Sherman ML, et al. Bilateral eventration of the diaphragm with perforated gastric volvulus in an adolescent. J Pediatr Surg 2000; 35:1824–1826.
9. Goonetilleke G. Chronic volvulus of the stomach with eventration of the diaphragm. Ceylon Med J 1995; 40:158–159.
10. Kim HS, Yoo JS, Han SJ, et al. Chronic recurrent volvulus of the colonic splenic flexure associated with the eventration of left diaphragm. Korean J Gastroenterol 2007; 49:37–40.
11. Nason LK, Walker CM, McNeeley MF, et al. Imaging of the diaphragm: anatomy and function. Radiographics 2012; 32:E51–70.

12. Cohn D, Benditt JO, Eveloff S, McCool FD. Diaphragm thickening during inspiration. J Appl Physiol 1997; 83:291–296.
13. Kiryu S, Loring SH, Mori Y. Quantitative analysis of the velocity and synchronicity of diaphragmatic motion: dynamic MRI in different postures. Magn Reson Imaging 2006; 24:1325–1332.
14. American Thoracic Society/European Respiratory Society. ATS/ERS statement on Respiratory Muscle Testing. Am J Respir Crit Care Med 2002; 166:518–624.
15. Gharagozloo F, McReynolds SD, Snyder L. Thoracoscopic placation of the diaphragm. Surg Edosc 1995; 9:1204–1206.
16. Mouroux J, Padovani B, Poirier NC, et al. Technique for the repair of diaphragmatic eventration. Ann Thorac Surg 1996; 62:905–907.
17. Visouli AN, Mpakas A, Zarogoulidis P, et al. Video-assisted thoracoscopic plication of the left hemidiaphragm in symptomatic eventration in adulthood. J Thorac Dis 2012; 4:6–16.
18. Hwang Z, Shin JS, Cho YH, Sun K, Lee IS. A simple technique for the thoracoscopic plication of the diaphragm. Chest 2003; 376–378.
19. Dunning J. "Thoracoscopic diaphragm plication." Interact Cardiovasc Thorac Surg 2015; 20:689–690.
20. Moon SW, Wang YP, Kim YW, Shim SB, Jin W. Thoracoscopic plication of diaphragmatic eventration using endostaplers. Ann Thorac Surg 2000; 70:299–300.
21. Ikeda, Masaki, Sonobe M, Bando T, Date H.. "Reconstruction of recurrent diaphragmatic eventration with an elongated polytetrafluoroethylene sheet." Interact Cardiovasc Thorac Surg 2013; 17:433–435.
22. Takanami I. Hernia of the diaphragm with gastric ulcer and volvulus: an unusual complication after diaphragmatic resection by VATS. Interact Cardiovasc Thorac Surg 2003; 2:544–546.
23. Wu HH, Chen CH, Chang H, et al. A preliminary report on the feasibility of single-port thoracoscopic surgery for diaphragm plication in the treatment of diaphragm eventration. J Cardiothorac Surg 2013; 8:224.

Chapter 21 Surgery for pectus excavatum

Marco Scarci, Benedetta Bedetti

INTRODUCTION

Pectus excavatum is a congenital deformity of the anterior chest wall consisting in the concavity of the sternum and of the costal cartilages due to an abnormal growth of the bone and of the costal cartilage (**Figure 21.1**). In pectus excavatum, the growth of bone and cartilage in the anterior chest wall is abnormal, typically affecting 4–5 ribs on each side of the sternum. The appearance of the defect widely varies, from mild to very severe cases, and some patients present with significant asymmetry between the right and left sides. The severity of the pectus can be measured by the Haller index, obtained after dividing the side diameter by the anteroposterior diameter. Normal value is 2.56, a severe condition is considered to be when the value is > 3.25.[1]

The etiopathogenesis of this deformity is still unknown, but the researchers hypothesize that a genetic disorder of the connective tissue may be involved.[2] In fact pectus excavatum is commonly associated with connective tissue disorders such as Marfan and Ehlers Danlos syndromes.[3] Despite the lack of an identifiable genetic marker, the familiar occurrence of pectus deformity is reported in 37% of cases.[4]

Valvular abnormalities are common among patients with pectus excavatum, particularly mitral valve prolapse occurs in 20% of patients with pectus excavatum.[5] Pectus anomalies in more than 80% of all cases are identified within the first 1–2 years of life and the deformity typically becomes more prominent during adolescence or early adulthood. They are three times more common in males than in females.

Patients with severe pectus excavatum often suffer from limitations in physical activity, whereas patients with mild defects are mostly asymptomatic.

The inward concavity of the anterior chest wall can displace mediastinal structures, compromise cardiac output, or impair the pulmonary function. These can significantly alter the patients' functional capacity and exercise tolerance.[6] In severe cases or in patients in which the defect directly impinges on the right ventricle, pectus excavatum is more than a cosmetic deformity.[6]

The preoperative workout should include a radiographic evaluation (**Figure 21.2**) (e.g. chest CT scan, MRI), echocardiography (**Figure 21.3**), pulmonary function tests and cardiopulmonary exercise testing.[7]

The surgical repair is indicated when the deformity is severe and has a significant functional impairment for the patients. The psychosocial issues surrounding body image can be life-altering and can affect the emotional and psychological development, as most of the patients are children or adolescents, so the surgical repair can have a benefit also regarding the psychological dimension of the patients.

The pectus surgery is easily accomplished in teenagers, who are close to the age of skeletal maturity.[8] Repair during the later stage of teenage growth allow the patient to complete their growth and have a lower chance of recurrence. Younger children with significant compromise cardiopulmonary status may also be candidates for repair; however repair at too early of an age can result in improper growth

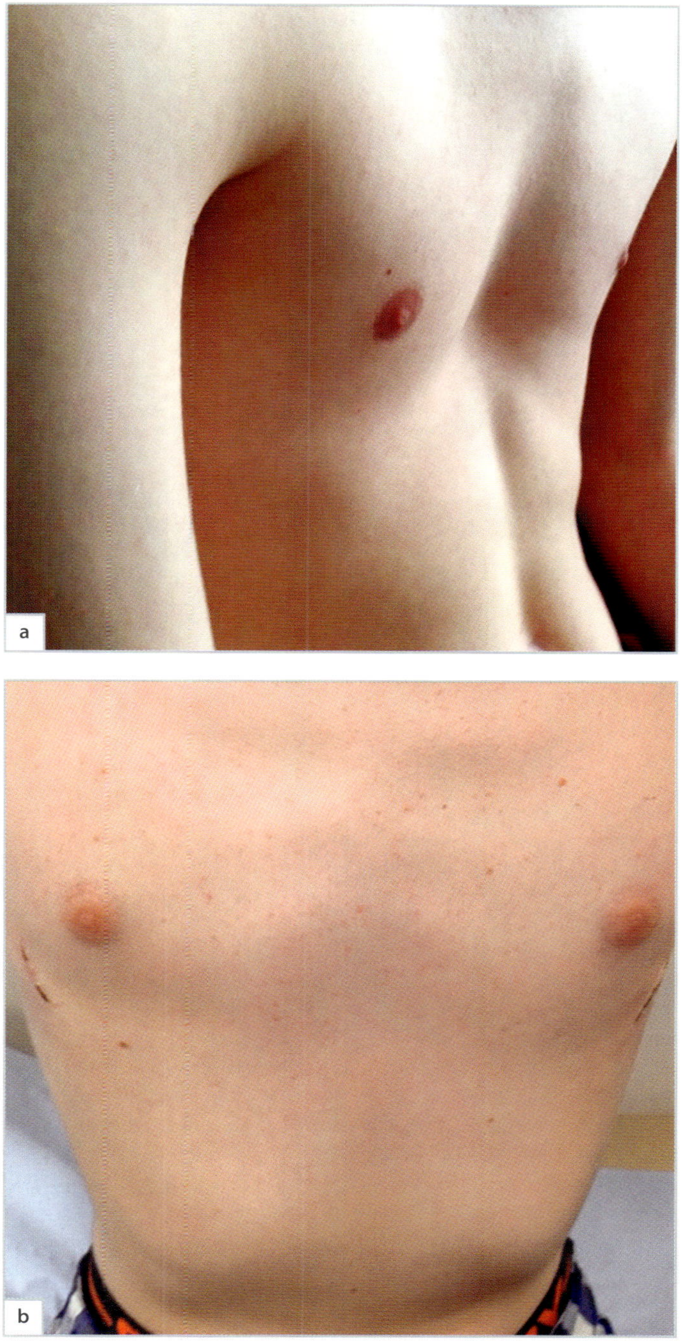

Figure 21.1 Severe pectus excavatum (a) preoperatively and (b) postoperatively.

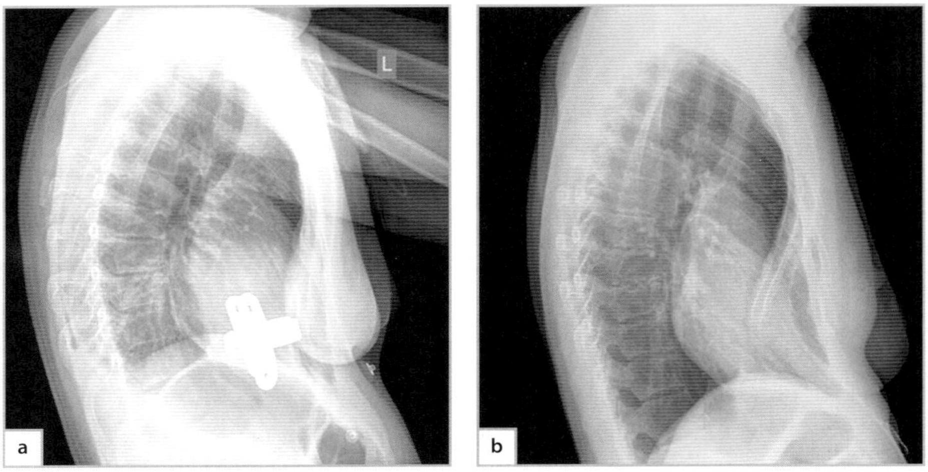

Figure 21.2 Chest X-ray of a severe pectus excavatum (a) preoperatively and (b) postoperatively.

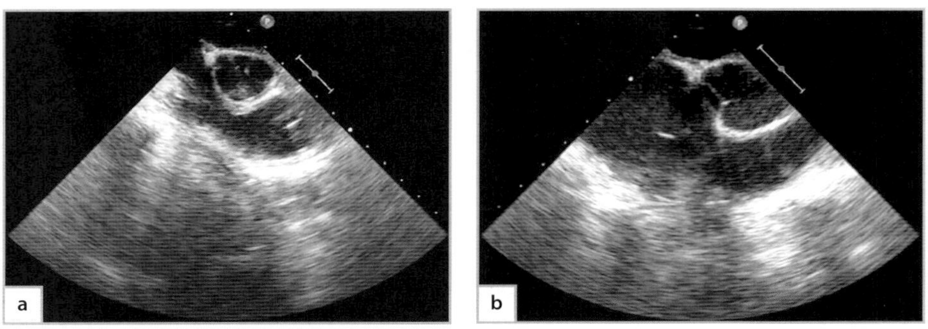

Figure 21.3 (a) Preoperative echocardiogram showing the collapsed right ventricle outflow. (b) Postoperative echocardiogram showing the RV reexpansion.

of the chest wall and other complications, including recurrences.[7] Adult repair is also feasible and has been reported in patients as old as 78 years.[9]

MEDICAL CARE

Many non-operative management strategies have been attempted to correct severe pectus excavatum but none has been proved to be curative. Several exercise programs have been suggested. However, no substantial scientific evidence has determined that they are effective in achieving anatomical correction.

External braces have also been used, but good results are unlikely to be achieved with this technique.

The magnetic mini-mover procedure (3MP) uses a magnetic implant coupled with an external magnet to generate force sufficient to gradually remodel pectus excavatum deformities. The 3MP technique appears to be a safe, minimally invasive, outpatient, cost-effective alternative treatment of pectus excavatum, but the project is still in phase II of the clinical trial and the results have not been reported yet.[10]

The vacuum bell is a promising useful alternative in selected cases of pectus excavatum, providing that the thorax is flexible. Treatment duration is directly linked to age, severity and the frequency of use. It is becoming a well-recognized therapy, which improves the self-image of those patients whose anterior chest wall is still pliable. The cup suction can be used for pediatrics and young adults waiting for a treatment, possibly surgery, however, the long-term effect of this procedure remains unclear.[11] The vacuum bell can also be used in preparation to surgery.[12]

SURGICAL MANAGEMENT

There are a variety of techniques in the surgical management of pectus excavatum, but the two most common methods include modifications of the open approach, first described by Ravitch[13] and minimally invasive approach (Nuss technique).[14]

Plastic surgeons are also involved with the treatment of these patients from a purely morphological perspective with custom-made implants or with the lipofilling.

MINIMALLY INVASIVE CORRECTION (NUSS TECHNIQUE)

The minimally invasive repair is currently the preferred method of pectus excavatum repair, most of all in younger patients, but good results can be achieved in adults as well.[15] It was introduced by Donald Nuss in 1988 and since then has undergone some modifications. Instrumentation for Nuss pectus excavatum surgery is seen in **Figure 21.4**.

The patient is placed in supine position with the right arm wrapped around a T-shaped bar and the left arm on an arm board. The reason for this position is to allow easy access to both sides of the chest should the need arises. After draping, the chest is marked with a sterile marking pen in the deepest portion of the pectus on the corresponding intercostal spaces on the right and left sides where the bar is to be inserted. Then the measurement of the pectus bar is performed, using the marks made on the chest. In the technique initially described by Dr Nuss, the length of the bar should be measured from the mid-axillary

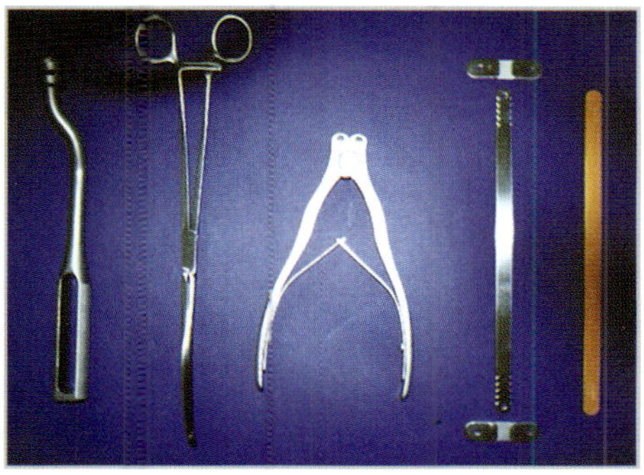

Figure 21.4 Instrumentation for Nuss pectus excavatum surgery. From left to right: aluminium template, pectus bar and stabilizers, bar bender, clamp and bar clipper.

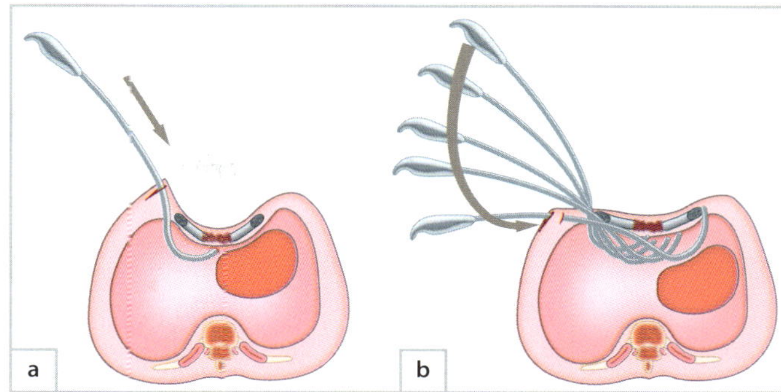

Figure 21.5 Use of the introducer. (a) The introducer is advanced in the direction of the arrow (from right to left) in the retrosternal plane. The point of the instrument is always in contact with the sternum and so away from the heart. (b) Dissection of the retrosternal plane. Once the introducer is passed behind the sternum, the tip is pushed through the intercostal space at the top of the pectus ridge on the left side and brought out through the left skin incision.

line in one side to the opposite mid-axillary line. Today there is the tendency to use shorter bars to reduce the chances of bar dislodgement, especially in older patients. The bar is bent from the center out to either end, making small gradual bends with the bar bender. The curvature of the bar is shaped to fit each individual patient's chest using an aluminium template as a reference.

A transverse 2-cm skin incision is made at the level of the skin marks in line with the deepest point of the depression on the right and left sides. A skin tunnel is raised anteriorly from both incisions to the top of the pectus ridge at the previously selected intercostal space. This can be accomplished by introducing a large clamp through the small incisions in the mid axillary line bilaterally. If multiple bars are to be placed, any bar above the level of the nipples is placed between the pectoralis and serratus muscles; otherwise the position of the bar is subcutaneous. Such technique allows easier bar removal as the osteogenic reaction is reduced compared to when the bar is directly on the ribs, but it is less comfortable, especially for lean patients, as they are more able to feel the ends of the bar.

Then a 5-mm trocar is placed one or two intercostal spaces below the space that has been chosen for the pectus bar on the patient's right side. A 30° thoracoscope is inserted at this point and this provides excellent visualization of the pleural cavity, lung, and mediastinal structures. If necessary, the scope can be used bilaterally.

Once the lateral ridge of the defect is reached, an introducer is advanced from the right side to the left in the retrosternal plane and the sternum is elevated. Retrosternal dissection is performed under direct thoracoscopic vision to avoid injury to the pericardium and pleura.

Always face the point of the instrument anteriorly (away from the heart) and maintain contact with the sternum to avoid injury to mediastinal structures (**Figure 21.5**). Once the instrument is passed behind the sternum, the tip is pushed through the intercostal space at the top of the pectus ridge on the left side and brought out through the left skin incision.

Some surgeons also employ transesophageal echocardiogram for further monitoring of mediastinal structures during bar insertion.

Double tapes are tied to the introducer tip and passed from side to side while removing the introducer from the left side. Finally, the pectus bar is passed from side to side along the plane guided by the tapes. The bar is inserted with its concavity facing forward and is flipped over when correctly positioned. This maneuver pushes up the depressed sternum against the downward force of the chest. The ends of the bars are placed in the subcutaneous tissue, anterior to the muscle fascia.

To prevent bar displacement, unilateral or bilateral stabilizing bars are placed at either end of the Nuss bar and attached to the chest wall with heavy sutures. Reinforcement wires placed around the ribs have also been proposed to prevent bar migration. This can be repeated as many times as necessary. Typically, only one bar is necessary to correct the deformity, but occasionally, a second bar may be necessary. The second bar can be placed above or below the first one. Adult patients are more likely to require two bars. The thoracoscope and trocar are removed at this point.

A chest tube can be placed on one or both sides of the chest. This is not mandatory, but we believe that ensuring full lung expansion is beneficial in these patients.

The subcutaneous tissue and skin are reapproximated with absorbable sutures. Chest radiography is performed as soon as possible to confirm good lung expansion and to reveal the final positioning of the bar.

The advantages of the Nuss approach include avoiding an anterior chest wall incision, resection of rib cartilages and no sternal osteotomy. The incorporation of thoracoscopic techniques has made the operation safer. Bar displacement is one of the most serious complications after the Nuss procedure. Incidence rates of bar displacement vary from 1.8 to 16.6%.[16]

The combination of general endotracheal anesthesia and a thoracic epidural is considered ideal. The epidural catheter is left in place for up to 3 days following the operation, providing excellent adjuvant therapy to pain management techniques. Medications and therapies depend on the patient's response to pain and may include an epidural catheter, opioids, patient-controlled analgesia and non-steroidal anti-inflammatory drugs. The patient is discharged home when able to walk unassisted (average length of stay: 3–5 days). Regular activity is permitted as pain reduces and mobility increases. Heavy lifting is not permitted for 4–6 weeks following surgery; contact sports should be avoided for at least 3 months. The bar is usually removed after 2–3 years.

REFERENCES

1. Haller JA Jr, Shermeta DW, Tepas JJ, et al. Correction of pectus excavatum without prostheses or splints: objective measurement of severity and management of asymmetrical deformities. Ann Thorac Surg 1978; 26:73–79.
2. Crump HW. Pectus excavatum, Am Fam Physician 1992; 46:173–179.
3. Creswick HA, Stacey MW, Kelly RE, et al. Family study of the inheritance of pectus excavatum. J Pediatr Surg. 2006; 41:1699–703.
4. Shamberger RC. Congenital chest wall deformities. Curr Probl Surg 1996; 33:469–542.
5. Schamberger RC, Welch KJ. Incidence of mitral valve prolapse associated with pectus excavatum. J Pediatr 1987; 111:404–407.
6. Malek MH, Fonkalsrud EW, Cooper CB. Ventilatory and cardiovascular responses to exercise in patients with pectus excavatum. Chest 2003; 124:870–882.
7. Jaroszewski D, Notrica D, McMahon L, et al. Current management of pectus excavatum: a review and update of therapy and treatment recommendations. J Am Board Fam 2010; 23:230–239.
8. Kim do H, Hwang JJ, Lee MK, et al. Analysis ofthe Nuss procedure for pectus excavatum in different age groups. Ann Thorac Surg 2005; 80:1073–1077.
9. Aronson DC, Bosgraaf RP, van der Horst C, Ekkelkamp S. Nuss procedure: pediatric surgical solution for adults with pectus excavatum. World J Surg 2007; 31:26–29.
10. Harrison MR, Curran PF, Jamshidi R, et al. Magnetic mini-mover procedure for pectus excavatum II: initial findings of a Food and Drug Administration-sponsored trial. J Pediatr Surg 2010; 45:185–191.
11. Lopez M, Patoir A, Costes F, et al. Preliminary study of efficacy of cup suction in the correction of typical pectus excavatum. J Pediatr Surg 2016; 51:183–187.
12. Elsayed H. Crane technique with the vacuum bell device for improving accesss in the Nuss procedure. J Thorac Cardiovasc Surg 2015; 150:1372–1373.
13. Ravitch MM. The operative treatment of pectus excavatum. Ann Surg 1949; 129:429–444.
14. Nuss D, Kelly RE, Croitoru DP, et al. A 10-year review of a minimally invasive technique for the correction of pectus excavatum. J Pediatr Surg 1998; 33:545–552.
15. Sacco Casamassima MG, Gause G, Goldstein SD, et al. Patient Satisfaction After Minimally Invasive Repair of Pectus Excavatum in Adults: Long-Term Results of Nuss Procedure in Adults. Ann Thorac Surg 2016; 101:1338–1345.
16. Sa YJ, Lee J, Jeong JY, et al. A clinical decision-making model for repeat surgical treatment of pectus Bar displacement: distance measurement after nuss procedure. J Cardiothorac Surg 2016; 11:16.

Chapter 22 Robotic-assisted mediastinal surgery

Carmelina Zirafa, Federico Davini, Ilenia Cavaliere, Vittorio Aprile, Roberta Ricciardi, Alfredo Mussi, Franca Melfi

INTRODUCTION

The mediastinum is considered a virtual area, delimited by the chest cavity, the thoracic inlet on the upper part and the diaphragm on the lower side. According to Fraser et al.'s classification, based on a lateral projection of chest X-rays, the mediastinum is divided into anterior, middle and posterior compartments.[1]

For many years, surgery of the mediastinum was performed by open surgery, usually a median sternotomy, but also by posterolateral thoracotomy, hemi-clamshell (unilateral anterior thoracotomy with partial sternotomy) or clamshell incision (bilateral anterior thoracotomy with transverse sternotomy). These approaches have been associated with high morbidity and postoperative pain, long hospital stay and poor cosmesis. In the late 1980s, the minimally invasive technique, video-assisted thoracic surgery (VATS) and several other combined approaches, such as subxiphoid video-thoracoscopic surgery, were introduced to treat mediastinal lesion.[2,3]

Since then many papers have demonstrated the benefits of video-assisted thoracic surgery (VATS) compared with traditional open surgery. However, this technique is not accepted worldwide and concerns still remain in terms of a lack of radical resection. The limited surgical working space of the mediastinum, containing vital structures, as well as the 2D vision, the long and rigid instruments with few articulations and occasionally the inverted movements, represent the main concerns of the VATS procedure.

To overcome these a surgical robot system was developed in the mid-1990s; and in 2000 two systems, Zeus (Computer Motion Inc.,Goleta, CA, USA) and Da Vinci (Intuitive Surgical, Sunnyvale, CA, USA), were introduced. Today only one system, the Da Vinci Surgical System, exists as a complete surgical system which is applied to a wide range of surgical procedures, including mediastinal resections.

Robotic surgery is considered an evolution of conventional minimally invasive surgery (MIS) characterized by three-dimensional (3D) vision where the magnification of the images is up to ten times the normal size, greater range of motion (7DOF) for human hands, and filtration of any physiological tremor from the surgeon's hand movements.

The first robotic resection of a mediastinal lesion was reported by Yoshino et al. and robotic surgery is now the standard technique in mediastinum, performed by most thoracic surgeons.[4]

ROBOTIC SURGERY IN ANTERIOR MEDIASTINUM

The anterior mediastinum is bound anteriorly by the sternum, posteriorly by the pericardium, aorta and brachiocephalic vessels, superiorly by the thoracic inlet and inferiorly by the diaphragm. This mediastinal compartment contains the thymus gland, fat, lymph nodes and also, rarely, the thyroid and parathyroid glands.

Primary anterior mediastinal tumors represent approximately half of all mediastinal lesions.

The anterior mediastinal masses can be composed of:

- Thymic lesions
- Germ cell tumors
- Parathyroid adenoma
- Intrathoracic goiter

Thymic lesions

The principal surgical indications in the anterior mediastinum are constituted by thymic disorders such as myasthenia gravis (MG) and thymomatous disease. Even though the most common surgical approach to anterior mediastinum remains median sternotomy, minimally invasive surgery (and particularly robotic surgery) is now considered an effective alternative. The robotic system by means of 3D vision and CO_2 insufflation in the thoracic cavity, increasing the mediastinal space, allows an adequate visualization of the surgical area, which is mandatory to obtain a radical resection. The radicality of a thymectomy is vital in the resection of the thymic neoplasm, and in the treatment of myasthenia gravis, to achieve a completely stable remission. According to Masaoka criteria, in myasthenic patients an extended thymectomy with the resection of the whole thymus and the peri-thymic fat tissue, between the two phrenic nerves, is necessary to ensure removal of all ectopic thymic tissue.[5]

An extended thymectomy is indicated in those MG patients with positive AChRAb, mild-moderate MG according to the MGFA classification (including ocular forms of MG), or where a chest CT scan has detected thymic hyperplasia or thymic residue associated with AChRAb-positive MG (in patients under 50 years). Severe MG based on the MGFA classification, AchRAb-negative MG patients (including ocular forms), anti-MuSK positive MG patients, presence of important cardiac and respiratory comorbidities, severe obesity and patients older than 50 years with MG who are responsive to medical therapy all fall into the exclusion criteria for robot-assisted thymectomy.[6]

Minimally invasive thymectomy can be performed from either the right side, left side or bilaterally. The robotic system can also guarantee a radical thymectomy if it is performed from one side only. The choice of the side is guided by points that include safety of trocar placement, mediastinal dissection, anatomic considerations for the distribution of thymic tissue and surgeon's preference.

Reasons for left-sided approach:

1. The thymus sometimes descends posteriorly, totally or partially, rather than anteriorly to the innominate vein.
2. The left thymic portion is usually larger, with the phrenic nerve situated in a deeper position then the right thymic portion.

3. The aortopulmonary window is a frequent site for ectopic thymic tissue and is accessed better from the left side

Reasons for right-sided approach:

1. Better visualization of the venous confluence from the right side following the superior vena cava
2. The visualization and dissection of the aortocaval groove
3. The right side is a more effective ergonomic position in order to accomplish dissection from caudal to cephalad direction

Identifying the contralateral phrenic nerve is vital to safely achieve an extended thymectomy. Robotic system technology limits the possibility of nerve injury by using near-infrared (NIR) imaging combined with 3D high-definition vision.

The first application of NIR imaging during robotic thymectomy to identify contralateral phrenic nerve was reported by Wagner et al. NIR imaging requires a contrast agent containing a fluorophore, that releases NIR fluorescent light after being excited by a NIR light source; Indocyanine green (ICG) is the most commonly used fluorophore in surgery.

During the procedure a 5 mg bolus injection of ICG is prepared with a sterile ICG solution into a peripheral venous catheter, immediately followed by a 10 mL bolus of saline solution.

After activating the Firefly system (fluorescence imaging) a fluorescence response was visible in the mediastinal blood vessels.

This technique allows the surgeon to identify the phrenic neurovascular bundle showing the exact lateral borders of the extended thymectomy. NIR is useful in patients with a very thick adipose mediastinal tissue, helping to reduce the operating time.[7]

The use of the Da Vinci Robotic system in the resection of a mediastinal lesion was first published in 2001. In the last decade, robotic-assisted surgery for treatment of mediastinal mass has become the routine procedure and several studies report excellent results, which demonstrate a low conversion rate, low morbidity and relatively shorter operative time.[8] Other authors, however, have reported that neurological outcomes in myasthenic patients following robotic thymectomy are similar to those following traditional open technique, hence focusing the attention on the important target of extended thymectomy. Cakar et al. described the first study in which neurological results of robotic thymectomy were compared to the transsternal thymectomy in patients with myasthenia gravis. The authors observed good results particularly in patients who had undergone the robotic procedure in terms of improvements in neuro-muscular symptoms, dose reduction therapy, and lower rates of complications and re-intervention, compared with patients who had undergone standard trans-sternal surgery.[9]

In a single center comparison between thoracoscopic and robotic thymectomy, Ruckert et al., evaluating neurological outcome in 153 myasthenic patients, showed a cumulative complete remission rate of myasthenia gravis for robotic and thoracoscopic thymectomies respectively of 39.25% and 20.3%, confirming the superiority of the robotic procedure in order to guarantee a radical thymectomy. Both minimally invasive procedures showed no differences in intraoperative and postoperative complications, operative time, conversion rate and mortality.[10]

Another indication for robotic thymectomy is in the case of noninvasive thymoma, a neoplastic lesion sized < 5 cm without infiltration of the capsule or the surrounding structures. Removing the thymic neoplasm with the robotic system allows an easier 'no touch' dissection technique, which is recommended in the guidelines of the International Thymic Malignant Group, to prevent rupture of the tumor capsule and tumor cells seeding. In the case of noninvasive thymoma robot-assisted exeresis appeared feasible and safe, characterized by a short drainage period and reduced hospital stay. A multicenter European study, which reviewed the data of 134 patients undergoing robotic thymectomy for clinically defined early-stage thymoma (Masaoka stages I and II), showed good surgical results, with no mortality, low morbidity, and short hospital stays and good oncological results. There was only one disease relapse reported in a patient with initial Masaoka stage IVa and 5-year thymoma-related survival rates were 100%.[11]

Ectopic mediastinal parathyroid adenoma

Primary hyperparathyroidism is the most common cause of hypercalcemia. Usually, the culprit gland or glands are located in the cervical region, but in 15% to 20% of patients they can be found in ectopic locations (including the mediastinum) which were usually reached through a median sternotomy or thoracotomy.

Some case series, however, have reported the use of the robotic system to resect ectopic parathyroid glands located in the mediastinum. Despite the limited number of cases using this technique, robotic exeresis surgery of an ectopic parathyroid gland appear to be feasible and safe, thanks to the magnification of the image and better management of the vascular and nervous mediastinal structures, compared to the VATS technique.

Surgical technique

General anesthesia with single lung ventilation is required. The patient is positioned supine, with a pillow under the spine, to expose the left or right side of the thorax. The first incision is performed in the 5th intercostal space along the anterior–axillary line. The other two incisions are performed under camera vision and CO_2 insufflation, starting with low pressure 5 mmHg (ranging between 5 mmHg and 8 mmHg) to increase the operating space and to help perform the other port incisions safely, the first at the 3rd intercostal space along the anterior–axillary line and the last at 5th intercostal space on the mid-clavicular line (**Figure 22.1**). A Permanent Cautery Spatula (EndoWrist; Intuitive Surgical) with electric cautery function is generally utilized on the right arm, while a Fenestrated Bipolar Forceps (EndoWrist; Intuitive Surgical) placed on the left arm. An atraumatic bipolar instrument is also used to grasp the lesion.

In the left-sided approach the dissection starts following the mammary artery, first from the right side (the retrosternal area) while finding the right mediastinal pleura and the right phrenic nerve to allow a safe dissection of the right inferior horn under direct vision of the nerve.

Then on the left side at the pericardio phrenic angle, the dissection continues caudo-cephalically to the left part of the anonymous vein.

Currently, the thymic veins are isolated and clipped separately. The specimens are removed with an endoscopic bag from the cavity

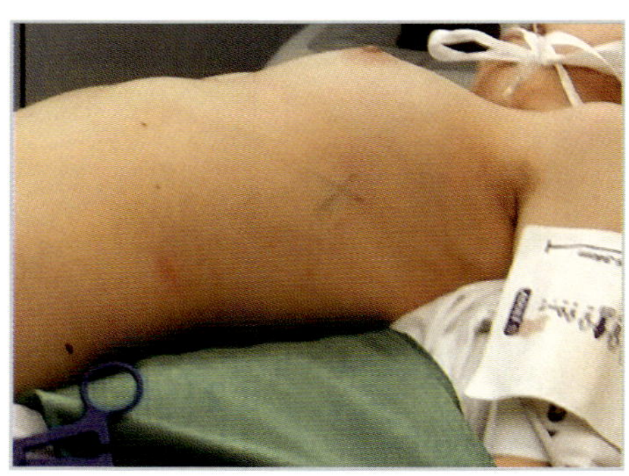

Figure 22.1 Robotic port-mapping for mediastinal surgery (anterior mediastinum).

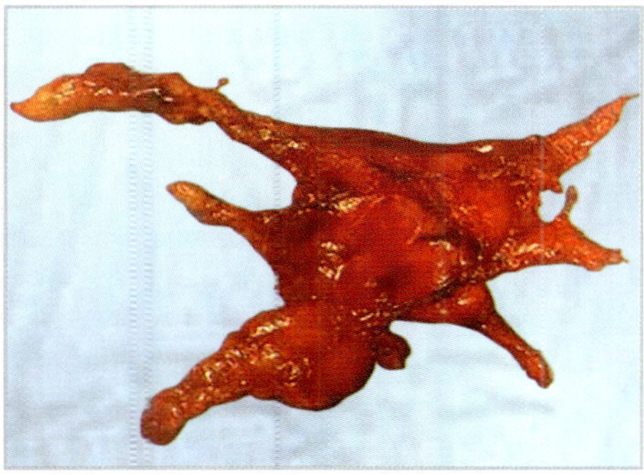

Figure 22.2 Thymic gland of myasthenic patient, underwent robotic extended thymectomy.

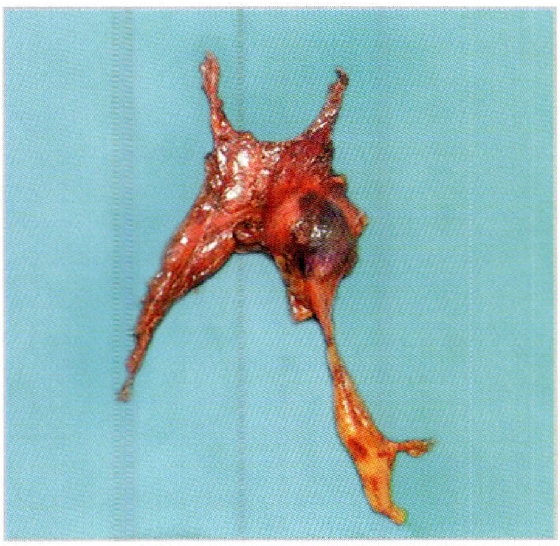

Figure 22.3 Thymoma en-bloc with thymus and adjacent fat.

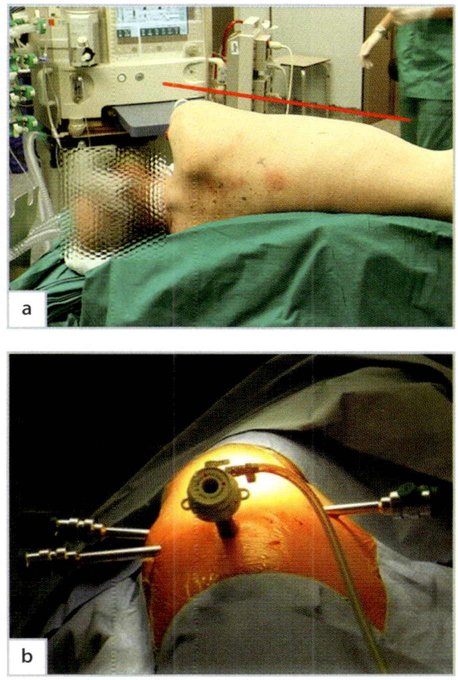

Figure 22.4 (a) Patient position for posterior mediastinal tumor. (b) Patient port-mapping for posterior mediastinal tumor.

through the port incision in the mid-axillary region (**Figures 22.2** and **22.3**). No additional utility incision is used. A 24-F drainage tube is inserted in to the left thoracic cavity.

Posterior mediastinal lesion resection

The most frequent lesion in the posterior mediastinum (75% of all tumors of the posterior mediastinum) is the neurogenic tumor. Neurogenic tumors are often asymptomatic and diagnosed accidentally. These tumors are usually benign and well defined, located in the paravertebral area and arising often from intercostal nerves. In the past, thoracotomy was the traditional surgical approach, but now the minimally invasive technique is considered the gold standard for the removal of posterior mediastinal lesions. Minimally invasive surgery minimises the trauma of the incision and reduces complications and length of time in hospital.[13] Only a few authors have reported robotic-assisted exeresis of a posterior-mediastinal mass, highlighting the safety and effectiveness of the procedure, when the tumor is located in an uncomfortable position and difficult to reach by VATS, for example, the thoracic apex or the inferior area of chest cavity, near the diaphragm.[14] Features of the Da Vinci Robotic System, such as depth perception and 7-degree articulation of the instrumentation with tremor filtration, allow a precise maneuver and safe isolation.

Surgical technique

As for all thoracic surgical procedures general anesthesia and double lumen intubation is required. In case of robotic procedure for the removal of neurogenic tumor, the patient is positioned in lateral decubitus, as in the posterolateral thoracotomy (**Figure 22.4a**). The port mapping is well standardized.

The first-port is placed in the 7th or 8th intercostal space on the midaxillary line for the camera (30° angled down scope).

The second-port incisions (8 mm) can be made in the same intercostal space, not less than 6 cm from the anterior port at 6th intercostal usually immediately over the diaphragm. The use of the 4th arm, located in the auscultatory area can be optional, depending on the surgeon's experience (**Figure 22.4b**).

A Permanent Cautery Spatula or a Permanent Cautery Hook (EndoWrist; Intuitive Surgical) with electric cautery function is generally utilized on the right arm, while a Fenestrated Bipolar Forceps (EndoWrist; Intuitive Surgical), is placed on the left arm. An atraumatic bipolar instrument is also used to grasp the lesion (**Figure 22.5**).

OUR SERIES

We began using robotic surgery in 2001. Between then and April 2016 we have used the procedure on 1030 patients.

Between January 2012 and April 2016 161 patients underwent robotic surgery for an anterior mediastinal mass excision and/or for myasthenia gravis. 82 (50.9%) patients suffered from myasthenia gravis.

All patients had a general anesthesia with double-lumen intubation. All procedures were performed with CO_2 insufflation. Almost all procedures were performed using the left-sided approach, and only 24 (14.9%) were operated using the right-sided approach (due to surgical requirements). The mean operative time was 137.4 minutes (range 35–335 minutes); no intraoperative complications occurred (no vessel or nerve injuries) and there were no mortalities. Conversion to open surgery was performed in 2 cases (1.2%) due to an unexpected tumor invasion in both cases.

The mean postoperative stay was 4 days (range 3–6 days) and mean chest drainage was 1.4 days (range 1–3 days). Postoperative morbidity occurred in 10 patients (6.2%): two patients due to pleural effusions (who were treated with medical therapy), three patients due

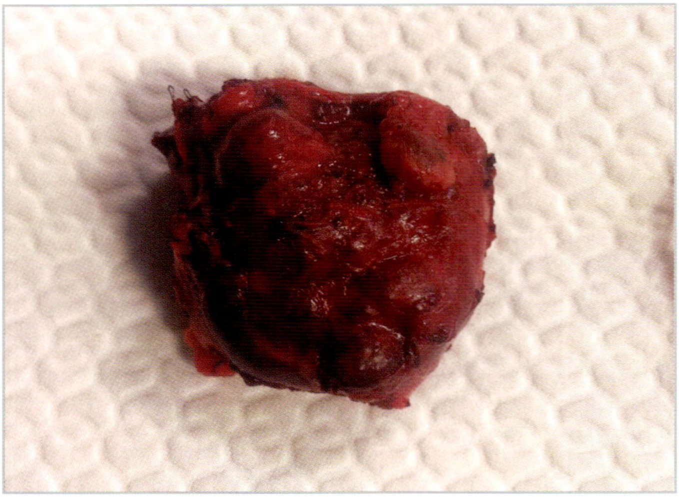

Figure 22.5 Neurinoma located in the left apex of thoracic cavity, laterally subclavian vessels.

to postoperative anemia (one treated with transfusion), two patients due to chylothorax (who were both treated quickly with surgery), two patients due to pneumothorax (one treated with chest drainage) and one patient due to left arm hematoma.

Histopathologic analysis revealed 80 thymic hyperplasia, 27 thymomas, 23 thymic cysts, 11 pleuropericardial cysts, 4 parathyroid adenomas, 2 thymolipomas and 14 others (i.e. thyroid cancer metastasis, Hodgkin lymphoma, etc).

Between January 2012 and April 2016 32 patients underwent robotic surgery for posterior mediastinal mass. All patients had a general anesthetic with double-lumen intubation which was performed with CO_2 insufflation. 18 (56.3%) were operated on using the right-sided approach and 13 (40.7%) with the left-sided approach according to surgical requirement. The mean operative time was 115.6 minutes (range 50–230 minutes); no intraoperative complications occurred and no mortality occurred. No conversion was observed.

The mean postoperative hospital stay was 4 days (range 2–17 days) and mean chest drainage was 2.6 days (range 1–14 days).

Morbidity occurred in 4 patients (12.5%): 2 left arm hematomas, 1 postoperative anemia (treated with transfusion) and 1 chylothorax (treated with fast and medical therapy).

Histopathologic analysis revealed 21 neurinomas, 3 mesothelial cysts, 3 teratomas, 2 bronchogenic cysts, 1 Castelman's disease, 1 cavernous hemangioma, and 1 solitary fibrous tumor of the pleura.

CONCLUSION

In recent decades, minimally invasive surgical approaches have been developed for the removal of mediastinal masses, guaranteeing less postoperative pain, better cosmetic results, reduction of morbidity and shorter hospitalization. Robotic surgery is considered the latest evolution in minimally invasive surgery, without the limitations of VATS (i.e. 2D- vision, a lack of depth perception, limited maneuverability of thoracoscopic instruments, and where the ribs act as a fulcrum area).

Features of the Da Vinci System (high-definition 3D vision, tremor filtration and 7-degree articulation of instruments inside the chest cavity) offer an effective and reliable technical support to the surgeon operating on the mediastinal region.

Randomized controlled studies are required to support the advantages of robotic surgery for the treatment of mediastinal lesions, to evaluate long-term neurological outcomes in myasthenic patients and oncological outcomes in patients with mediastinal tumors.

REFERENCES

1. Fraser RS, Paré JA. Synopsis of diseases of the chest. Philadelphia: WB Saunders Company, 1994.
2. Mack MJ, Landreneau RJ, Yim AP, et al. Results of video-assisted thymectomy in patients with myasthenia gravis. J Thorac Cardiovasc Surg 1996; 112:1352–1359.
3. Yim AP. Video-assisted thoracoscopic management of anterior mediastinal masses. Preliminary experience and results. Surg Endoscop 1995; 9:1184–1188.
4. Yoshino I, Hashizume M, Shimada M, et al. Thoracoscopic thymectomy with the da Vinci computer-enhanced surgical system. J Thorac Cardiovasc Surg 2001; 122:783–785.
5. Masaoka A, Yamakawa Y, Niwa H, et al. Extended thymectomy for myasthenia gravis patients: a 20-year review. Ann Thorac Surg 1996; 62:853–859.
6. Ricciardi R, Melfi F, Maestri M, et al. Endoscopic thymectomy: a neurologist's perspective. Ann Cardiothorac Surg 2016; 5:38–44.
7. Wagner OJ, Louie BE, Vallières E, et al. Near-infrared fluorescence imaging can help identify the contralateral phrenic nerve during robotic thymectomy. Ann Thorac Surg 2012; 94:622–625.
8. Melfi F, Fanucchi O, Davini F, et al. A Ten-year experience of mediastinal robotic surgery in a single referral centre European Journal of Cardio-Thoracic Surgery 2012; 41:847–851.
9. Cakar F, Werner P, Augustin F, et al. A comparison of outcomes after robotic open extended thymectomy for myasthenia gravis. Eur J Cardiothorac Surg 2007; 31:501–505.
10. Ruckert JC, Swierzy M, Ismail M. Comparison of robotic and nonrobotic thoracoscopic thymectomy: a cohort study. J Thorac Cardiovasc Surg 2011; 141:673–677.
11. Marulli G, Maessen J, Melfi F, et al Multi-institutional European experience of robotic thymectomy for thymoma. Ann Cardiothorac Surg 2016; 5:18–25.
12. Harvey A, Bohacek L, Neumann D, et al. Robotic thoracoscopic mediastinal parathyroidectomy for persistent hyperparathyroidism: case report and review of the literature. Surg Laparosc Endosc Percutan Tech 2011; 21:e24–27.
13. Li Y, Wang J. Experience of video-assisted thoracoscopic resection for posterior mediastinal neurogenic tumours: a retrospective analysis of 58 patients. ANZ J Surg 2013; 83:664–668.
14. Cerfolio RJ, Bryant AS, Minnich DJ. Operative techniques in robotic thoracic surgery for inferior or posterior mediastinal pathology. J Thorac Cardiovasc Surg 2012; 143:1138–1143.

Chapter 23 Robotic-assisted lobectomy

Benjamin Wei, Robert Cerfolio

INTRODUCTION

Minimally invasive lobectomy has traditionally been performed using video-assisted thoracoscopic surgery (VATS) techniques. The first robotic lobectomies were reported in 2003 by Morgan et al. and Ashton et al.[1,2] Since then, the use of robotic technology for lobectomy has become increasingly common.

INITIAL EVALUATION

The evaluation of candidates for robotic lobectomy includes the standard preoperative studies for patients undergoing pulmonary resection. For patients with suspected or biopsy-proven lung cancer, whole-body positron emission tomography–computed tomography (PET-CT) scan is currently the standard of care. Pulmonary function testing including measurement of carbon monoxide diffusion capacity (DL_{CO}) and spirometry is routine. Mediastinal staging can consist of either endobronchial ultrasound guided fine-needle aspiration (EBUS-FNA) biopsy or mediastinoscopy, depending on expertise. Certain patients may warrant additional testing, including stress test, brain MRI if concern exists for metastatic disease, and/or dedicated CT scan with intravenous contrast or MRI if concern exists for vascular or vertebral/nerve invasion, respectively.

Investigators have shown that thoracoscopic lobectomy is safe in patients with a predicted postoperative forced expiratory volume 1 (FEV_1) or DL_{CO} < 40% of predicted.[3] We consider robotic lobectomy feasible in these patients as well.

At present, we view vascular invasion, locally invasive T4 lesions, Pancoast tumors, and massive tumor (> 10 cm) as contraindications for a robotic approach to lobectomy. The need for reconstruction of the airway, chest wall invasion, presence of induction chemotherapy and/or radiation, prior thoracic surgery, and hilar nodal disease are not contraindications for robotic-assisted lobectomy for experienced surgeons.

OPERATIVE PROCEDURE

Preparation

A well-trained team that communicates effectively is a priority for successful performance of robotic lobectomy. Criteria for a well-trained team include: documented scores of 70% or higher on simulator exercises, certificate of robotic safety training and cockpit awareness, weekly access to the robot, familiarity with the robotic and the instruments, and a mastery of the pulmonary artery from both an anterior and posterior approach. Currently, the Da Vinci surgical system console (Intuitive Surgical, Sunnyvale, CA) is the only FDA-approved device available for robotic lobectomy. Proper location of the robot should be established prior to the operation. The third robotic arm will need to be located so that it will approach the patient from the posterior. The robot is driven from over to patient shoulder at a 15° angle off the longitudinal access of the patient. The patient will need to be turned so that the axis of the patient is 90° away from the typical position (i.e. head near the anesthesia workstation) to facilitate this (**Figure 23.1**). The use of long ventilator tubing and wrapping up this and other monitoring lines with a towel secured to the side of the bed is helpful to minimize interference with the surgeon/assistant. Precise placement of the double lumen endotracheal tube and the ability to tolerate single-lung ventilation should be established prior to draping the patient, as repositioning the tube will be virtually impossible once the robot is docked.

Patient positioning/port placement

The patient is positioned in lateral decubitus position. Axillary rolls and arm boards are unnecessary (**Figure 23.2**). The robotic ports are inserted in the 7th intercostal space for upper/middle lobectomy and in the 8th intercostal space for lower lobectomy. Typical port placement is shown in **Figure 23.3** for a right robotic lobectomy. The ports are marked as follows: robotic arm 3 (5 mm port) is located 1–2 cm lateral from the spinous process of the vertebral body, robotic arm 2 (8 mm) is 10 cm medial to robotic arm 3, the camera port (we prefer the 12 mm camera) is 9 cm medial to robotic arm 2, and robotic arm 1(12 mm) is placed right above the diaphragm anteriorly. The assistant port is triangulated behind the camera port and the most anterior robotic port, and as inferior as possible without disrupting the diaphragm. We use a zero-degree camera for this operation. Insufflation of the camera or assistant port with carbon dioxide is used to depress the diaphragm, decrease bleeding, and compress the lung.

Mediastinal lymph node dissection

After examining the pleura to confirm the absence of metastases, the next step during our performance of robotic lobectomy is removal of the mediastinal lymph nodes, for staging and also to help expose the structures of the hilum.

- **Right side:** The inferior pulmonary ligament is divided.Lymph nodes at stations 8 and 9 are removed. Robotic arm 3 is used to

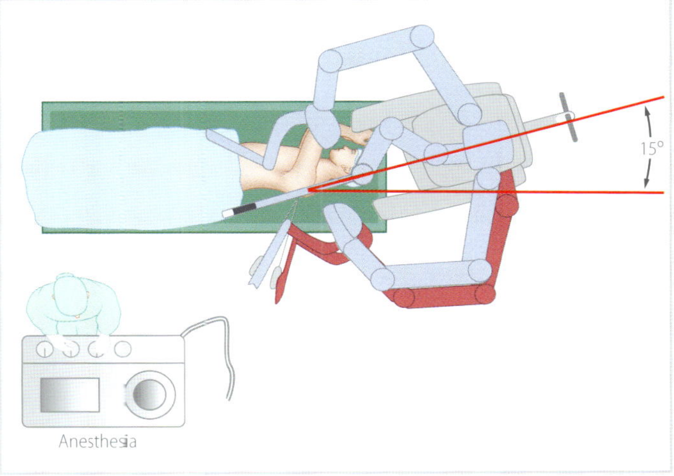

Figure 23.1 Docking for robotic lobectomy (left-sided).

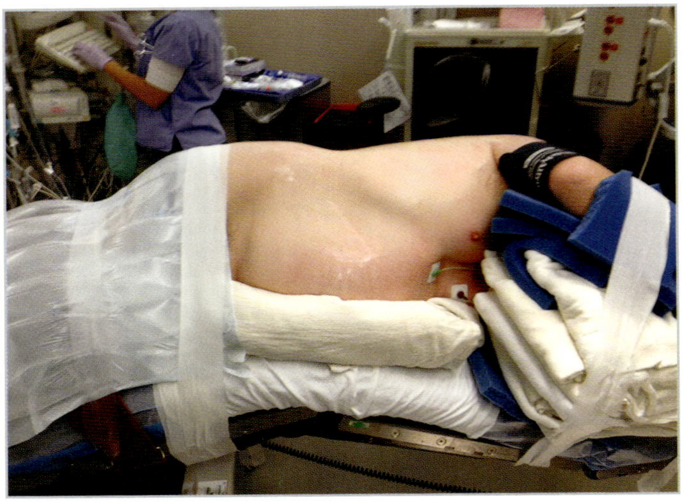

Figure 23.2 Patient positioning for robotic lobectomy (right-sided).

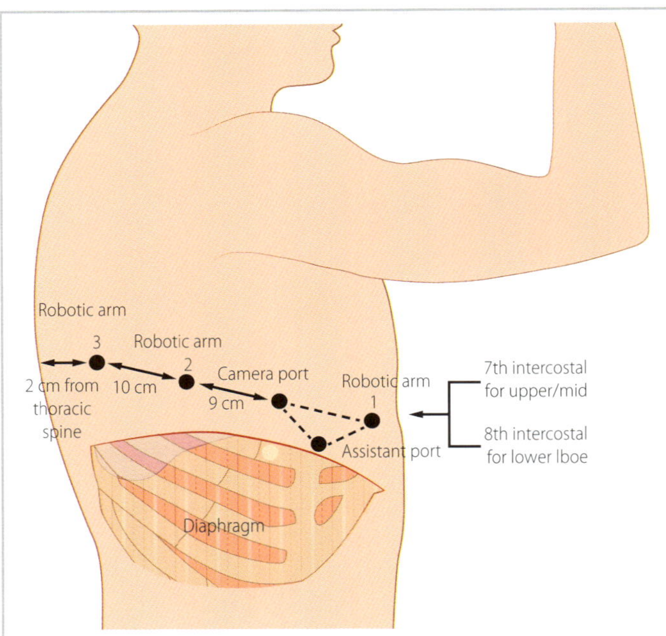

Figure 23.3 Port positioning for robotic lobectomy (right-sided).

retract the lower lobe medially and anteriorly in order to remove lymph nodes from station 7. Robotic arm 3 is used to retract the upper lobe inferiorly during dissection of stations 2R and 4R, clearing the space between the SVC anteriorly, the esophagus posteriorly, and the azygos vein inferiorly.Avoiding dissection too far superiorly can prevent injury to the right recurrent laryngeal nerve that wraps around the subclavian artery.

- **Left side:** The inferior pulmonary ligament is divided to facilitate the removal of lymph node station 9. The nodes in station 8 are then removed. Station 7 is accessed in the space between the inferior pulmonary vein and lower lobe bronchus, lateral to the esophagus. The lower lobe is retracted medially/anteriorly with robotic arm 3 during this process. Absence of the lower lobe facilitates dissection of level 7 from the left. Finally, robotic arm three is used to wrap around the left upper lobe and pressed it inferior to allow dissection of stations 5 and 6. Care should be taken while working in the aorto-pulmonary window to avoid injury to the left recurrent laryngeal nerve. Station 2L cannot typically be accessed during left-sided mediastinal lymph node dissection due to the presence of the aortic arch but the 4L node is commonly removed.

Wedge resection

Wedge resection of a nodule may be necessary to confirm the presence of cancer prior to proceeding with lobectomy. Because the current iteration of the robot does not offer tactile feedback, special techniques may be necessary to identify a nodule that is not obvious on visual inspection. An empty ring forceps may be used via the assistant port to palpate the nodule. Alternatively, preoperative marking of the nodule with a dye marker injected via navigational bronchoscopy can help facilitate location of the nodule. Preoperative confirmation of a cancer diagnosis with tissue biopsy is helpful to avoid being unable to locate the nodule intraoperatively.

THE FIVE LOBECTOMIES

A certain degree of adaptability is necessary for performance of robotic lobectomy. Structures may be isolated and divided in the order that the patient's individual anatomy permits. What follows is a description of an outline of the typical conduct of each lobectomy.

Right upper lobectomy

- Retraction of the right upper lobe laterally and posteriorly with robot arm 3 helps expose the hilum
- The bifurcation between the right upper and middle lobar veins is developed by dissecting it off the underlying pulmonary artery
- The 10R lymph node between the truncus branch and the superior pulmonary vein should be removed or swept up toward the lung, which exposes the truncus branch
- The superior pulmonary vein is encircled with the vessel loop and then divided. The truncus branch is then divided
- The right upper lobe is then reflected anteriorly to expose the bifurcation of the right main stem bronchus. There is usually a lymph node here that should be dissected out to expose the bifurcation. The right upper lobe bronchus is then encircled and divided. Care must be taken to apply only minimal retraction on the specimen in order to avoid tearing the remaining pulmonary artery branches
- Finally, the posterior segmental artery to the right upper lobe is exposed, the surrounding N1 nodes removed, and the artery encircled and divided
- The upper lobe is reflected again posteriorly, and the anterior aspect of the pulmonary artery is inspected to make sure that there are no arterial branches remaining. If not, then the fissure between the upper and middle lobes, and the upper and lower lobes, is then divided. This is typically done from anterior to posterior, but may be done in the reverse direction if the space between the pulmonary artery and right middle lobe is already developed. During completion of the fissure the right upper lobe should be lifted up to ensure that the specimen bronchus is included in the specimen

Right middle lobectomy

- Retraction of the right middle lobe laterally and posteriorly with robot arm 1 helps expose the hilum

- The bifurcation between the right upper and middle lobar veins is developed by dissecting it off the underlying pulmonary artery. The right middle lobe vein is encircled and divided
- The fissure between the right middle and lower lobes, if not complete, is divided from anterior to posterior. Care should be taken to avoid transecting segmental arteries to the right lower lobe.
- The right middle lobe bronchus is then isolated. It will be running from left to right in the fissure. Level 11 lymph nodes are dissected from around it. It is encircled and divided, taking care to avoid injuring the right middle lobar artery that is located directly behind it.
- Dissection of the fissure should continue posteriorly until the branches to the superior segment are identified. Then the one or two right middle lobar segmental arteries are isolated and divided.
- Stapling of middle lobar structures may be facilitated by passing the stapler from posterior to anterior, to have a greater working distance.
- The fissure between right middle and upper lobes is then divided.

Right lower lobectomy

- The inferior pulmonary ligament should be divided to the level of the inferior pulmonary vein
- The bifurcation of the right superior and inferior pulmonary veins should be dissected out. The location of the right middle lobar vein should be positively identified to avoid inadvertent transection
- A subadventitial plane on the ongoing pulmonary artery should be established. If the major fissure is not complete then it should be divided. The superior segmental artery and the right middle lobe arterial branches are identified. The superior segmental artery is isolated and divided. The common trunk to right lower lobe basilar segments may be taken as long as this does not compromise the middle lobar segmental artery/arteries; otherwise, dissection may have to extend further distally to ensure safe division.
- The inferior pulmonary vein is divided
- The right lower lobe bronchus is isolated, taking care to visualize the right middle lobar bronchus crossing from left to right. The surrounding lymph nodes, as usual, are dissected and the bronchus divided. If there is any question of compromising the right middle lobe bronchus, the surgeon can ask the anesthesiologist to hand-ventilate the right lung to confirm that the middle lobe expands.

Left upper lobectomy

- Retraction of the left upper lobe laterally and posteriorly with robot arm 3 helps expose the hilum
- The presence of both superior and inferior pulmonary veins is confirmed, and the bifurcation dissected
- The lung is then reflected anteriorly with robotic arm 3 and interlobar dissection is started, going from posterior to anterior
- If the fissure is not complete then it will need to be divided. Reflecting the lung posteriorly again and establishing a subadventitial plane will be helpful.The branches to the lingula are encountered and divided in the fissure during this process. The posterior segmental artery is also isolated and divided. Division of the lingular artery or arteries can be done before or after division of the posterior segmental artery
- The superior pulmonary vein is isolated then divided. Because the superior pulmonary vein can be fairly wide, it may require that the lingular and upper division branches be transected separately
- Often the next structure that can be divided readily will be the left upper lobar bronchus, as opposed to the anterior and apical arterial branches to the left upper lobe. The upper lobe bronchus should be encircled and divided, often passing the stapler from robotic arm 1 in order to avoid injuring the main pulmonary artery.
- Finally, the remaining arterial branches are encircled and divided.

Left lower lobectomy

- The inferior pulmonary ligament should be divided to the level of the inferior pulmonary vein. The lower lobe is then reflected posteriorly by robotic arm 3
- The bifurcation of the left superior and inferior pulmonary veins should be dissected out
- The lung is reflected anteriorly by robotic arm 3. The superior segmental artery is identified. The posterior ascending arteries to the left upper lobe are frequently visible from this view also. The superior segmental artery is isolated and divided. The common trunk to left lower lobe basilar segments may be taken as long as this does not compromise the middle lobar segmental artery or arteries; otherwise, dissection may have to extend further distally to ensure safe division. If the fissure is not complete, this will need to be divided to expose the ongoing pulmonary artery to the lower lobe
- After division of the arterial branches, the lung is reflected again posteriorly. The inferior pulmonary vein is divided
- The left lower lobe bronchus is isolated. The surrounding lymph nodes, as usual, are dissected and the bronchus divided
- For left lower lobectomy, it may be simpler to wait until after resection is performed before targeting the subcarinal space for removal of level 7 lymph nodes

EXPERT SITUATION

Prior thoracic surgery, induction therapy or hilar nodal disease

Previous thoracic surgery can create adhesions, most commonly from the location of prior incisions but also more troublesomely, from the apex, along the mediastinal surface, or around the hilum. If the robotic ports can be placed, lysis of adhesions with the robot is feasible. Thin filmy adhesions can often be dealt with blunt dissection or a sweeping motion of the robotic instruments. More vascular or fibrous adhesions should be divided with bipolar cautery. If adhesions are dense and prevent insertion of robotic ports, VATS techniques may be necessary to establish enough room to do so. These ports may need to be located in different positions than the future robotic ports; the robotic ports cannot be inserted through a larger incision, as they will be improperly moved during operation of the robotic arms. Avoidance of structures such as the phrenic nerve, innominate artery, and internal mammary artery is critical to prevent complications.

Induction therapy can also create problems during lobectomy, more typically in the area surrounding the tumor. Dissection of segmental and lobar structures can be more difficult in this situation. The presence of tumor-bearing or otherwise enlarged or calcified hilar lymph nodes can also make dissection more difficult. Meticulous identification and removal of lymph nodes is facilitated by the dexterity of robotic instruments in these cases. Resection of these nodes should be performed prior to any attempt to isolate vascular and airway structures.

Chest wall resection

The use of robotic assistance for lobectomy combined with chest wall resection may be helpful in some instances. In situations where an appropriately located thoracotomy (4th through 6th intercostal space) can be incorporated into the chest wall resection, robotic assistance may be less useful. However, a minimally invasive approach can be useful to access hilar structures that may be difficult to maneuver around with a chest-wall invading tumor in place, or when invasion of more superior ribs is present. Robotic division of the branches of the pulmonary artery, vein, and bronchi can be accomplished, followed by a muscle-sparing approach to resecting the chest wall that approaches the ribs and intercostal muscles from inside the chest rather than outside.[4]

Sleeve and bronchoplastic techniques

Robotic sleeve lobectomy or bronchoplasty is possible for very experienced surgeons. Bronchoplastic closure of the airway is accomplished as in an open operation, but with robotic instruments instead. Generally, a long-term absorbable suture is used. A robotic needle driver is used in the right hand, and a robotic Debakey or similar instrument is used in the left hand. Placement of interrupted or continuous sutures is acceptable, although it should be noted that the power of the robot can lead to fraying of the suture when a continuous technique is used, especially with a monofilament suture. Minimally invasive knot tying is facilitated greatly by the robot compared to VATS techniques. When performing robotic sleeve lobectomy, division of the airway is done after the remaining structures are isolated and divided. A robotic Potts scissors is used. The airway is then reconstructed with an interrupted technique using long-term absorbable suture. The anterior and posterior walls are completed separately, using robotic arm 3 to help retract the remaining lobe(s) in the appropriate direction to expose the anastomosis. The lung is then ventilated with the anastomosis submerged under saline, and any necessary repair sutures are placed.

INTRAOPERATIVE COMPLICATIONS

Intraoperative complications can be minimized and managed by following certain rules and guidelines.

- The passing of vascular staplers around fragile structure such as the pulmonary artery and or vein deserves special attention. Carefully orchestrated moves and clear communication is needed between the bedside assistant and the surgeon. We have developed our own communication system between the bedside assistant and the surgeon to prevent iatrogenic injuries. This uses the anvil of the stapler as the hour hand of a clock and the degree of articulation is also quantified and communicated.
- Robotic instruments should be initially inserted under direct vision during thoracic surgery for their initial placement. Once safely positioned instruments then can be quickly and safely inserted or changed for other instruments by properly using the memory feature of the robot that automatically inserts any new instruments to a position that is exactly 1 cm proximal to its latest position. However, if this feature is used it is incumbent on the surgeon to ensure that no vital structure have moved into the path of that newly placed instrument. The most common structure would be the lung.
- A rolled-up sponge should always be immediately accessible when working around vascular structures. If an injury occurs, the first step should be to tamponade the structure with the sponge. A minor injury may respond to this packing alone. If bleeding is massive or persists, a thoracotomy will be necessary. Lap pads should be inserted via the assistant port and packed around the injury to control bleeding. The robot is then de-docked and a thoracotomy made.

Table 23.1 Troubleshooting of common problems during robotic lobectomy

Problems	Solutions
Robotic arms are not responding to hand movement	• Ensure trocar's remote center is in chest • Ensure trocar's docked properly to robotic arms • Ensure sterile plastic gown covering robotic arms is not interfering with wheeled mechanism of robot • Ensure surgeons' hand not maximized at console
The camera is fogging	• Place humidified CO_2 insufflation through non-robotic access port (and not through the camera port) • Pre-heat the camera • Evacuate smoke from intraoperative field
There are conflicts between robotic arms 3 & 1 or 2	• Ensure at least 10 cm between robotic arm 3 and closest robotic arm (robotic arm 1 or 2) • Use 5 mm thoracic lung grasper as the instrument of choice through the most posterior robotic arm • After docking, ensure the link 2's of robotic arms are aligned parallel to one another • When surgeon toggles between robotic arm 3 and 2 or 1, ensure the non-active instrument is placed anteriorly toward chest wall
The bipolar cautery or thoracic dissector is not working.	• Ensure bipolar: • source is connected to robot • energy source is functioning • cord is not damaged
There is a sudden loss of working space	• Ensure DLET is properly positioned • Inflate more air in bronchial cuff • Ensure no leaks out of ports if using a completely portal technique • Ensure all valves are closed on ports • Do not place sucker in chest on suction unless immersed under water or blood
You are unable to achieve proper of angle of stapler to come across vessels or fissures.	• Try placing stapler through robotic access port or robotic arm 1 or 2 to achieve best angle • Use a stapler which maximizes the degrees of rotation and articulation • Do not force the stapler; tie vessels with suture or • Use 8 mm robotic clips on vessel
There is difficulty in bagging specimen	• Use a bag that provides easy opening and closing by bed side assistant • Place bag under trocar prior to deployment • Place bag in the most anterior superior aspect of chest to maximize use of gravity, space and keep bag away from stapled hilar structures • Use robotic arm 3 to place specimen into bag and then hold back of the bag in place while stuffing specimen into bag with robotic arms 1 & 2

Abbreviation: DLET, double lumen endotracheal tube

- The 'drop zone' for the specimen should be well away from the pulmonary artery, which can be injured during this process if care is not taken.
- To remove the specimen, the assistant non-robotic port is enlarged posteriorly to avoid injuring the diagram.
- The robotic arms are removed under direct vision with insufflation discontinued in order to confirm the absence of bleeding.

Table 12.1 shows how to trouble shoot common problems encountered during robotic lobectomy.

CONCLUSION

Robotic lobectomy can be done with very low morbidity and mortality, as we and other investigators have demonstrated (**Table 12.2**), and is clearly advantageous when compared to open lobectomy with regards to short-term outcomes, both in community and academic settings.[5,6] Long-term oncologic results, although not yet extensively studied, are thus far consistent with prior reports for VATS and open lobectomy.[7] With proper training and experience, robotic lobectomy can become part of the fundamental armamentarium of the modern thoracic surgeon.

Table 23.2 Results reported in series of robotic-assisted lobectomies

Study	Year	n	Conversion rate (%)	Morbidity (%)	Perioperative mortality (%)	Median LoS (days)	Other notes
Cerfolio et al.[6]	2011	168	7.7	27	0	2	Decreased morbidity, improved QoL, shorter LoS than open lobectomy
Park et al.[7]	2006	30	12	26	0	4.5	
Veronesi et al.[8]	2009	54	13	20	0	4.5	Shorter LoS than open lobectomy
Gharagozloo et al.[9]	2009	100		21	3	4	

Abbreviations: LoS, length of stay; QoL, quality of life; n, number of patients

REFERENCES

1. Burt BM, Kosinski AS, Shrager JB, Onaitis MW, Weigel T. Thoracoscopic lobectomy is associated with acceptable morbidity and mortality in patients with predicted postoperative forced expiratory volume in 1 second or diffusing capacity for carbon monoxide less than 40% of normal. J Thorac Cardiovasc Surg 2014; 148:19–28.
2. Cerfolio RJ, Bryant AS, Minnich DJ. Minimally invasive chest wall resection: sparing the overlying, uninvolved extrathoracic musculature of the chest. Ann Thorac Surg 2012; 94:1744–1747.
3. Kent M, Wang T, Whyte R, et al. Open, video-assisted thoracic surgery, and robotic lobectomy: review of a national database. Ann Thorac Surg 2014; 97:236–242.
4. Adams RD, Bolton WD, Stephenson JE, et al. Initial multicenter community robotic lobectomy experience: comparisons to a national database. Ann Thorac Surg 2014; 97:1893–1898.
5. Park BJ, Melfi F, Mussi A, et al. Robotic lobectomy for non-small cell lung cancer (NSCLC): long-term oncologic results. J Thorac Cardiovasc Surg 2012; 143:383–389.
6. Cerfolio RJ, Bryant AS, Skylizard L, Minnich DJ. Initial consecutive experience of completely portal robotic pulmonary resection with 4 arms. J Thorac Cardiovasc Surg 2011; 142:740–746.
7. Park BJ, Flores RM, Rusch VW. Robotic assistance for video-assisted thoracic surgical lobectomy: technique and initial results. J Thorac Cardiovasc Surg 2006; 131:54–59.
8. Veronesis G, Galetta D, Maisonneuve P, et al. Four-arm robotic lobectomy for the treatment of early-stage lung cancer. J Thorac Cardiovasc Surg 2010; 140:19–25.
9. Gharagozloo F, Margolis M, Tempesta B, et al. Robot-assisted lobectomy for early-stage lung cancer: report of 100 consecutive cases. Ann Thorac Surg 2009; 88:380–384.

Chapter 24 Needlescopic and biportal VATS lobectomy

Alan DL Sihoe, Robert S George

INTRODUCTION

The advent of video-assisted thoracic surgery (VATS) has undoubtedly been the single greatest advance in thoracic surgery of this generation.[1,2] By significantly reducing pain, hastening recovery, minimizing complications, and improving postoperative quality of life for patients compared to open thoracotomy,[3,4] VATS is now well established as the approach of choice for almost every common thoracic operation – including lobectomy for early stage lung cancer.[5]

VATS has achieved success through a combination of eschewing rib-spreading and use of smaller access wounds. The standard technique of VATS is commonly via a 4–6 cm utility incision supplemented by two other smaller ports for placement of a video-thoracoscope and an instrument respectively.[6] This has been thoroughly detailed elsewhere in this book.

Nonetheless, VATS surgeons have not rested on their laurels. The last two decades have witnessed a progressive evolution of the standard three-port VATS approach. The underlying assumption is that if VATS is 'better' than open surgery because it inflicts less trauma upon the patient, then further reducing surgical access trauma by using smaller or fewer wounds would be even 'better' still.

This evolution in turn has taken two paths (*see* Figure 2.1). The first path is that of robot-assisted thoracic surgery. This has been typically characterized by high capital and consumables costs, but also by considerable ease-of-use and permitting fine tremor-free dissection. The pros and cons of robot-assisted thoracic surgery are beyond the scope of this chapter, and readers are referred to the relevant chapter dealing with this approach elsewhere in this book.

The second path of VATS evolution is the progressive advancement of surgical technique from the standard three-port strategy to 'next generation' VATS. These approaches include needlescopic, two-port and uniportal VATS. The hallmark of these 'next generation' techniques is that they are all essentially developments from the basic three-port approach, and hence employ similar skills and instruments. This has significant implications for how these new approaches are learned.[7] In this author's experience, progressing in a step-wise fashion from conventional three-port VATS, to needlescopic VATS, to two-port VATS, and then to uniportal VATS was a smooth, easy-to-master process because each incremental step involved only a relatively small adaptation. It may be misconstrued by some that this sequential progression means that uniportal VATS may be the goal or 'end point', and hence should by something to strive for. Despite now using the uniportal technique for almost all operations, this author does not agree with that view. Instead, needlescopic and two-port VATS have proven to be very useful and versatile techniques in themselves. They offer easier operations in the hands of many surgeons, and uniportal VATS has never been shown to hold any significant advantage over them.

This chapter will describe these two important offspring of the VATS evolution: needlescopic and two-port VATS. The lessons learned from their development and use have implications for the practice of three-port VATS as well as for the increasingly popular uniportal VATS approach. These two approaches also provide excellent, viable alternatives to three-port and uniportal VATS.

NEEDLESCOPIC VATS

To operate in the human thorax, a surgeon must place three things into it: a right hand; a left hand; and a pair of eyes to look inside.[4] With open surgery, one must forcibly retract the ribs for up to several hours for a major operation to allow these three things to be placed. VATS greatly reduces surgical access trauma by replacing the right and left hands with surgical instruments, and direct vision through the wound with a video-thoracoscope – thereby obviating the need for any rib-spreading and minimizing the size of the wounds.

Although many variations exist in how VATS lobectomy is performed, the most common approach uses three ports.[1] An 8–12 mm camera port is typically placed in about the 7th or 8th intercostal space in the mid-axillary line, and another 8–12 mm posterior instrument port just anterior the tip of the scapula. A 4–6 cm utility port is usually placed in the anterior axillary line to take advantage of the naturally wider intercostal space towards the front of the chest to facilitate specimen retrieval. The utility port is typically sited in the 4th intercostal space for an upper lobectomy or 5th intercostal space for a lower lobectomy. This triangulation strategy of port placement allows the 'axis' of the operation to follow the natural longitudinal axis of the patient from feet towards the head. The right and left hands straddle this axis on both sides and reduced fencing between instruments and camera.[4,7]

Over time, the port placement strategy has been modified slightly (**Figure 24.1**). The camera port was brought more anterior to the anterior axillary line and the posterior port was lowered from anterior to the scapula tip to a lower intercostal level. The utility port position remained unchanged. Effectively, this was a posterior rotation of the 'baseball diamond',[4,7] allowing a more comfortable umbilicus-toward-shoulder axis of dissection and the use of the lower posterior port for inserting staplers at an easier (more shallow) angle for tackling hilar vessels during upper lobectomies.

However, studies have shown that even with conventional VATS as above, up to 32% of patients still have some residual discomfort for up to years after surgery.[8] We have also found that 53% of patients still feel chest wall paresthesia distinct from nociceptive wound pain at 19 months after VATS.[9]

To further reduce surgical morbidity, one approach was to make the VATS wounds even smaller.

Instead of the 10 mm tools used in conventional VATS equipment, very fine thoracoscopes and instruments are employed in needlescopic VATS (with diameters of 2–3 and 3–5 mm, respectively).[10] The technique was first applied in sympathectomy, to treat patients who had palmar hyperhidrosis and sympathetic chain disorders.[11] The reduction in wound size not only reduced pain but also gave excellent cosmetic results: within a few weeks incisions were all but invisible. Use of this technique was then extended to treatment of pneumothorax, with considerable success.[12]

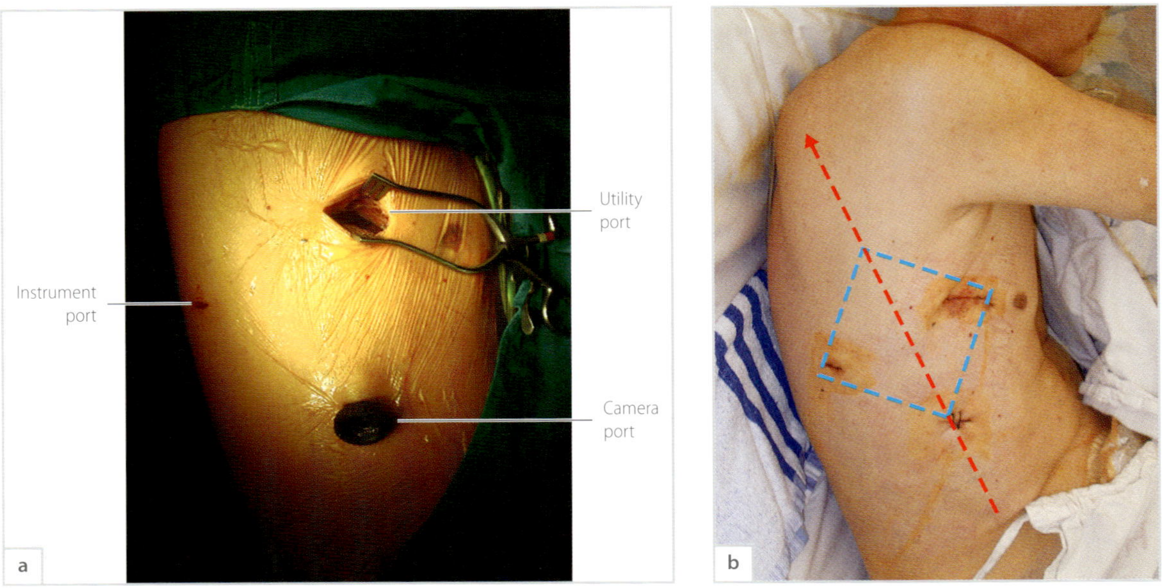

Figure 24.1 Port strategy for conventional three-port VATS lobectomy. This is a classic 'baseball diamond' strategy (blue square): the camera port is at 'home base', the target or the video monitor is toward '2nd base', and the utility and posterior ports are at '1st and 3rd base'. The 'axis' of the operation (red arrow) goes through home and 2nd base, and placing the 1st and 3rd bases on either side of the axis reduces fencing of instruments. Notice that the baseball diamond has rotated so that the axis runs slightly anterior-to-posterior, making instrumentation more ergonomic for the surgeon.

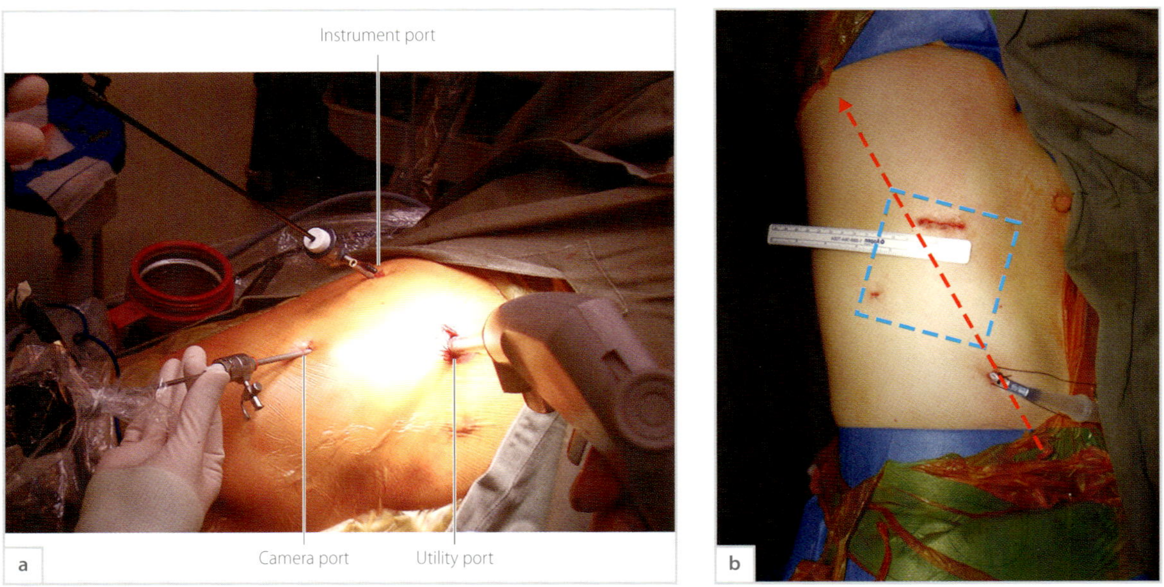

Figure 24.2 Port strategy for needlescopic VATS lobectomy. Notice that the port placement, orientation of the 'baseball diamond' (blue square) and 'axis' of the operation (red arrow) are all similar to that for conventional VATS as shown in Figure 24.1. The key difference is the reduction in size of the camera and posterior instrument ports to only 3 mm in diameter, resulting in excellent cosmesis (right).

Subsequently, needlescopic VATS was used in treatment of patients with lung cancer.[4,7] The ports are positioned as in the modified three-port strategy described above (**Figure 24.2**). The utility port is unchanged, needing to be 3–5 cm to allow the resected lobe to be extracted. The size of the other two ports is altered: the posterior port is reduced to 3 mm (from 10 mm); the camera port is 3 mm, produced by puncturing the skin with a no. 11 scalpel. A 3 mm 30° video-thoracoscope is fed through the incision with the aid of a trocar. There is an alternative approach for camera placement, which is to use a small mosquito forceps to create a tract into the pleural space and to place a 5 mm 30° video-thoracoscope directly through this tract. Within the chest, lens tip can be wiped using a pledget lightly soaked with anti-fogging solution held on a Roberts' forceps and inserted via the chest tube thoracostomy wound. In the author's experience, a 3 mm scope can be broken by a careless or overzealous camera-assistant, whereas a 5 mm scope tends to be harder and more resistant to bending and breaking in the hands of the surgeon. The small caliber of scope is not a problem for visualization: modern high-definition surgical video cameras have such good light sensitivity and superb resolution that in practice the view is not far short of a 10-mm scope.

The smaller camera and posterior instrument port sizes confer significant advantages. A problem with the conventional 10 mm thoracoscope is that, given the narrowness of the human intercostal space, the thoracoscope can pivot against and cause blunt trauma to the intercostal bundles. Using much finer thoracoscope and instruments means that the effect of hinging at the wound is reduced and cosmesis is of course much better. Additionally, because three ports are still being utilised, the conduct of needlescopic VATS is essentially the same as with conventional VATS, which means the experienced VATS surgeon can learn the technique quickly. Furthermore, complete lymph node dissection is also eminently feasible with needlescopic VATS.

When performing a typical lobectomy using the needlescopic approach, the surgeon can use exactly the same instruments as with conventional three-port VATS via the utility incision. These include open instruments such as ring forceps for retraction, open scissors and energy devices for dissection, and so on. The basic technique of dissection is therefore essentially the same as in conventional VATS. The posterior port only admits a 3-mm needlescopic instrument. An atraumatic, rounded-tip 3 mm grasper can be used for gentle retraction of the lung – ideally by retracting rather than grasping. Given that the 3 mm instruments are small and can potentially cause inadvertent puncturing of the lung parenchyma, any grasping should be limited to the lobe of lung to be resected. Soft tissue to be dissected (such as lymph nodes or fascia around hilar vessels) can be grasped by 3 mm instruments in the same way that they are grasped by Debakey (or similar) tweezer forceps during open surgery (**Figure 24.3**). Lifting of such fascia via a 3-mm grasper through the posterior port facilitates fine dissection with any conventional instrument via the utility port.

The biggest difference with conventional three-port VATS is that staplers can now only be admitted via the utility incision. The loss of the posterior port for introduction of the stapler is compensated for by better understanding of how to maneuver the lung (**Figure 24.7**). Simple retraction of the lung toward the posterior or anterior utility port can result in the wrong angle of approach for the stapler, with medial or posterior structures impeding the passage of the anvil. For example, when trying to pass the stapler around a superior pulmonary vein, the utility port is sited immediately over the vein so that a stapler inserted directly will be blocked against the hilum posteriorly. The trick is to fully reticulate the stapler so that the anvil is made to pass behind the vein from an inferior-to-superior direction. The lung must then be retracted in a cephalad and slightly anterior direction, creating more space behind the vein for the anvil to pass. The cephalad distraction also creates a less acute angle for the stapler to approach the superior vein in a more horizontal direction without hitting the hilar structures behind the vein (**Figure 24.4**). The use of curved tip stapler reloads also greatly helps to negotiate vessels in this situation. In a similar way, the retraction of the lung becomes very important to present the right angles for the stapler to approach via the utility port when dividing any vessel or bronchus of any lobe.

At the end of the procedure, the utility port is closed in the usual layered fashion. The 3 mm posterior port can be closed using adhesive strips alone. However, the author's experience is that closing with a 5/0 nylon stitch (which can be removed in clinic a week later) provides better cosmesis. The author places a 16F or 20F chest drain via the camera port – which is a snug fit if a 5-mm in diameter thoracoscope was used. Unless there is a large air leak, this smaller caliber drain is usually sufficient for a lobectomy. The cosmetic result is usually excellent (**Figure 24.2**), with the posterior and camera ports healing to only very small (sometimes barely visible) pinpoint scars within 2 weeks after surgery.

TWO-PORT (BIPORTAL) VATS

Once the three-port needlescopic VATS approach had been used for a while, it became clear that the posterior port was not always needed. The obvious development was to omit it altogether, retaining the camera and utility ports. The result is called the two-port, or biportal, VATS technique. The biportal technique does have a disadvantage: when there is only a single utility port for all the instrumentation, this demands heightened surgical dexterity because the surgeon must control all the instruments coaxially through the shared port.

The camera port is placed in the same site as for conventional and needlescopic VATS. As with the latter approach, the author uses a 30-degree 5 mm video-thoracoscope placed without a trocar as above. This means that for the camera assistant, all camera handling and viewing angles are unchanged, making his/her job relatively easy to get used to (**Figure 24.5**). This is a key advantage of the two-port approach over a uniportal approach. If the surgical team does not have an experienced camera assistant, this can impede on the learning curve.

For the chief surgeon, the loss of the posterior port takes a little getting used to. Most importantly the lung retraction must be performed via the same incision as the dissection. It is for this reason that long, curved lung graspers (usually ring forceps) become highly useful. The curvature of the grasper allows the lung to be better distracted away from the site of dissection, reducing fencing between the surgeon's own hands/instruments. Other than this, the dissection is done similarly to conventional and needlescopic VATS, using similar instruments (**Figures 24.6–24.11**). The same tips regarding passage of staplers via the utility port (as described for needlescopic VATS above) still apply. It is emphasized again that successful passage of staplers around hilar structures requires a two-handed approach. Much more than with conventional three-port VATS as the passage of the staplers requires the constant manipulation of lung with the non-dominant hand to provide the right angle for the passage of the stapler which itself is controlled with the dominant hand. If the non-dominant retracting hand is kept

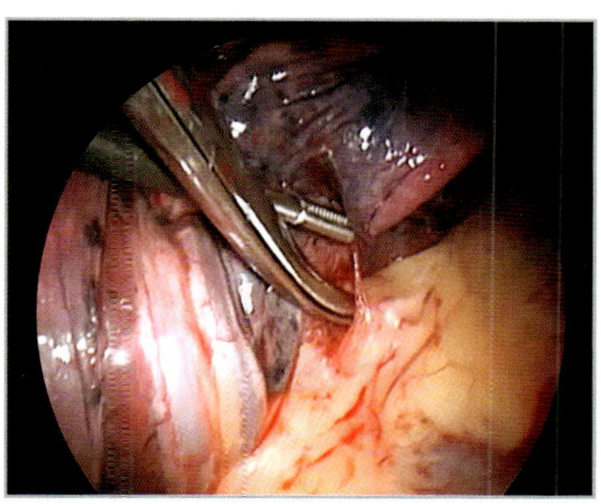

Figure 24.3 Intraoperative view during a needlescopic VATS right upper lobectomy. The 3 mm grasper is inserted via the posterior port. The shaft helps provide retraction of the lung, while the tip grasps the fascia around the anterior hilum allowing dissection by the open Metzenbaum scissors (inserted via anterior utility port).

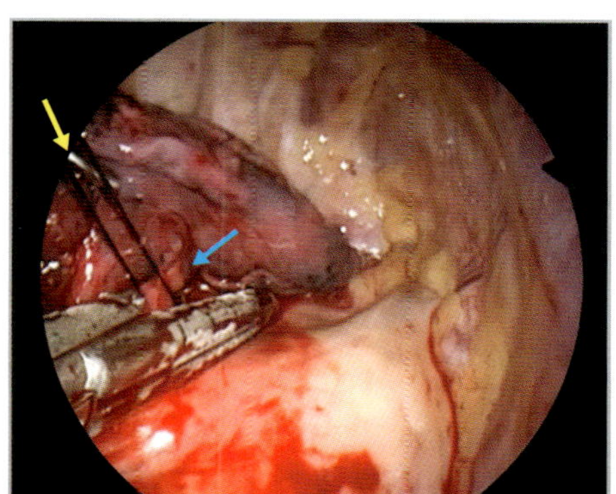

Figure 24.4 Intraoperative view during a needlescopic VATS right upper lobectomy. The 3 mm grasper is inserted via the posterior port (yellow arrow). The right upper lobe is retracted laterally and cephalad so that the superior pulmonary vein (blue arrow) is running perpendicular to the mediastinum: this allows the reticulated stapler to be passed across the vein very easily from left-to-right. At this angle of approach, the stapler does not point down into the mediastinum, and the anvil can emerge from behind the vein without impinging on any structure. The slight anterior retraction of the upper lobe also provides more room behind the vein for the stapler anvil to pass through.

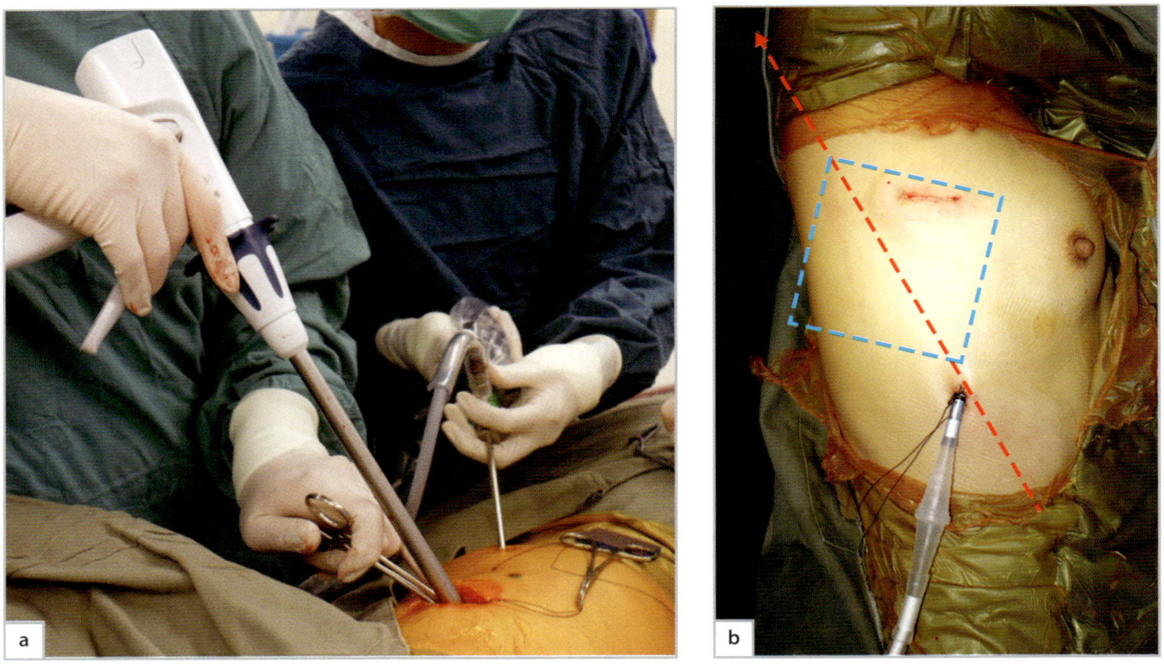

Figure 24.5 Port strategy for two-port VATS lobectomy. Notice that the port placement, orientation of the 'baseball diamond' (blue square) and 'axis' of the operation (red arrow) are similar to that for conventional and needlescopic VATS, but the posterior port has been deleted. The surgeon performs the operation using all instruments inserted coaxially via the utility port (left), and again the cosmesis is excellent (right).

still, and one tries too aggressively to simply insert the stapler through with the dominant hand, trauma to the hilar structures such as catastrophic bleeding from vessel avulsion can occur.

Closure of the utility incision and placement of a chest tube via the camera port is the same as with needlescopic VATS.

It should be noted that variations of the two-port approach have been well reported. The most well-known of these is that of Thomas D'Amico of Duke University.[13] Coming to two-port VATS directly from open surgery – without going through an evolution through three-port VATS – D'Amico's port strategy differs from the author's as described above. In particular, the camera port is sited quite posteriorly – at the mid or posterior axillary line. This is used to pass a 10-mm video-thoracoscope with a trocar. Although this approach uses a larger camera port, it retains the possibility of passing the stapler in via that camera port if necessary. More recently, the Duke approach has been further modified. The standard utility incision is created, but the camera port is now sited via a second skin incision along the same intercostal space.[14] This two-incision but single intercostal space approach is said to potentially offer the same benefits as a uniportal approach whilst reducing some of its difficulties, such as with camera handling and chest drain wound complications.

A word of caution should be given to the term 'single operating port VATS' or "single utility port VATS".[15] This has been used in some countries – particularly in Asia – to describe when the operation is performed by instrumentation via a single incision (the 'single operating port') but with an additional small camera port also created. If that sounds like the two-port approach described above, that is because it is the same. This author would advise against using the 'single operating/utility port VATS' terminology, as it would create confusion between it and proper uniportal VATS. As the thoracic committee seeks to create databases and prospective studies to evaluate the different 'next generation' approaches, it is important to have clear definitions of and distinctions between the various approaches so that their strengths, weaknesses and roles can be clinically well investigated.

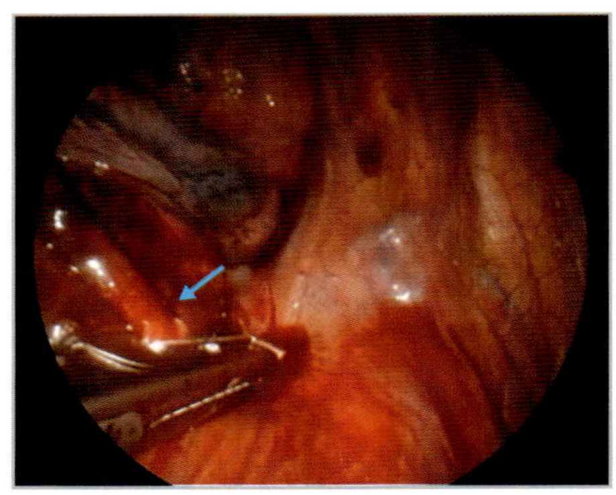

Figure 24.6 Intraoperative view during a two-port VATS right upper lobectomy. Notice the striking similarity to the view in Figure 24.4. The right upper lobe is retracted laterally and cephalad so that the superior pulmonary vein (blue arrow) is running almost perpendicular to the mediastinum: this allows the roticulated stapler to be passed across the vein very easily from left-to-right. The slight anterior retraction of the upper lobe also provides more room behind the vein for the stapler anvil to pass through.

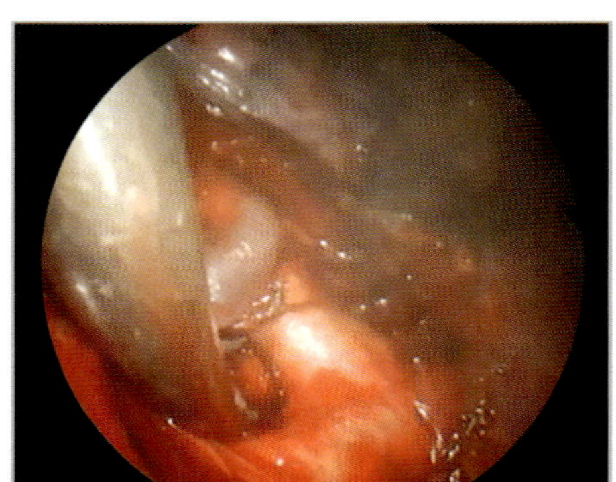

Figure 24.7 Intraoperative view during a two-port VATS right upper lobectomy. The pulmonary artery truncus anterior to the right upper lobe is readily dissected using the same open instruments as would be used in conventional VATS or even open thoracotomy (in this case, a simple Rumel type curved forceps).

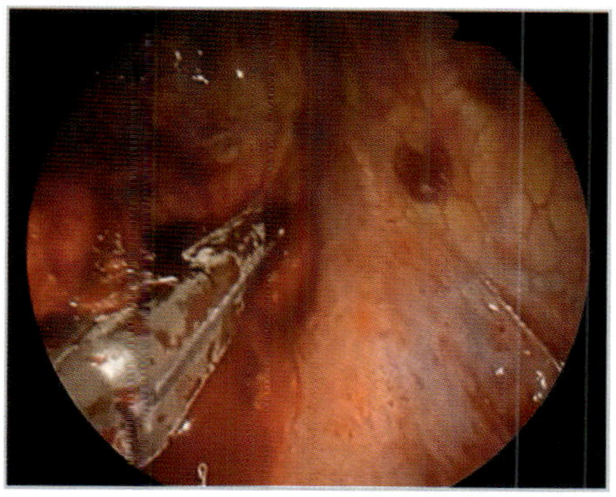

Figure 24.8 Intraoperative view during a two-port VATS right upper lobectomy. The pulmonary artery truncus anterior to the right upper lobe is staple divided. Notice the similarity with Figure 24.6: a similar retraction is used as with the superior pulmonary vein. The lateral, cephalad and slightly anterior retraction allows the reticulated stapler to be passed across the artery easily without impinging on any structures as the anvil exits.

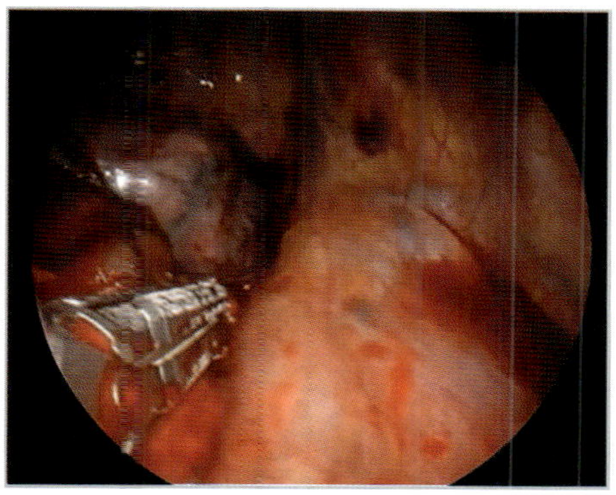

Figure 24.9 Intraoperative view during a two-port VATS right upper lobectomy. The lobar bronchus to the right upper lobe is readily dissected using the same open instruments as would be used in conventional VATS or even open thoracotomy (in this case, a simple Rumel type curved forceps).

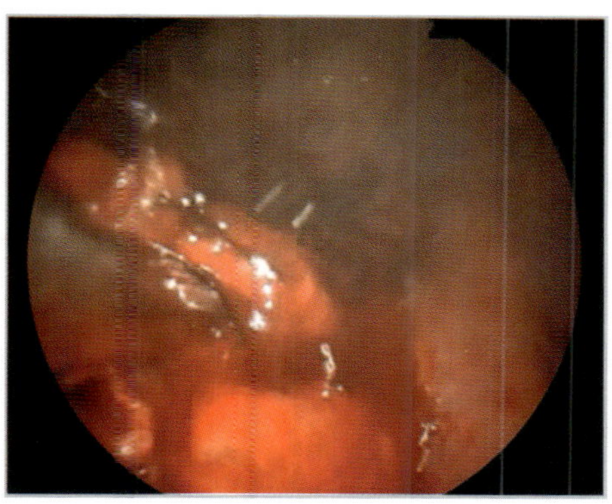

Figure 24.10 Intraoperative view during a two-port VATS right upper lobectomy. The right upper lobe bronchus is stapled. Notice the similarity with Figure 24.6: a similar retraction is used as with the superior pulmonary vein. The lateral, cephalad and slightly anterior retraction allows the reticulated stapler to be passed across the bronchus easily without impinging on any structures as the anvil exits.

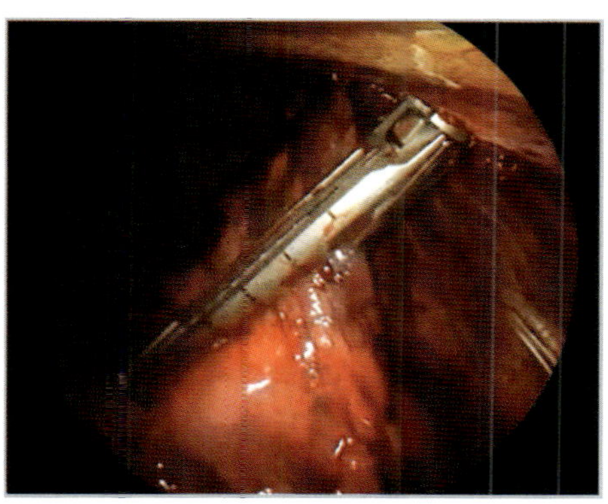

Figure 24.11 Intraoperative view during a two-port VATS right upper lobectomy. The horizontal fissure between the upper and middle lobes is completed by staple-division using a 'fissure-last' (or 'fissureless') approach.

PERIOPERATIVE CARE

The author's unit employs general anesthesia and one-lung ventilation when performing needlescopic and biportal VATS. Patient positioning is identical as for conventional three-port VATS: lateral positioning with gentle 'bridging' of the operating table to lower the hip and open up the intercostal spaces on the operation side.[1,2] A pre-incisional paravertebral blockade with bupivacaine bolus injections is given percutaneously after induction of GA. For most lobectomies, further intercostal blockade or insertion of catheters for postoperative blockade infusion is unnecessary.

Postoperatively, all patients receive regular oral paracetamol (acetaminophen) 1 g 6-hourly, supplemented by oral tramadol 50 mg 4–6-hourly as required only for breakthrough pain.

Chest drains are routinely connected to a digital chest drainage system (Medela Thopaz, Medela AG, Baar, Switzerland).[16] A negative pressure of 15 cmH_2O is applied initially, then reduced to gravity mode (8 cmH_2O) on the morning after surgery. Drains are removed when the air flow is less than 40 mL/min for 6 hours with no 'spikes' of air leak during that time.

It is strongly recommended that a bespoke perioperative management protocol – a clinical pathway – be designed to complement any program of 'next generation' VATS. This is necessary to ensure the patient receives the maximum benefit of the surgical technique in terms of expedited recovery. The pathway should incorporate all aspects of perioperative management, including: chest drainage; analgesia; mobilization; physiotherapy; investigations; communications with patient and family, etc. Failure to adopt a bespoke pathway can result in failure to see any benefit of 'next generation' approaches compared to traditional ones. At the University of Hong Kong, the average length of stay after lobectomy with the 'next generation approaches is now 3 days.

KEY LESSONS FROM NEEDLESCOPIC AND TWO-PORT VATS

Step-wise training

For a thoracic surgeon used to operating via conventional VATS, starting to learn uniportal VATS may feel uncomfortable. The jump to uniportal involves having to place the instruments from both right and left hands through the same port, and furthermore having to share that port with a video-thoracoscope. One would think that this is a technique that required considerable time to master. However, in reality, the author's learning curve was surprisingly short.[7] This author's learning curve with uniportal VATS lobectomy was less than 15 cases. The key to obtaining good results so quickly was not in the personal skill of the author, but in the fact that uniportal VATS was because of a step-wise progression from conventional VATS to needlescopic VATS to two-port VATS to uniportal VATS.[7]

The transition from conventional three-port to needlescopic VATS approach was a relatively small step. One first needed to get used to the view with a 3 mm or 5 mm video-thoracoscope. However, as already described, with modern high-definition video systems, the view obtained is barely inferior to that via a standard 10 mm scope – especially, if one uses the 5 mm scope. The next issue was that of placing the stapler via the utility port because the posterior and camera ports were no longer available for this. This required a greater appreciation of how to retract the lung using the nondominant hand to allow the correct angles for the stapler to be applied around the hilar structures using the dominant hand. The Needlescopic approach trains the surgeon to be more reliant on displaying good angles for dissection and stapling, and less reliant on using an extra port.

The transition from Needlescopic VATS to two-port VATS was another small step, because in reality the posterior port was no longer highly useful and its loss would not matter greatly. Also, the stapling via the utility port has been mastered. The surgeon is now required to simply become accustomed to placing right and left hand instruments via the utility port only during two-port VATS. During this time, a greater appreciation of using curved or right-angled instruments (such as long curved ring forceps, or simply Roberts and Rumel forceps) to facilitate dissection through a shared port is quickly gained. Because the utility port is in the same place as with conventional and needlescopic three-port VATS, most of the very same instruments could also be used – including standard Metzenbaum scissors, Debakey forceps, hand-control diathermy devices with long-tip extensions, and so on. This proved invaluable by allowing a familiar set of instruments to be maintained without the surgeon having to learn to use new ones alongside learning a new technique. With the instruments largely unchanged, the surgeon can focus of getting used to having both hands work coaxially, rather than coming in from two opposite sides. A great advantage of the needlescopic and two-port technique is that the camera port is the same as with conventional three-port VATS. This means that while the surgeon is practising the new manual skills required, the camera assistant has a relatively easy job providing the same visualization as with conventional VATS.

Once one has mastered using right and left hand instruments via the same shared utility port using the two-port approach, proceeding to a uniportal VATS approach merely becomes the transferral of the video-thoracoscope to the same port. Provided the surgeon has already mastered the coaxial instrumentation via the utility port, the only thing left to do now is to have the video-thoracoscope is brought up to the utility port. The same right and left hand instrumentation as with two-port VATS is maintained, and the surgeon now can focus on learning the visual element: looking in the same direction as the instruments rather than from an angle. Of course, along with that, the surgeon must also get used to sharing the only port with the camera – including coping with twister-like intimacy with the camera assistant.

This author highly recommends that learning uniportal VATS should take this step-wise approach. By breaking down the progression into steps, defined learning objectives at each step can be clearly seen as described above. This makes it much easier for the surgeon to learn and progress to uniportal if he/she may so wish. It also makes the process safer for patients, as the surgeon need not progress too adventurously but instead take small incremental steps.

Instruments

As suggested above, the gradual progression from conventional VATS to needlescopic VATS to two-port VATS to uniportal VATS means that there is no rush to immediately buy new instruments. The use of the same utility port essentially means that most – if not all – the instruments the surgeon is already comfortable with can be used unchanged when moving up to the next step along the evolution. The implication of this is that it is not necessary to purchase any expensive new instruments to 'allow' one to start performing uniportal VATS. Instead, it is better to first try the new technique using familiar instruments. Not only will this make it easier to learn, but it will allow the surgeon to gradually understand exactly where the old instruments may or may not be inadequate when performing uniportal VATS. There are many wonderful 'VATS' instruments available, some of which are very good but many of which are quite expensive. This author has witnessed many instances where a unit beginning to perform 'next generation' VATS mistakenly believed that purchase of a fancy set of tools will enable them to instantly do it. Not only is this fantasy invariably proved wrong, but the unit is left with a set of instruments that they seldom use again thereafter. It is advised that the surgeon should gain some experience with the technique and understand the specific areas where an expensive new instrument may help before splurging on a new purchase.

A vital 'instrument' that is often neglected is the operating table. Rotation of the operating table can facilitate exposure of the hilar structures and nodal stations when retraction alone is not enough. The exposure of the superior pulmonary vein can be facilitated by tilting the table posteriorly, and approaching the upper mediastinum by tilting it 'head up', for example. The subcarinal nodal station in particular is better accessed by rotating the table forwards.

Troubleshooting

Because the `next generation' VATS techniques are developments of minimally invasive thoracic surgery (MITS), the solutions that are used in other forms of VATS can be applied just as effectively when difficulties are encountered.[1,2] Examples of this are:

- **Mild and severe bleeding:** Topical hemostats and compression can effectively control mild bleeding. Endoscopic suturing is done for more severe bleeding.
- **Fused interlobar fissure:** The 'fissure-less' (or 'fissure last') approach to a lobectomy, commonly used in conventional VATS,[4,17] can be employed in needlescopic and two-port VATS.
- **Air leaks detected during surgery:** Major leaks can be repaired using endoscopic suturing. For minor leaks topical sealants are applied. The author's experience is that the time for which a chest drain is needed and the duration of hospital stay can both be reduced after VATS lung surgery if aerosolized fibrin sealant is sprayed onto areas of small air leaks (the sealant cost is usually easily offset by reduced postoperative hospital cost).
- **Large tumors:** It is essential that a resected specimen can be delivered through the intercostal space; conversion to a thoracotomy or use of forcible rib-spreading to deliver an especially large specimen cancels out the pain-reducing advantages of any type of VATS. Thus, when the resected specimen is too large, the technique the author uses is controlled cutting of a rib anteriorly to allow the intercostal space to be widened using minimal force.[18] Originally developed for multi-port VATS, this technique is applicable in needlescopic, two-port and uniportal VATS.

The step-wise evolution is also useful if the need to convert should arise. If during any operation some difficulty is encountered, the surgeon may also choose to revert to a previous step instead of converting immediately to open thoracotomy. For example, if the patient is stable, one could convert from uniportal to a two-port approach, or from a needlescopic to a conventional three-port approach instead of immediately going to an open thoracotomy.

Dealing with critics

One of the painful lessons from the early days of VATS was that whenever a new approach is developed, there will be many conservative surgeons who will attack it vehemently. Critics would first argue whether the new technique is safe. To this, the reasonable response is that these 'next generation' VATS approaches represent step-wise modifications only of an already well-established approach of VATS.

Furthermore, needlescopic and two-port VATS has already been practiced safely with adequate literature documentation.[7,15]

The next argument from the critics is not so easy to deflect. They would ask 'what is the advantage of the new approach?' In fairness, the only real answer to that is that there is no clinical advantage at all in performing needlescopic, two-port, or uniportal VATS when compared to conventional VATS. At the time of this writing, only a couple of limited studies have compared these approaches for lobectomy, and thus far there is no convincing evidence that the 'next generation' approaches offer any benefit to patients compared with conventional VATS.[19-21] On the other hand, results to date show that the newer approaches do not put the patients at any added risk or compromise their outcomes. It can be crudely summarized therefore that current evidence says that we 'can' safely perform the new techniques, but is insufficient to say that everyone 'should' perform these techniques. That is perhaps enough for the pioneers and 'early adapters' to continue their work, so that their results can subsequently define the role of these techniques and prove the doubters right or wrong.

CONCLUSION

In this chapter, 'next generation' VATS has been portrayed as a stepwise evolution from conventional VATS to needlescopic to two-port and finally to uniportal VATS. If this has somehow led the reader into concluding that uniportal is the 'end of the line' or the final destination of this process, then this author apologizes. Uniportal VATS is by no means the 'holy grail' of MITS. The last 20-odd years of VATS has taught us that progress is unrelenting, and there will be many new advances to come in the years ahead. These include new surgical technologies, novel methods of perioperative care, infusion of the latest immunophysiology and molecular oncology philosophies into surgical practice, and many others.

It is therefore too simplistic and naive for surgeons to simply think that any mode of VATS alone – be it three-port or uniportal – should be the ultimate goal of our specialty. To do so would cause at least two harmful effects. First, this attitude would engender complacency in those who feel they have 'mastered' VATS. This in turn would leave our specialty ill-prepared for the coming assault on our specialty by pulmonologists, oncologists and other specialties armed with such 'patient-friendly' alternatives to surgery, such as medical thoracoscopy, percutaneous ablation, stereotactic body radiation therapy, targeted therapy, and so on. Second, this attitude would trivialize the role of needlescopic and two-port VATS. To the conservative, who sees no point in moving beyond open thoracotomy or conventional three-port VATS, these may seem worthless upstarts. To the dedicated uniportalist, these seem like minor waypoints along the path to the final destination of single-port surgery.

We as thoracic surgeons must guard against such attitudes. Instead, we should take these waypoints very seriously. They are indeed waypoints, but not simply to uniportal VATS. Needlescopic and two-port VATS are steps along the never-ending path to creating better surgery for patients. Indeed, conventional and uniportal VATS are just other steps along that same path. Viewed in this light, Needlescopic and two-port VATS are not 'inferior' to uniportal VATS. Evidence for that does not currently exist. If a surgeon feels that uniportal VATS is not the right approach for him/her for any reason, there is nothing wrong with sticking to needlescopic and two-port VATS (or conventional VATS for that matter). This is because the fact that the surgeon has embarked upon the path to try to improve surgery for patients is in itself the most important thing. It is the striving for improvement that will provide thoracic surgery with the best defence against the above onslaught from other specialities. If this chapter has stirred some interest in the reader to try any form of 'next generation' VATS as a first-step to improving surgery for patients, then it has fulfilled its primary mission.

REFERENCES

1. Sihoe ADL, Yim APC. Video-assisted pulmonary resections. In: Thoracic Surgery (3rd edn). Patterson GA, Cooper JD, Deslauriers J, et al. (Eds). Elsevier, Philadelphia, USA, 2008:970–988.
2. Sihoe ADL, Yim APC. VATS as a diagnostic tool. In: General Thoracic Surgery (7th edn). Shields TW, Locicero J, Ponn RB, Rusch VW (Eds). Lippincott Williams & Wilkins, Philadelphia, USA, 2009:313–332.
3. Li WWL, Lee TW, Lam SSY, et al. Quality of life following lung cancer resection: video-assisted thoracic surgery versus thoracotomy. Chest 2002; 122:584–589.
4. Sihoe ADL. The Evolution of VATS Lobectomy. In: Topics in Thoracic Surgery. Cardoso P (Ed). Intech, Rijeka, Croatia, 2011:181–210.
5. Howington JA, Blum MG, Chang AC, Balekian AA, Murthy SC. Treatment of stage I and II non-small cell lung cancer. Chest 2013; 143:e278S–313S.
6. Swanson SJ, Herndon JE 2nd, D'Amico TA, et al. Video-assisted thoracic surgery lobectomy: report of CALGB 39802 – a prospective, multi-institution feasibility study. J Clin Oncol 2007; 25:4993–4997.
7. Sihoe ADL. The evolution of minimally invasive thoracic surgery: implications for the practice of uniportal thoracoscopic surgery. Journal of Thoracic Disease 2014; 6:S604–617.
8. Passlick B, Born C, Sienel W, Thetter O. Incidence of chronic pain after minimal invasive surgery for spontaneous pneumothorax. Eur J Cardiothorac Surg 2001; 19:355–359.
9. Sihoe ADL, Au SS, Cheung ML, et al. Incidence of chest wall paresthesia after video-assisted thoracic surgery for primary spontaneous pneumothorax. Eur J Cardiothorac Surg 2004; 25:1054–1058.
10. Yim APC, Sihoe ADL, Lee TW, Arifi AA. A simple maneuver to detect airleak on-table following 'needlescopic' VATS. J Thorac Cardiovasc Surg 2002; 124:1029–1030.
11. Sihoe ADL, Cheung CS, Lai HK, Lee TW, Thung KH, Yim APC. Incidence of chest wall paresthesia after needlescopic video-assisted thoracic surgery for palmar hyperhidrosis. Eur J Cardiothorac Surg 2005; 27:313–319.
12. Sihoe ADL, Yu PA, Wong JCC, et al. Needlescopic video-assisted thoracic surgery for primary spontaneous pneumothorax. Respirology 2012; 17:17–24.
13. Burfeind WR, D'Amico TA. Thoracoscopic lobectomy. Oper Tech Thorac Cardiovasc Surg 2004; 9:98–114.
14. Kara HV, Balderson SS, D'Amico TA. Modified Uniportal Video-Assisted Thoracoscopic Lobectomy: Duke Approach. Ann Thorac Surg 2014; 98:2239–2241.
15. Ng CSH. Uniportal VATS in Asia. J Thorac Dis 2013; 5:S221–225.
16. Pompili C, Detterbeck F, Papagiannopoulos K, et al. Multicenter international randomized comparison of objective and subjective outcomes between electronic and traditional chest drainage systems. Ann Thorac Surg 2014; 98:490–497.
17. Sihoe ADL, Tan HY. Complete video assisted thoracic surgery major lung resection for lung cancer: the impact of tuberculosis and post-inflammatory adhesions on outcomes. Respirology 2011; 16:138.
18. Sihoe AD, Chawla S, Paul S, et al. Technique for delivering large tumors in video-assisted thoracoscopic lobectomy. Asian Cardiovasc Thorac Ann 2014; 22:319–328.
19. Jutley RS, Khalil MW, Rocco G. Uniportal vs standard three-port VATS technique for spontaneous pneumothorax: comparison of post-operative pain and residual paraesthesia. Eur J Cardiothorac Surg 2005; 28:43–46.
20. McElnay PJ, Molyneux M, Krishnadas R, et al. Pain and recovery are comparable after either uniportal or multiport video-assisted thoracoscopic lobectomy: an observation study. Eur J Cardiothorac Surg 2015; 47:912–915.
21. Chung JH, Choi YS, Cho JH, et al. Uniportal video-assisted thoracoscopic lobectomy: an alternative to conventional thoracoscopic lobectomy in lung cancer surgery? Interact Cardiovasc Thorac Surg 2015; 20:813–819.

Chapter 25 Single-port video-assisted thoracoscopic lobectomy

Diego Gonzalez-Rivas, Carlos Velasco

INTRODUCTION

Video-assisted thoracic surgery (VATS) anatomic lobectomy for lung cancer was initially described more than 20 years ago.[1] Since then, many surgical units have successfully adopted this technique – its precise definition, however, varies.[2]

The final step in the evolution of the technique is the use of a single-port approach. The uniportal access for minor procedures was first described in 2004.[3] The first uniportal VATS lobectomy was described by Gonzalez-Rivas and colleagues in 2010.[4] With the development of ultra-high definition cameras, increasingly narrow and more articulated staplers and purposely-designed instruments, it is easier to perform major pulmonary resections through a single-incision approach. The growing number of surgical videos which have been posted on specialized websites, live surgery events and experimental courses have contributed to the rapid development of the uniportal approach worldwide. This chapter describes the technique for single-port VATS major pulmonary resections.

MATERIAL

Although uniportal VATS lobectomy can be performed with conventional instruments, the use of specially adapted conventional material, such as instrumentation with both proximal and distal articulation (**Figure 25.1**), seems to be more effective for successful single-incision lobectomy. The experience we acquired with the uniportal technique, as well as other technological improvements have made this approach safer, incrementing the indications for single-port thoracoscopic resections. The use of videolaparoscope with the distally mounted CCD design and antifog system facilitates the instrumentation (**Figure 25.1**).

POSITIONING AND INSTRUMENTS

The surgeon and the assistant must to be positioned in front of the patient in order to have the same thoracoscopic vision during all steps of the procedure (**Figure 25.1b**). Even though the field of vision is only obtained through the anterior access site, the combined movements of the thoracoscope along the incision will create different angles of vision (in this context, a 30-degree thoracoscope is recommended to achieve a panoramic view). The advantage of using the thoracoscope in coordination with the instruments is that the vision is directed to the target tissue, bringing the instruments to address the target lesion from a direct, sagittal perspective.[5]

Instruments must be long and curved to allow the insertion of 2–3 instruments simultaneously (**Figure 25.1**). Optimal exposure of the lung is vital in order to facilitate the dissection of the structures and to avoid instrument interference.

The patient is placed in a lateral decubitus position as is normal for a conventional VATS. The incision, about 3–4 cm long, is performed preferably in the 5th intercostal space in the anterior position. This location of the incision provides a better angle for hilar dissection and insertion of staplers. This incision is the same size as the utility incision we would use for a double- or triple-port VATS technique. There is no need to use a trocar for the thoracoscope.

It is helpful to rotate the surgical table away from the surgeons during the hilar dissection and division of structures, and toward the surgeons for the subcarinal lymph node dissection.

We recommend inserting staplers with angulation, through the anterior part of the incision. The curved tip load is very helpful to transect the upper lobe vein, which is the most difficult hilar structure to divide through a single-port (**Figure 25.2**). It is important to dissect

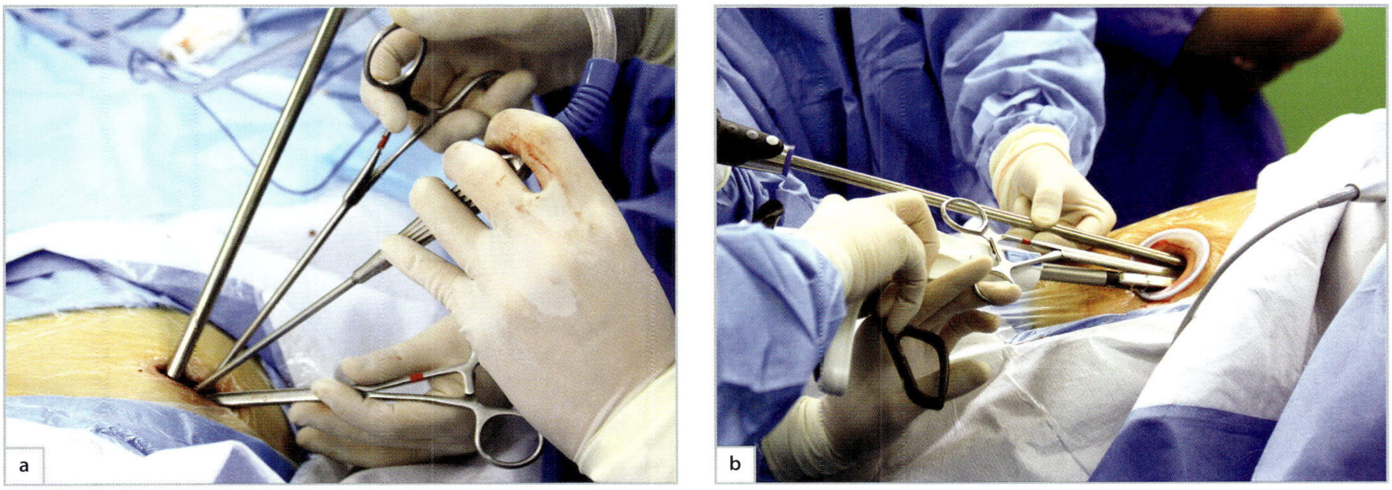

Figure 25.1 (a) Bimanual instrumentation during anatomic resections (camera is on the posterior part of the incision). (b) Photo showing the use of a wound protector and the position of surgeon and assistant, who are both in front of the patient.

the vessel as distal as possible in order to achieve a better angle for stapler insertion. When the angle is difficult for stapler insertion, the use of vascular clips (click aV, Grena) or ligatures is recommended. We recommend using one or two proximal clips and energy devices for distal division of the vessel (using distal clips avoids interference with the stapler when dividing the fissure at the end of the procedure).

It is crucial to always keep the thoracoscope placed at the posterior region of the utility incision while working with the instruments in the anterior region (**Figure 25.1**). The only time we position the camera down is for division of the anterior part of the minor fissure (with the staplers placed above).

For lower lobectomies the normal sequence of dissection is as follows: inferior pulmonary ligament, inferior pulmonary vein, pulmonary artery, bronchus and finally completion of the fissure. In the case of upper lobectomies, the pulmonary artery is normally divided first, followed by the vein, bronchus and fissure (**Figure 25.3**).

When the lobectomy is completed, the lobe is removed in a protective bag and a systematic lymph node dissection is performed. The intercostal spaces are infiltrated with bupivacaine at the end of the surgery under a thoracoscopic view. A single chest tube is placed in the posterior part of the incision.

SURGICAL TECHNIQUE

Lower lobectomy

The lobectomy may be technically different depending on whether the fissure is complete or not. If the fissure is complete we try to dissect and staple the artery in the fissure. Sometimes, it is easier to individually divide the arterial branches of the superior and basilar segments. The vein is usually dissected and divided easily. Then, the lower lobe bronchus is exposed, dissected and stapled in the same way as we discussed for the vein. The last step is to staple the fissure and remove the lobe in a protective bag.

In the presence on an incomplete fissure or no visible artery, the technique is different. Our preferred method is to not involve dissection within the fissure, so as to avoid postoperative air leaks. In this case, the lobectomy must be performed from caudal to cranial leaving the fissure stapling as the final step (fissure-less technique). Once the lobe is retracted cranially the sequence of the dissection should be as follows: inferior pulmonary ligament; inferior vein; inferior bronchus. Subsequently, a plane is created between the bronchus and the artery; the artery is taken thus leaving the fissure to be divided last (**Figure 25.3**).

The strategy for right lower lobectomy is similar to that of the left side except that when the artery is exposed in the fissure the origin of superior segmental artery must be dissected in the posterior and superior portion of the fissure.

Care must be taken to identify and avoid the damage of the bronchus or artery of the middle lobe. Once the inferior pulmonary vein has been stapled, the lower lobe bronchus is exposed, dissected and divided from its inferior aspect to its bifurcation with the middle lobe bronchus. Dissection of the bronchus with development of the plane between the bronchus and artery is performed leading to the visualization of the artery. We recommend removal of the interbronchial lymph nodes to better define the anatomy. Once identified, the segmental arterial branches of the lower lobe (basilar artery and superior segmental artery) are divided, with the fissure being stapled at the end of the procedure.

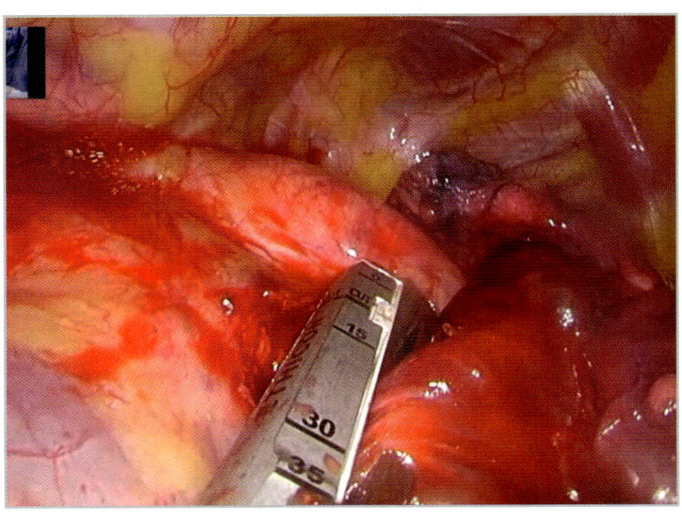

Figure 25.2 Use of curved tip angulated stapler for left upper vein división.

Upper lobectomy

The operative procedure for left upper lobectomies is similar to a conventional VATS. The uniportal approach provides a direct view and facilitates the dissection and division of upper anterior and apical segmental trunks, which are usually hidden by the superior vein when we use a conventional VATS view. We recommend to divide the upper anterior and apical segmental trunk first, in order to facilitate the insertion of the endostaplers in the upper lobe vein (**Figure 25.4a,b**). Once this arterial branch is stapled, the vein is easily exposed (**Figure 25.4c,d**). It is important to dissect the vein as distal as possible for optimal stapler insertion. The use of a curved-tip stapler facilitates improved positioning around the superior pulmonary vein and bronchus through a single-incision (**Figure 25.2**). Another option for management of the upper lobe vein is to firstly open the fissure as the first step from a hilar view, and then dissect the plane between upper and lower vein, identifying the bronchus and artery. The stapler is inserted over the artery, dividing the fissure, and the lobe is mobilized to allow stapling of the vein from a different angle.

The management of bronchus during left upper lobectomies is more difficult because care must to be taken with the lingular artery which usually lies behind the bronchus. We have four different ways of managing the upper lobe bronchus. The easiest option is to expose the lingular artery and subsequently divide it in the fissure (which is easier when the fissure is complete). At this point, the insertion of an endostapler for the bronchus is easy. In the second option, a TA stapler is used for division of the left upper lobe bronchus in certain cases of incomplete fissure to avoid injury of the lingular artery. The third option is to divide the bronchus with scissors and close it at the end of the surgery (by manual suture or with a stapler). The final and fourth option is to insert an endostapler after division of superior arterial trunk (and optionally posterior ascending artery) and vein. This last option should only be attempted by experienced uniportal VATS surgeons due to the risk of lingular artery injury.

For right upper lobectomy, sometimes it is helpful to partially divide the minor fissure as the first step (the anvil of the stapler is placed between the upper and middle lobe vein, pulling the parenchyma into the jaws of the stapler) in order to achieve a better angle for the insertion of the staplers into the upper vein (**Figure 25.5**). This maneuver provides a much better field of vision to dissect and transect the right upper lobe bronchus or the ascending arteries. Care must be taken when dissecting and dividing the ascending artery (laceration

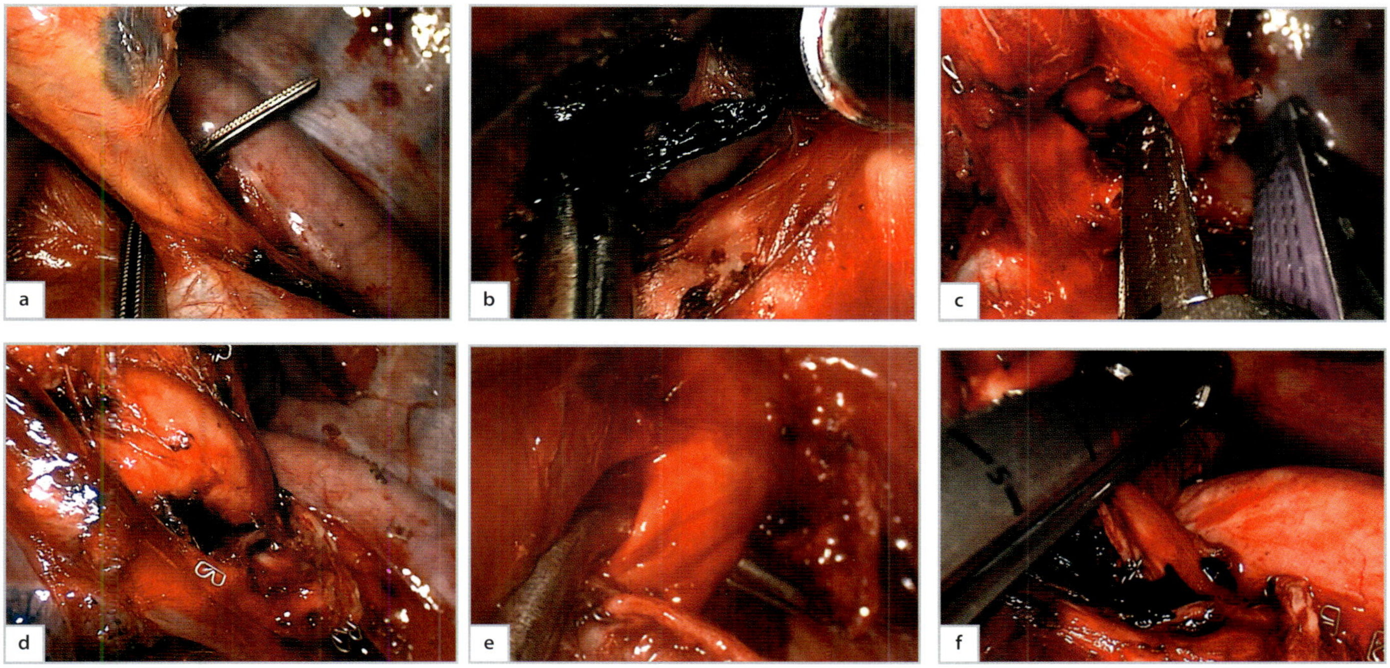

Figure 25.3 Sequence of left lower lobectomy from bottom to top. (a) dissection of inferior vein. (b) Removal of peribronchial lymph nodes to expose the plane between bronchus and artery. (c) Division of lower lobe bronchus. (d) Photo showing the lingular vein, the artery and the stump of the bronchus. (e) Dissection of the artery for lower lobe. (f) Division of fissure as the last step (fissureless technique).

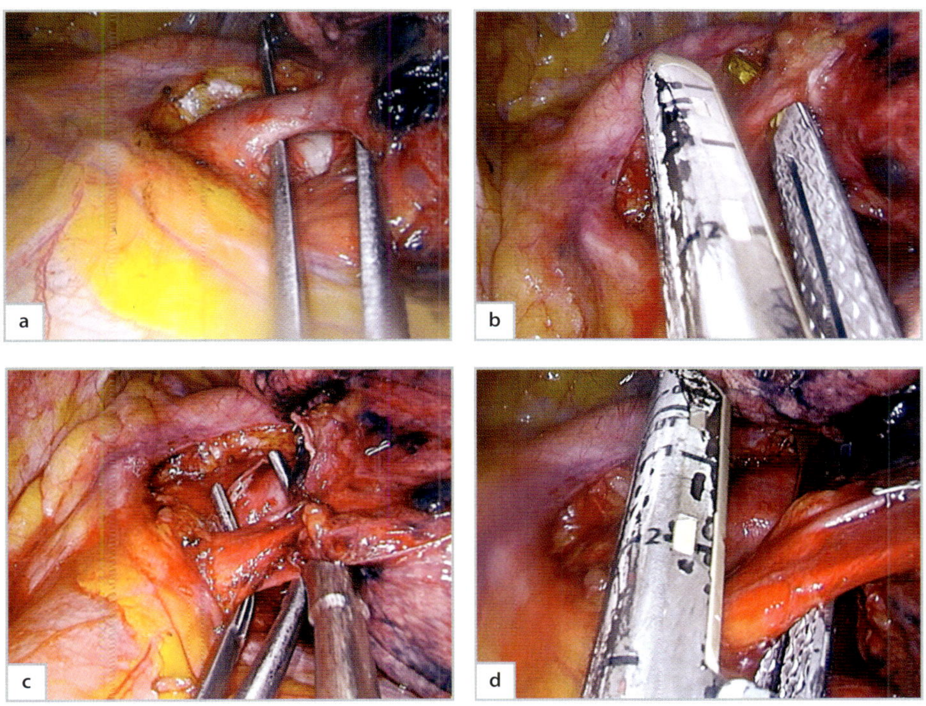

Figure 25.4 (a) Dissection of the artery for left upper lobectomy and (b) division by using an angulated curved tip stapler. (c) Dissection of the left upper lobe vein and (d) division using an angulated curved tip stapler.

of the posterior ascending artery is one the most frequent reasons for conversion).

The last step would be to complete the fissure (anvil of the stapler placed over the artery). After transecting the vein, artery and bronchus and after identifying the artery for the middle lobe, we can continue to divide the fissure by placing the stapler over the interlobar artery, pulling the parenchyma anteriorly and making sure the middle lobe artery is not included in the stapler line. The vascular and bronchial stumps should also avoid the stapler's jaws.

Occasionally, it is better to divide the bronchus after the division of the Boyden trunk to facilitate stapling of the upper lobe vein. We recommend exposing the posterior bifurcation between the upper

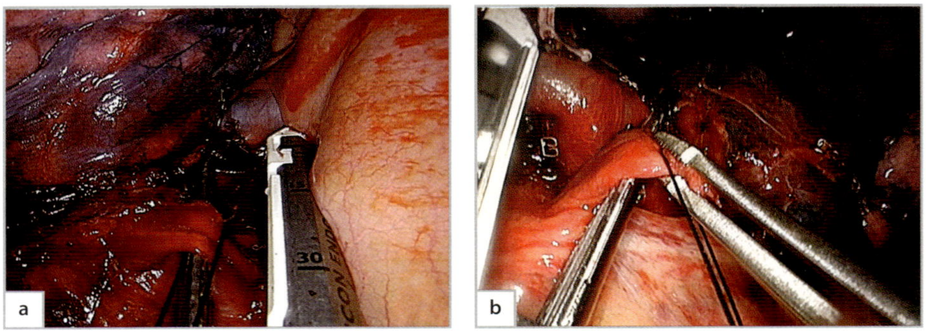

Figure 25.5 Two different angles for stapler insertion during division of the right upper lobe vein. (a) Division of the vein following division of the artery. (b) Division of the vein after division of the anterior part of a minor fissure.

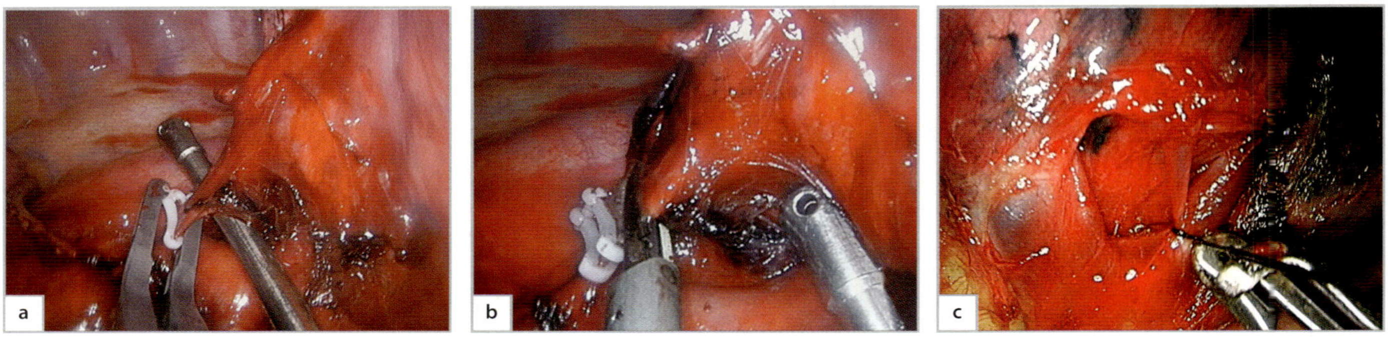

Figure 25.6 (a) Use of curved 45° applier to place polimer clips (click aV, Grena) to the segmental artery (S6) during right lower lobectomy and (b) division of the distal part of the segmental atery using energy devices. (c) Ligation of the segmental vein (S3) on the left upper lobe using a thoracoscopic knot pusher.

lobe and intermediate bronchus first, by dividing the posterior pleural reflection. This maneuver facilitates the following anterior bronchial dissection and the subsequent insertion of staplers to divide the vein.

The use of vascular clips is helpful in the division of segmental branches of the pulmonary vessels. The angulated 45° curved applier facilitates the placement of the clips through a single-incision approach (**Figure 25.6a**). We recommend using one or two clips for proximal control, and energy devices for distal division of the vessel (**Figure 25.6b**). Another option is to tie off the segmental branches by using a thoracoscopic knot pusher (**Figure 25.6c**).

Middle lobectomy

We recommend performing the middle lobectomy from caudal to cranial: anterior portion of the major fissure, vein, bronchus, artery, anterior portion of minor fissure and finally the posterior portion of fissure. The identification of medium lobe vein (MLV) and lower lobe vein (LLV) shows where to place the stapler to divide the anterior portion of the major fissure. The anvil of the stapler is then placed between the MLV and LLV, and the parenchyma is pulled into the jaws of the stapler. This maneuver facilitates the dissection and insertion of stapler to transect the vein.

Once the vein is divided, the middle lobe bronchus is exposed, dissected and stapled. After bronchus division the middle lobe artery is exposed and divided more easily. Finally, the fissures are divided.

Lymphadenectomy

With high definition view, long and specifically adapted instruments and energy devices, the uniportal technique is an excellent approach to perform radical lymph node dissection. For paratracheal dissection the anti-Trendelenburg position should be adopted because it naturally makes the lung 'fall down'. For subcarinal dissection the Trendelenburg position and the anterior table rotation facilitate exposure. Preliminary division of the pulmonary ligament gives a better access to the subcarinal space.

It is mandatory to place the camera in the posterior part of the incision. We can insert three or four instruments below the camera to complete the systematic dissection of the subcarinal and paratracheal space on the right side and subcarinal and aortopulmonary window on the left side. The use of bimanual instrumentation by using a long, curved instrument in the left hand and energy devices in the right hand, facilitates the radicality of the procedure and diminishes the incidence of bleeding during dissection. For hilar and N1 station lymphadenectomy, it is important to rotate the operating table posteriorly in order to place the lung in the back position.

Segmentectomies

Single-port VATS segmentectomy follows the principles of major pulmonary resections by VATS: individual dissection of segmental veins, segmental arteries and lobar segmental bronchus with a no rib-spreading, video-assisted thoracoscopic approach (**Figure 25.7**). The size of the utility incision is comparable to those commonly used for double- or triple-port approaches[6] and it is usually smaller than for a lobectomy (about 2–3-cm long). The most frequent and easy anatomic segmental resections are the superior lingulectomy and the superior segment of the lower lobe because there are constant anatomical landmarks (S6) (**Figure 25.7a**).

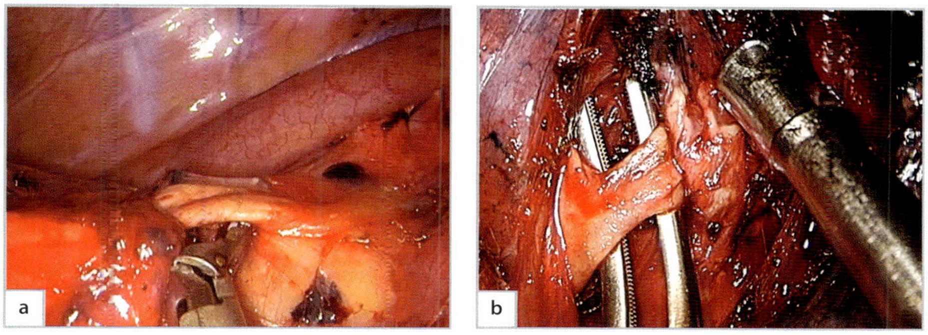

Figure 25.7 (a) Dissection of the segmental artery (S6) on the right lower lobe using energy devices. (b) Exposure of the segmental artery (S3) on the left upper lobe using a thoracoscopic dissector.

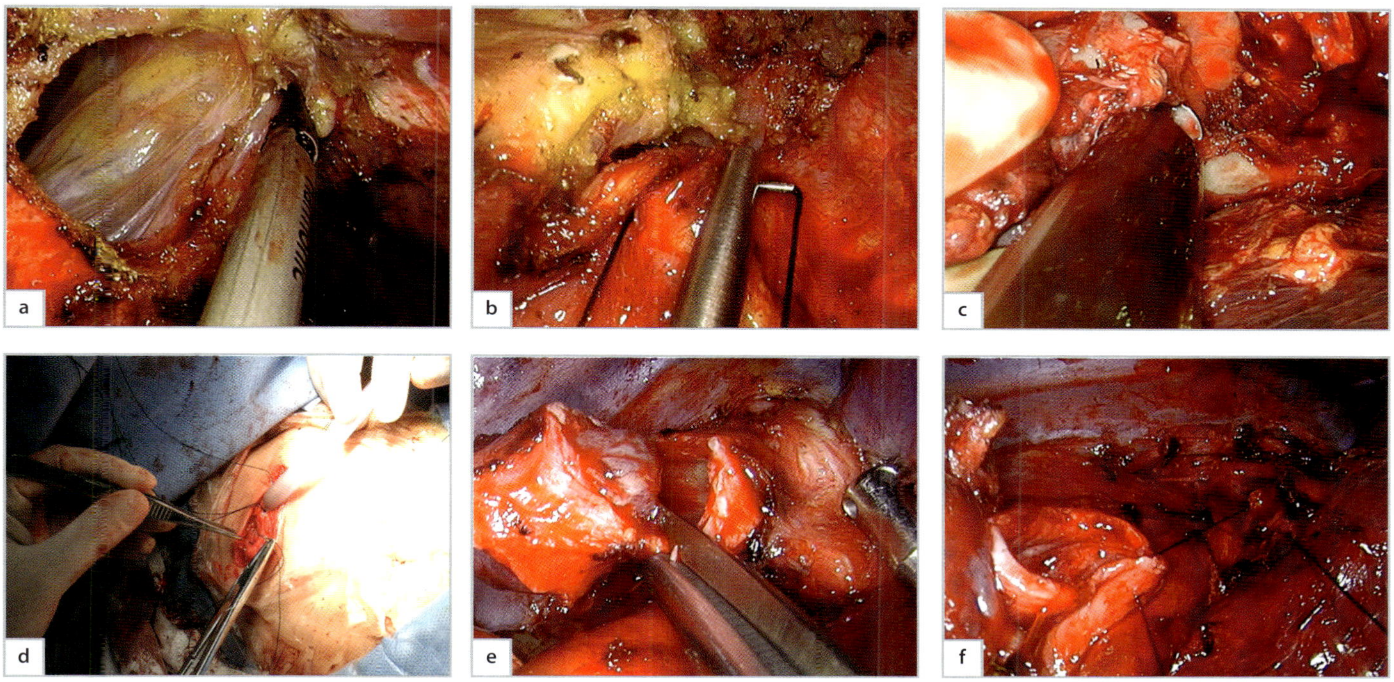

Figure 25.8 (a) Diaphragmatic resection by using energy devices. (b) Closure of diaphragm by using double interrupted silk sutures. (c) Use of thoracoscopic rib cutter for chest wall resection – (d) Closure of single incision after uniportal VATS lobectomy with en bloc chest wall resection. (e) Bronchus intermedius sleeve resection (lung sparing) for a carcinoid tumor. (f) Bronchial sleeve anastomosis (bronchus intermedius).

Pneumonectomies

The uniportal thoracoscopic resection of the whole lung is technically easier to perform than a lobectomy because the fissure does not need to be managed. However, extra care must to be taken during dissection and division of the main artery and transection of the main bronchus. The procedure on the right side is similar to that of the left, apart from the anatomical differences of the right pulmonary artery and its relationship to the main bronchus and superior vena cava. On the left side, the bronchus should be elevated by pulling up the whole lung and then transected as proximal as possible following division of the vascular elements. Once the stapler is inserted to divide the bronchus, it is recommended that the lung is pulled down before firing to achieve a short bronchial stump. Once the lung is removed a radical mediastinal lymph node dissection is performed.[7]

Complex resections: sleeve, chest wall or diaphragm resection

The uniportal technique allows us to make other complex procedures, such as tumors with diaphragm invasion (**Figure 25.8a,b**),[8,9] chest wall involvement (**Figure 25.8c,d**), sleeve resections (**Figure 25.8e,f**), superior sulcus or pan-coast tumors (hybrid approach is necessary) or complex cases after chemoradiotherapy. The geometrical explanation of the approach, and the direct view and bimanual parallel instrumentation could explain the benefits of this approach for complex resections.[10]

As we have become more experience in the single-port VATS approach we have increased the rate of thoracoscoscopic sleeve bronchovascular procedures and decreased the incidence of pneumonectomies.[11]

When performing bronchial suturing using single-port VATS, it is important to maintain the camera on the posterior part of the incision, operating with both hands below the camera. Here we apply the same principle as when performing an anterior thoracotomy in open surgery: to ensure a direct view so the surgeon's eyes are above his/her hands. Using a wound protector is helpful when dealing with obese patients as fatty tissue can interfere with the suture threads.

The operating table's position makes the lung exposure easier to perform the anastomosis (the anterior rotation of the table at 45° to the surgeon places the lung on an anterior position and makes the posterior bronchial suture easier, especially the membranous portion).

The use of material with proximal and distal articulation is crucial. The surgeon ties the knot outside of the chest with the right hand, holding both ends of the thread with the left hand's index and little fingers and pushing down the knots using a thoracoscopic knot pusher. The suture may be either a single-stitch or continuous suture (prolene 3/0). Monofilament sutures make thread movement - and tying - easier. We usually don't buttress the suture except in cases of preoperative radiotherapy. In these cases, we use an intercostal muscle flap, a pericardial pedicle or mediastinal fat pad. The bronchial edge must be assessed during the operation. The suture is checked for integrity at the end of surgery using insufflation under water and bronchoscopic control.

THE FUTURE

The future of thoracic surgery is based on the development of surgical procedures and innovations to further reduce surgical and anesthetic trauma. The combination of nonintubated or awake thoracoscopic surgery and the single-port VATS technique currently represent the least invasive procedures for pulmonary resections. Due to the limited use of intubation, mechanical ventilation and muscle relaxants, the anesthetic side effects are minimal and most patients avoid the intensive care unit. Given that only one intercostal space is opened, the use of local anesthesia and blockade of a single intercostal space is enough for pain control throughout surgery. This nonintubated major pulmonary resections must only be performed by experienced anesthesiologists and uniportal thoracoscopic surgeons (preferably skilled in VATS). In our experience, the quality of the pulmonary collapse obtained by iatrogenic pneumothorax via VATS under spontaneous breathing is at least as good as in mechanical ventilation using a double-lumen endotracheal tube. The mechanism of performing this lung collapse is more physiological via small intercostal incision than via one-lung mechanical ventilation and results in less lung inflammation and stress, with possible better postoperative recovery and outcomes. It is important to reduce the surgical and anesthetic trauma in high risk patients, such as elderly patients or those with poor pulmonary function. The influence of mediastinal and diaphragmatic movement do not usually interfere with hilar dissection for experienced VATS surgeons, especially when the cough is inhibited by using a correct vagus blockade.

Further development of new sealing device technologies for all vessels and fissure, robotic arms that open inside the thorax and wireless cameras, will allow the uniportal approach combined with robotic technology to become the standard surgical procedure for major pulmonary resections in most thoracic departments.

REFERENCES

1. Roviaro G, Rebuffat C, Varoli F, et al. Videoendoscopic pulmonary lobectomy for cancer. Surg Laparosc Endosc 1992; 2:244–247.
2. Rocco G, Internullo E, Cassivi SD, Van Raemdonck D, Ferguson MK. The variability of practice in minimally invasive thoracic surgery for pulmonary resections. Thorac Surg Clin 2008; 18:235–247.
3. Rocco G, Martin-Ucar A, Passera E. Uniportal VATS wedge pulmonary resections. Ann Thorac Surg 2004; 77:726–728.
4. Gonzalez D, Paradela M, Garcia J, de la Torre M. Single-port video-assisted thoracoscopic lobectomy. Interact Cardiovasc Thorac Surg 2011; 12:514–515.
5. Gonzalez-Rivas D, Fernandez R, de la Torre M, Martin-Ucar AE. Thoracoscopic lobectomy through a single incision. Multimed Man Cardiothorac Surg 2012; 2012:mms007.
6. Gonzalez-Rivas D. Single incision video-assisted thoracoscopic anatomic segmentectomy. Ann Cardiothorac Surg 2014; 3:204–207.
7. Gonzalez-Rivas D, Delgado M, Fieira E, et al. Uniportal video-assisted thoracoscopic pneumonectomy. J Thorac Dis 2013.
8. Gonzalez-Rivas D, Fernandez R, Fieira E, Rellan L. Uniportal video-assisted thoracoscopic bronchial sleeve lobectomy: First report. J Thorac Cardiovasc Surg 2013; 145:1676–1677.
9. Gonzalez-Rivas D, Fernandez R, Fieira E, Mendez L. Single-incision thoracoscopic right upper lobectomy with chest wall resection by posterior approach. Innovations 2013; 8:70–72.
10. Bertolaccini L, Rocco G, Viti A, Terzi A. Geometrical characteristics of uniportal VATS. J Thorac Dis 2013:S214–216.
11. Gonzalez-Rivas D, Delgado M, Fieira E, Fernandez R. Double sleeve uniportal video-assisted thoracoscopic lobectomy for non-small cell lung cancer. Ann Cardiothorac Surg 2014.
12. Gonzalez-Rivas D, Fernandez R, de la Torre M, et al. Single-port thoracoscopic lobectomy in a nonintubated patient: The least invasive procedure for major lung resection? Interactive Cardiovasc Thoracic Surg 2014; 19:552–555.
13. Gonzalez-Rivas D, Bonome C, Fieira E, et al. Non-intubated video-assisted thoracoscopic lung resections: the future of thoracic surgery? Eur J Cardiothorac Surg 2015.

Chapter 26 Single-port (uniportal) VATS for benign disease

Michele Salati, Gaetano Rocco, Robert S George

PRINCIPLES OF UNIPORTAL VATS

Uniportal VATS is the less invasive surgical technique which is used to treat intrathoracic pathologic conditions.

It is performed using a single thoracic incision of 2–2.5 cm in length on the lateral chest wall, between the anterior and posterior axillary lines. The intercostal space level may vary depending on the intrathoracic target lesion.[1,2]

As all the instruments enter the chest cavity through a single-port, this technique is a radical change to the traditional multiportal (three-portal) video-assisted thoracic surgery. In fact, in the uniportal VATS, the instruments diverge from the fulcrum, represented by the unique thoracic access, and approach the action point with a linear cranio-caudal perspective. In this setup the camera, the operative instruments and the target lie within the same line conversely to the traditional three-portal VATS where the target is reached using a lateral perspective.

Despite the fulcrum of all instruments being placed externally of the thoracic cage, the uniportal VATS offers the highest grade of spatial movement inside the thoracic cavity. Also, acces to the target is much easier as the tools diverge from the fulcrum. So the use of curved and reticulating instruments (and a 30-degree videocamera) facilitate each stage of the operative procedure. The potential to adopt 5 mm operative instruments enhances the possibility of greater movement within the incision port, while avoiding mutual interference.

The geometrical arrangement of the instruments and optical source ensemble using the uniportal technique automatically offers optical and practical benefits to the surgeon.[3] In fact the use of a craniocaudal perspective maintains the depth of the intraoperative visualization similar to that of the normal vision during the open surgery.

Over the last decade, several papers have described the versatility of the uniportal VATS for treating all intrathoracic pathological conditions, usually by traditional video-assisted minimally invasive techniques.[4]

Many authors have discussed the effectiveness of the uniportal VATS in treating benign disease, and there is growing evidence that the technique is becoming increasingly widespread.[15]

PRIMARY SPONTANEOUS PNEUMOTHORAX

Primary pneumothorax can be effectively treated in most cases by uniportal VATS.[5,6] The unique 2–2.5 cm incision is usually placed in the 5th intercostal space between the median and posterior axillary line. This port, without the aid of any retractor, is used for introducing a 5-mm 30° video-thoracoscope and the articulating, curved and rotating instruments. Pulmonary resections for removing blebs, bullae or dystrophic parenchyma are performed using endo-staplers. The following abrasion of the parietal pleura is done using a scratch pad mounted on a curved endo-clamp. At the end of the procedure an intercostal drain is left in place through the same surgical incision.

Several studies have shown the advantages of the uniportal VATS in comparison to the three-portal standard approach.[5,7,8] The uniportal VATS technique offers a reduction in early postoperative pain and a lower incidence of chronic neurologic symptoms (such as numbness, swelling or pins and needles').

INTERSTITIAL LUNG DISEASE

Despite the small size of the pulmonary resection necessary to obtain a specimen, patients submitted to lung biopsy for the histopathological classification of a clinical-radiologically supposed interstitial lung disease (ILD) are often frail patients with a high operative risk.[9] Consequently, the use of the uniportal VATS, inducing the least surgical impact, is particularly indicated for the diagnostic phase of the ILD patients.

The 2 cm thoracic incision should be placed at the level of the 5th intercostal space along the anterior-median axillary line.[10] Through this port it is easy to approach all the lung lobes in both sides, with the possibility of performing more than one pulmonary resection from different lobes as indicated by the international guidelines.[11] Again the use of 5 mm 30° video-thoracoscope (positioned in the posterior edge of the surgical wound), endoscopic curve clamp and articulating endo-staplers increase the mutual movement of the instruments, resulting in a gentler manipulation of the underlying affected lung parenchyma and a lesser stress of the section line.

There is evidence on the effectiveness of uniportal VATS in obtaining a pathological diagnosis in ILD patients without major morbidity or mortality.[10]

SYMPATHECTOMY

The uniportal VATS approach can be used to divide the sympathetic chain at different levels bilaterally.[2] In this case, the patient is placed in a semilateral decubitus (with the chest inclined at 30–45°) and a shortened surgical incision (1–1.5 cm) is located at the level of the axillary hairline. The thoracoscope is inserted using a trocar which is then retracted along the stem allowing for more convenient allocation of the other instruments. Usually, the lung is completely deflated; alternatively, endograspers or endoclamps could be used to move and collapse to allow visualization of the sympathetic chain along the apical-posterior region of the chest cavity. Using a diathermy hook the parietal pleura is interrupted and the nerves are divided at the desired intercostal level, ensuring the nerve stumps are free from residual bridges and the Kuntz's fibers are included in the resection.

PERICARDIAL WINDOW

The uniportal VATS has been described as an effective option to treat large and recurrent pericardial effusions.[12]

The 2 cm incision is placed at the level of the 5th intercostal space along the middle axillary line on the side where the pericardium is most protruding in the pleural cavity, with the hemithorax elevated at 45°. After identifying the phrenic nerve, a circumferential window on the pericardium is opened anterior to the course of the nerve using an endograsper, diathermy hook or endoscissors.

At the end of the procedure a thoracic drain is left in the pleural cavity through the same uniportal incision.

EARLY EMPYEMA, PLEURAL EFFUSIONS AND TRAUMA

Given its versatility, uniportal VATS can be used for treating and managing many other intrathoracic conditions.[13]

A small incision at the 5th intercostal space along the axillary line with the patient in lateral decubitus is made for easy access of the entire thoracic cavity in case of early empyema or hemothorax after a chest trauma.

In case of empyema, the fluid can be aspirated and the loculations broken in order to obtain a complete debridement of the pleural cavity. Also, small specimens of the pleura can be taken for diagnostic purposes using an endograsper or an endoclamp. In patients with recurrent pleural effusion, pleurodesis can be performed by insufflating talc powder using the thoracoscopic insufflators.

In a hemodynamically stable patient following chest trauma, uniportal VATS exploration[14] primarily allows complete evacuation of the blood. The sources of bleeding can be identified and, if not massive, can be controlled using vascular clips or directly by cauterization. Foreign bodies can be removed using an endoclamp or endobags. It is also possible to assess potential concomitant lesions of the lung, diaphragm, ribs and others intrathoracic structures.

SUMMARY

Due to the specific technical features of uniportal VATS, this approach is likely to become the gold standard for the management of benign intrathoracic conditions.[15] Moreover, performing a significant volume of this surgery for benign pathologies, such as surgery for pneumothorax, may serve the purpose of developing the necessary expertise in this approach prior to embarking into more complex major uniportal VATS operations.

REFERENCES

1. Rocco G, Martin-Ucar A, Passera E. Uniportal VATS wedge pulmonary resections. Ann Thorac Surg 2004; 77:726–728.
2. Rocco G. Endoscopic VATS sympathectomy: The uniportal technique. Multimed Man Cardiothorac Surg 2007 doi:1 0.1510/mmcts.2004.000323
3. Bertolaccini L, Rocco G, Viti A, Terzi A. Geometrical characteristics of uniportal VATS. J Thorac Dis 2013; 5:S214–216.
4. Salati M, Brunelli A, Rocco G. Uniportal video-assisted thoracic surgery for diagnosis and treatment of intrathoracic conditions. Thorac Surg Clin 2008; 18:305–310.
5. Jutley RS, Khalil MW, Rocco G. Uniportal vs standard three-port VATS technique for spontaneous pneumothorax: comparison of post-operative pain and residual paraesthesia. Eur J Cardiothorac Surg 2005; 28:43–46.
6. Salati M, Brunelli A. Uniportal VATS for pneumothorax and interstitial lung disease. J Thorac Dis 2013; 5:S217–220.
7. Salati M, Brunelli A, Xiumè F, et al. Uniportal video-assisted thoracic surgery for primary spontaneous pneumothorax: clinical and economic analysis in comparison to the traditional approach. Interact Cardiovasc Thorac Surg 2008; 7:63–66.
8. Chen PR, Chen CK, Lin YS, et al. Single-incision thoracoscopic surgery for primary spontaneous pneumothorax. J Cardiothorac Surg 2011; 6:58.
9. Fibla JJ, Alessandro Brunelli A, Cassivi SD, et al. Aggregate risk score for predicting mortality after surgical biopsy for interstitial lung disease. Interact Cardiovasc Thorac Surg 2012; 15:276–279.
10. Rocco G, Khalil M, Jutley R. Uniportal video-assisted thoracoscopic surgery wedge lung biopsy in the diagnosis of interstitial lung diseases. J Thorac Cardiovasc Surg 2005;129:947–948.
11. Bradley B, Branley HM, Egan JJ, et al. Interstitial lung disease guideline: the British Thoracic Society in collaboration with the Thoracic Society of Australia and New Zealand and the Irish Thoracic Society. Thorax 2008; 63:v1–v58.
12. Rocco G, La Rocca A, La Manna C, et al. Uniportal video-assisted thoracoscopic surgery pericardial window. J Thorac Cardiovasc Surg 2006; 131:921–922.
13. Rocco G. Single-port video-assisted thoracic surgery (Uniportal) in the routine general thoracic surgical practice. Op Techn Thorac Cardiovasc Surg 2009; 14:326–335.
14. Jutley RS,. Cooper GJ, Rocco G. Extending video-assisted thoracoscopic surgery for trauma: The uniportal approach. J Thorac Cardiovasc Surg 2006; 131:1424.
15. Rocco G, Martucci N, La Manna C, et al. Ten-year experience on 644 patients undergoing single-port (uniportal) video-assisted thoracoscopic surgery. Ann Thorac Surg 2013; 96:434–438.

Chapter 27 Nonintubated VATS

Joanne Irons

INTRODUCTION

The use of general anesthesia (GA) with intubation and one-lung positive pressure ventilation has always been considered mandatory for thoracic surgery. However, with the introduction and development of minimally invasive surgical techniques, there has been increased interest in awake and nonintubated surgery in the last few years to further decrease the invasiveness of the procedures and limit the insult applied to the patient.

Nonintubated techniques allow thoracic surgery to be performed on patients who are spontaneously ventilating awake, under minimal sedation or under GA with the aid of local or regional anesthesia. Lung collapse and the provision of a cavity for safe surgical manipulation are delivered by the creation of a spontaneous iatrogenic pneumothorax as the surgeon enters the chest. This can provide excellent operating conditions without the need for intubation and positive pressure single-lung ventilation.

ADVANTAGES OF NONINTUBATED SURGERY

There are many potential advantages to nonintubated surgery and these are summarised in **Table 27.1**.

Awake and minimal sedation techniques allow a more physiological cardiopulmonary and neurological status and avoid postoperative nausea and vomiting. The avoidance of intubation and positive pressure ventilation aims to minimize the morbidity associated with intubation related injuries, ventilator-induced lung injury and residual neuromuscular blockade.

There is a growing field of evidence and data relating to thoracoscopic minor and major lung surgeries taking place nonintubated under spontaneous ventilation. Published results to date are positive and demonstrate that nonintubated techniques offer benefits to the patients including attenuation of stress hormone and immunologic responses, quicker recovery times, better pain scores, lower morbidity rates and shorter hospital lengths of stay compared with intubated surgery. There is no increase in complications, morbidity or mortality.

TYPES OF SURGERY

Early reports of nonintubated VATS involved patients for relatively minor procedures. More recently, however, there is increasing evidence that nonintubated techniques are safe and feasible in a variety of different minor and major thoracic procedures. These include:

- Drainage of pleural effusion
- Pleurodesis
- Pleural biopsy
- Drainage of empyema
- Decortication
- Treatment of pneumothorax
- Bullectomy
- Lung biopsy
- Lung volume reduction surgery
- Wedge resection
- Metastasectomy
- Segmentectomy
- Lobectomy
- Pneumonectomy
- Pericardial window
- Thymectomy
- Tracheal resection

PATIENT SELECTION FOR NONINTUBATED VATS

Initially the technique was performed on fit and healthy patients:

- American Society of Anesthesiologists grade 1 or 2
- Good airway
- Body mass index of less than 30
- Few comorbidities, especially no significant cardiorespiratory issues

Table 27.1 Advantages of nonintubated surgery

Technique features	Advantages
Avoid IPPV	Less barotrauma Less volutrauma Decrease atelectasis Improved VQ matching Less shunt Less ventilator associated lung injury
Avoid neuromuscular blockade	Decrease atelectasis Avoid residual blockade Decrease side effects in certain patients, e.g. myasthenia gravis
Avoid intubation	Avoid trauma to teeth Avoid mucosal ulceration Avoid laryngeal or tracheobronchial injury and rupture Avoid sore throat
Avoid general anesthesia	Lower mortality Less cardiovascular compromise Less postoperative cognitive dysfunction Less nausea and vomiting
Regional anesthesia	Less postoperative pain
Pulmonary complications	Lower incidence pneumonia Lower incidence of ALI/ARDS
Stress and immune response	Decrease stress hormones Decrease immunological response
Productivity	Decrease anesthetic time Decrease recovery time Quicker to eat, drink and mobilise Decrease hospital length of stay Decrease costs

There are now, however, increasing reports of higher risk patients undergoing nonintubated thoracic surgery including elderly patients, those with cardiorespiratory disease, interstitial lung disease, severe emphysema and neuromuscular disease. These patients may be the sub-populations who will benefit the most from a nonintubated technique and avoiding GA, muscle relaxation, intubation and positive pressure ventilation. Further training and research is required, however, to determine the true short- and long-term gains.

There are a few absolute and relative contraindications to a nonintubated technique and these are listed in **Table 27.2**.

TEAM DYNAMICS AND PREPARATION

Thorough patient selection, strict planning, preparation and vigilance are essential to a successful nonintubated VATS program. All team members, especially the anesthetist and the surgeon should be experienced in thoracic surgery. The surgeon should be skilled and expert in VATS surgery, preferably in advanced cases and bleeding control via VATS. The anesthetist must be comfortable and experienced with intubation and lung isolation in the lateral position, in case of the need for conversion to an intubated technique intraoperatively.

The anesthetic assistants and theater team must be well briefed in the technique and what equipment and protocols to follow should sudden conversion to GA and intubation be required. Complications should be anticipated and prevented if possible with good judgment to appropriately convert to conventional intubated GA as required.

Patient cooperation is vital if the awake technique is to be employed. Their understanding and preparation is paramount and they should be briefed on what to expect from the theater environment, planned technique and possible conversion to GA.

THE TECHNIQUE

There are a number of different options available when considering a non-intubated technique. These will depend upon the patient, the procedure and the institution.

Firstly, a nonintubated technique may be performed:

- Awake
- With light sedation
- Under deep sedation/GA

Table 27.2 Contraindications to non-intubated VATS

Absolute	Relative
Inexperienced team	Obesity
Expected difficult airway management	Hemodynamic instability
High risk of regurgitation	Persistent cough and secretions
Type 2 respiratory failure	Resting hypoxemia or hypercarbia
Requirement for lung isolation for protection from contamination	Neurological conditions, e.g. dementia, seizure risk, etc. if considering awake
High intracranial pressure	Coagulopathy
Contralateral phrenic nerve palsy	Extensive adhesions or previous surgery
Patient refusal	

Awake

These patients are fully conscious and responsive, although may have been premedicated with a benzodiazepine or opiate prior to surgery. The majority of reports of awake VATS surgery are performed under thoracic epidural blockade, although with the introduction of uniportal VATS, minor procedures may be performed under intercostal blocks or paravertebral blocks, however, these are better tolerated with the aid of sedation. Oxygen is delivered via nasal cannula or facemask.

Advantages of a fully awake technique include the total avoidance of sedative or anesthetic drugs. This technique, however, usually requires epidural placement to tolerate the procedure and may cause anxiety and distress to the patient with movement and coughing.

Sedation

The use of light sedation allows the patient to better tolerate the surgical procedure and decreases anxiety and discomfort. With the use of sedation, epidural blockade is not necessary and less invasive regional techniques, such as intercostal nerve blocks and paravertebral blocks, can be employed. Target-controlled sedation, using propofol and remifentanil either separately or together, is currently the most popular reported technique. These drugs are easily titratable to achieve the desired sedation level and provide anxiolysis without losing responsiveness when under the management of an anesthetist experienced in their use. Care must be taken not to compromise spontaneous ventilation and airway reflexes. Other drugs used for mild sedation include dexmedetomidine, an $\alpha 2$ agonist, which can have cardiovascular depressant effects and midazolam, a benzodiazepine, which is much less titratable.

During sedation, oxygen delivered via a facemask or nasal cannula is often sufficient and is most commonly used. Monitoring of airway patency and respiration rate and pattern by end tidal carbon dioxide monitoring is also recommended. This can be achieved by placing the detector in the patient's nostril or attaching to the facemask.

General anesthesia

General anesthesia (or 'deep sedation') has also been described in nonintubated VATS procedures. Patients under GA are unresponsive but without compromise of spontaneous ventilation. Airway support is mandatory and should be via a fitted facemask with formal airway maneuvers or adjuncts or a supraglottic airway device, with a closed circuit gas delivery system and end-tidal gas monitoring (**Figure 27.1**). Regional blockade can be performed once asleep and in the lateral position and epidural anesthesia is not necessary.

This technique prevents problems with patient anxiety and distress and minimizes coughing and movement during the procedure. GA with formal airway support provides excellent airway patency and control and allows for rescue positive pressure ventilation if required. The technique may also provide a smoother conversion to intubation with enhanced preoxygenation and no additional requirement for induction of GA. Disadvantages and morbidity associated with GA, however, include cardiorespiratory depression and the risk of postoperative neurocognitive dysfunction and nausea and vomiting.

REGIONAL TECHNIQUES

Various regional anesthesia techniques have been described for use in nonintubated VATS procedures. These include:

- Local wound infiltration

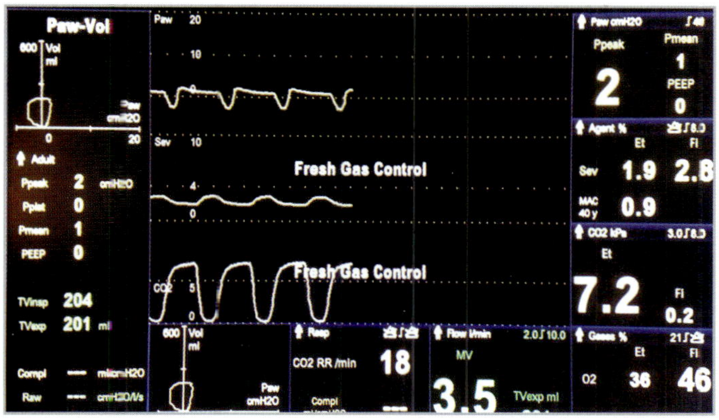

Figure 27.1 Ventilation monitoring during nonintubated VATS with a supraglottic airway device. Note the end tidal carbon dioxide trace and spirometry demonstrating regular uniform one-lung spontaneous ventilation with tidal volumes of 220 mL and respiratory rate of 18 during nonintubated VATS.

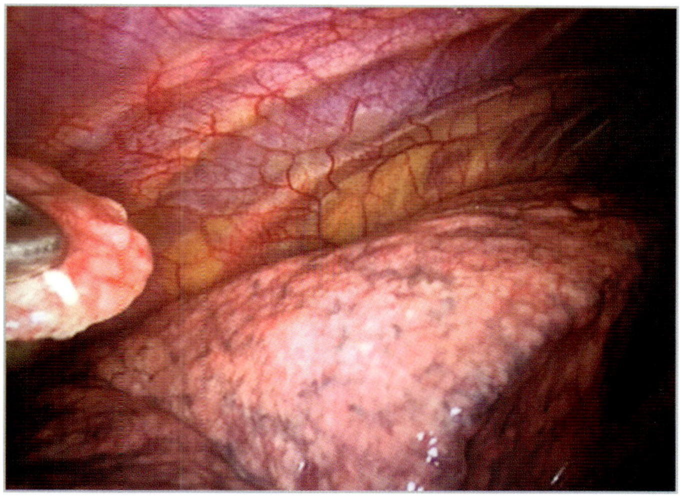

Figure 27.2 Lung isolation and the surgical field during a nonintubated VATS lung biopsy.

- Serratus anterior plane blocks
- Intercostal nerve blocks
- Thoracic paravertebral block
- Thoracic epidural block

Each of these techniques are described in more detail in Chapter 4

Early publications report the use of thoracic epidural blocks for the majority of nonintubated VATS cases. Thoracic epidural block allows the surgery to take place in patients who are awake or under minimal sedation and provides arguably the best pain relief for the procedure. There are, however, a number of rare but serious complications associated with their use including nerve injury, epidural abscess and hematoma. Other more common side effects include failure, inadequate block and sympathetic block and hypotension, which can lead to further invasive monitoring and delay in mobility, recovery and discharge.

With the drive to decrease invasiveness and to promote streamlining of the patient pathway, enhanced recovery programs for thoracic surgery now discourage the use of epidural blocks and encourage the use of alternative regional techniques such as intercostal nerve blocks and paravertebral block. This can still be achieved in nonintubated techniques providing adequate sedation or GA is used. Additionally, with the development of single-port VATS techniques, nonintubated major lung resection surgery is now being performed effectively under these less invasive regional techniques and sedation or GA

Regardless of the regional technique utilized, a multimodal approach to analgesia is recommended both intra- and postoperatively. Multimodal approaches are described in more detail in Chapter 4.

LUNG COLLAPSE AND RE-EXPANSION

Lung collapse

To facilitate nonintubated thoracic surgery, lung collapse is provided by the creation of a spontaneous pneumothorax during chest opening. This requires a patent airway and the preservation of spontaneous ventilation to provide a negative pressure in the pleural space. Lung collapse appears to be comparable to double lumen intubation and one-lung ventilation with adequate operating field for surgical manipulation (**Figure 27.2**). Surgical feasibility does not appear to be compromised in the majority of cases. Rarely, however, inadequate collapse and troublesome movements of the mediastinum and diaphragm may be problematic. Difficulty may also arise in the case of air trapping and severe adhesions as is equally the case during intubated surgery.

Re-expansion

Re-expansion of the collapsed lung occurs by asking the patient to breath deeply and cough or by applying positive pressure via a sealed facemask or supraglottic airway device while the patient continues to breath spontaneously.

INTRAOPERATIVE COMPLICATIONS

Hypoxia

To allow adequate conditions for surgical maneuvers, a pneumothorax is created with lung collapse as described above. The hypoxia which results from this is, however, usually minimal and can be easily treated using supplementary oxygen via nasal cannula, venturi mask or supraglottic airway devices.

Hypercapnia

Hypoventilation during nonintubated surgery can cause hypercapnia, which can be exacerbated by sedation or GA. This can be detrimental to a minority of patients with conditions such as elevated pulmonary pressures, raised intracranial pressures and arrhythmias; however, it is usually well tolerated and resolves immediately post-surgery. In addition, 'permissive hypercapnia' is a recognized ventilation technique in protective one-lung ventilation during thoracic surgery and may improve hemodynamics and ventilation/perfusion matching. In the event of patient compromise or the development of acidosis, positive pressure can be administered via a fitted mask or supraglottic airway device.

Cough and lung movements

Occasionally, unpredicted lung movements and cough can present problems to the surgeon during nonintubated VATS. Inadequate sedation or regional blockade and surgical manipulation of the bronchi may result in airway hyper-reactivity and a cough reflex. Epidural associated sympathetic block can also lead to an increase bronchial tone and hyper-reactivity.

Various techniques have been implemented and reported in an attempt to prevent this:

- Inhaled or nebulized lignocaine prior to the procedure
- Sedation with remifentanil with careful titration to avoid apnea
- Vagal nerve blockade performed under direct vision by the surgeon
- Lignocaine spray to the surface of the lung

Conversion to intubated thoracic anesthesia

The risk of intraoperative conversion to an intubated general anesthetic technique is one of the challenges nonintubated techniques present to the anesthetist and one of the reasons it is yet to gain widespread acceptance in thoracic surgery. The incidence of conversion is reported as 0% to 10% and is dependent on the procedure and team experience.

Reasons for conversion are listed in **Table 27.3**.

Indications and protocols for conversion should be discussed and agreed with the team prior to proceeding with nonintubated surgery. The ultimate decision to convert, however, will lie with the consultant surgeon and anesthetist. Elective conversion is always preferable during early, unexpected difficulties.

There are various conversion procedures reported in the literature and these will depend on the patient's anatomy, the reason for conversion and the anesthetist's preference. In our institution, the default plan is to preoxygenate via a supraglottic airway device and perform intubation with a double lumen tube in the lateral position with the chest remaining open. Other centers, however, proceed by closing the surgical wounds with sealed dressings and inserting a chest drain to aid lung expansion prior to induction and intubation. If in the lateral position, some centers advocate the use of a bronchoscope to guide single lumen tube intubation, followed by insertion of a bronchial blocker. To enable quick conversion to a supine position, one group suggests positioning an additional bed sheet at the back of the patient to allow rapid change of position following wound closure with a sterile transparent dressing.

Table 27.3 Reasons for conversion to intubated VATS

Anesthetic reasons	Surgical reasons
Patient anxiety	Inadequate lung collapse
Persistent hypercapnia and acidosis	Challenging mediastinal/lung/ diaphragm movement
Severe hypoxia	Dense adhesions
Airway compromise	Bleeding
Hemodynamic instability	Conversion to thoracotomy
Inadequate regional block	

Whatever the conversion technique, planning and preparation are paramount. Preoxygenation where possible should be performed, rapid acting induction and neuromuscular blocking drugs should be used and a selection of intubation aids should be available including a fibreoptic bronchoscope.

CONCLUSION

Nonintubated techniques are innovative and exciting and drive to reduce the invasiveness of VATS procedures. With training and further research in this field, it may mean that older and sicker patients are able to undergo more major thoracic surgery, avoiding the risks of GA, tracheal intubation and mechanical ventilation. This will provide greater benefit to the patient and a truly minimally invasive procedure.

FURTHER READING

Gonzalez-Rivas D, Bonome C, Fieira E, et al. Non-intubated video-assisted thoracoscopic lung resections: the future of thoracic surgery? Eur J Cardiothorac Surg 2016; 49:721–731.

Pompeo E. State of the art and perspectives in non-intubated thoracic surgery. Ann Transl Med 2014; 2:106.

Kiss G, Castillo M. Non-intubated anesthesia in thoracic surgery: general issues. Ann Transl Med 2015; 3:110.

Kiss G, Castillo M. Non-intubated anesthesia in thoracic surgery: technical issues. Ann Transl Med 2015; 3:109.

Chapter 28 Endobronchial ultrasound

Puja R Mehta, Nicholas R Carroll, Robert C Rintoul

ENDOBRONCHIAL ULTRASOUND

Endobronchial ultrasound (EBUS) makes use of a combination of bronchoscopy and ultrasonography to visualise structures in and around the main airways. EBUS combined with transbronchial needle aspiration (TBNA) allows visualization and accurate biopsying of lymph nodes and parabronchial lung lesions. Over the last decade, EBUS-TBNA has become the leading technique to assess the mediastinum and has been incorporated into a number of major clinical guidelines. Whilst EBUS-TBNA is used primarily for diagnosing and staging lung cancer, it can also be used for assessing isolated mediastinal lymphadenopathy in cases of *Mycobacterium tuberculosis*, sarcoidosis, and lymphoma.

There are two types of EBUS: radial EBUS and linear EBUS.

Radial probe EBUS

Radial probe EBUS uses a mechanical radial mini-ultrasound probe enclosed in a polyethylene sheath which is passed through the working channel of a flexible bronchoscope. Imaging at a frequency of 20 MHz allows a 360° image of the airway wall and surrounding structures. Radial probe EBUS is used:

- To identify the position of hilar and mediastinal lymph nodes prior to performing non-ultrasound-guided TBNA
- For the localization and biopsy of peripheral lung nodules
- For the examination of airway wall layers

Linear probe EBUS

Linear EBUS was first reported in 2003.[1] Over the last decade, it has progressed from being a research tool to entering routine clinical practice.

Linear EBUS uses an electronic curved linear array ultrasound transducer sited at the end of a flexible bronchoscope, covered with a water-inflatable balloon sheath (**Figure 28.1**). The bronchoscope permits simultaneous viewing of endobronchial and ultrasound imaging at between 5 MHz and 12 MHz allowing tissue penetration of up to 50 mm in order to identify lymph nodes (**Figure 28.2**). EBUS allows access to mediastinal lymph nodes 2R, 2L, 3P, 4R, 4L, 7 and hilar nodes 10R, 10L, 11R, and 11L (**Figure 28.3**). 21, 22, or 25 gauge needles are used to perform transbronchial needle aspiration.

Surgical mediastinal staging is usually performed by cervical mediastinoscopy and, more recently, video-mediastinoscopy. Using mediastinoscopy it is possible to access to stations 2 and 4 and the upper, anterior part of station 7. Lymph node stations 5 and 6 cannot be routinely accessed by either cervical mediastinoscopy or EBUS, and are best targeted using left anterior mediastinotomy or video-assisted thoracoscopic surgery. New surgical approaches to the mediastinum such as video-assisted mediastinal lymphadenectomy and transcervical extended mediastinal lymphadenectomy (TEMLA) have been described. Although they are reported to have high sensitivity and negative predictive value, complication rates are higher and at present they are restricted to a few specialist centers and have not been adopted into routine practice.

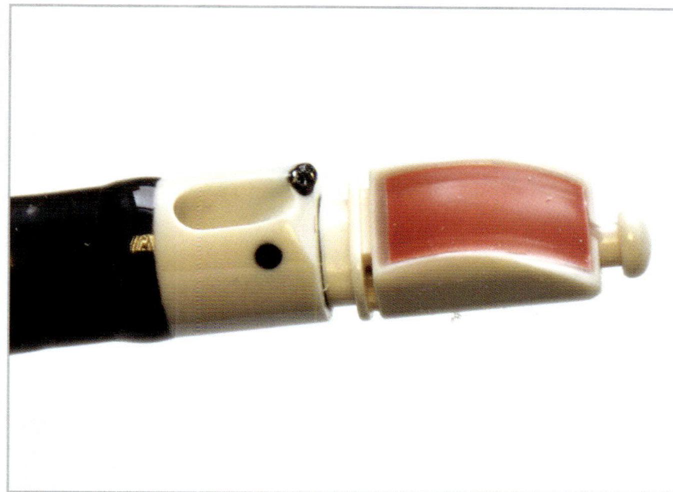

Figure 28.1 EBUS-TBNA bronchoscope (Olympus BF-UC180F).

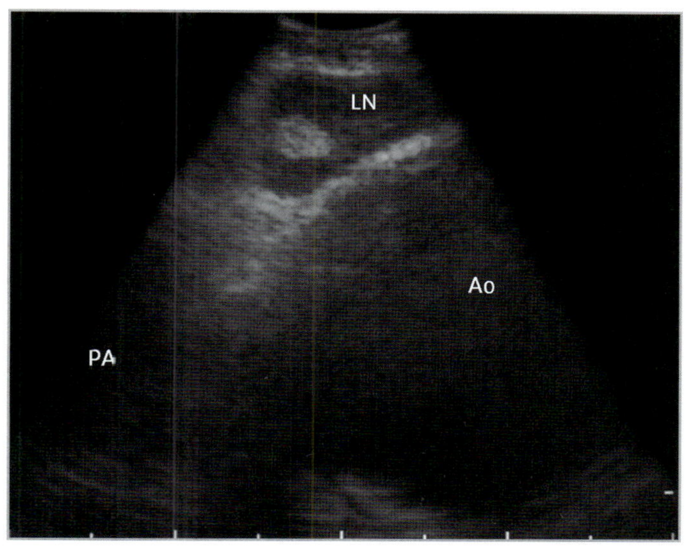

Figure 28.2 Endobronchial Ultrasound image of station 4L lymph node (containing a fatty centre) adjacent to the descending aorta.

THE EBUS-TBNA PROCEDURE

EBUS-TBNA can be performed under local anesthesia with sedation, or under GA. In most centers the former approach is adopted. Because the EBUS scope is slightly larger than a standard bronchoscope it is usually passed through the mouth with the patient lying supine and the operator standing behind. Once in the trachea, the EBUS scope is guided through the bronchial tree and each lymph node station is examined in a systematic fashion. A common ap-

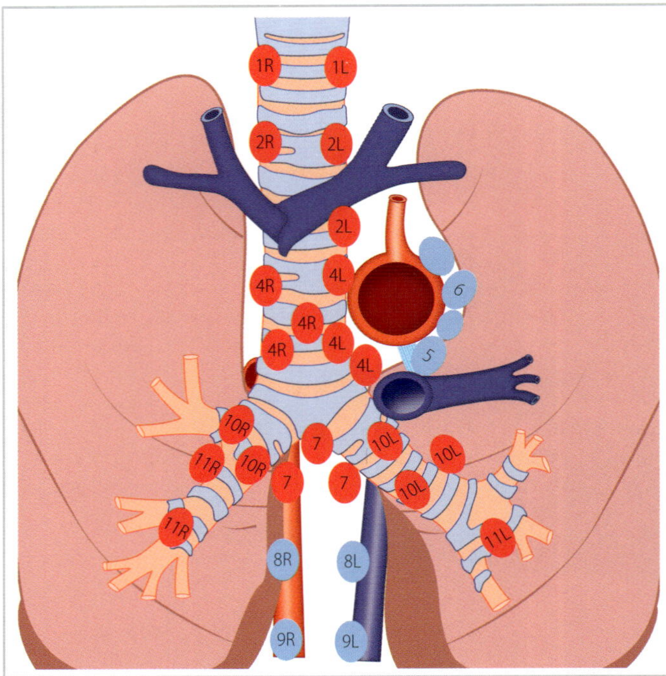

Figure 28.3 Lymph node regions and the procedures that are able to access each region. Lymph node stations accessible by transbronchial fine needle aspiration (TBNA) are shown in red. Nodes that cannot be sampled by TBNA are shown in blue.

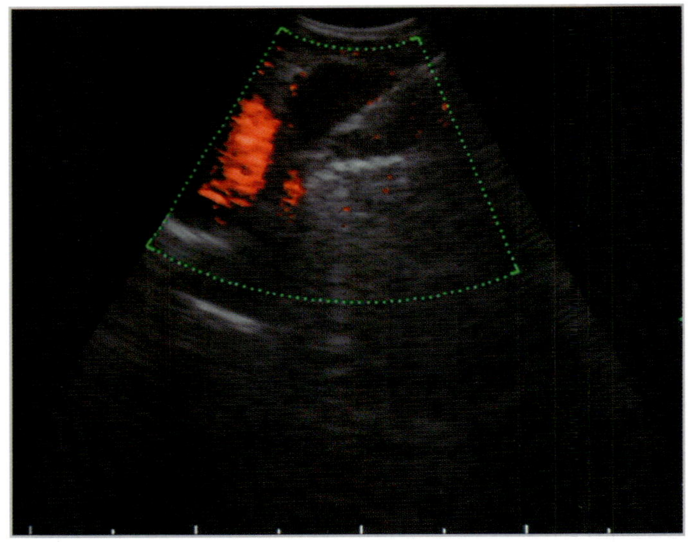

Figure 28.4 Ultrasound image showing 21-gauge needle within a lymph node adjacent to a branch of the pulmonary artery.

proach would be to start at right hilar lymph nodes (11R and 10R) and slowly withdraw the ultrasound transducer up the trachea examining the right paratracheal nodal stations 4R and 2R (**Figure 28.3**). The subcarinal station (7) can be examined from both the right and left main bronchi. Next, the left hilar nodes (11L and 10L) are examined before completing the evaluation by examining the 4L and 2L nodes. In order to sample lymph nodes, a needle is passed through the airway wall and into the target using real-time ultrasound guidance (**Figure 28.4**).

INDICATIONS FOR LINEAR PROBE EBUS

Linear EBUS with TBNA is used for:

1. The diagnosis and staging of lung cancer
2. Re-staging of the mediastinum following neoadjuvant chemotherapy
3. Investigation of isolated mediastinal lymphadenopathy:
   a. Diagnosis of suspected metastatic extrathoracic malignancy
   b. Diagnosis of suspected sarcoid
   c. Diagnosis of suspected *Mycobacterium tuberculosis*
   d. Diagnosis of suspected lymphoma

DIAGNOSIS AND STAGING OF LUNG CANCER

A number of groups published their initial experience with EBUS-TBNA between 2003-2006.[1-4] A few years later, following the publication of several larger nonrandomized prospective case series, Gu et al. published a meta-analysis that showed that the pooled sensitivity of EBUS-TBNA was 0.93 (95% CI 0.91–0.94).[5] In 2013 Dong et al. undertook a meta-analysis of 1066 patients who had had their EBUS-TBNA results confirmed by surgery. They found that the pooled sensitivity of EBUS-TBNA was 0.90 (95% CI 0.84–0.96) and the pooled accuracy was 0.96.[6] In the American College of Chest Physicians (ACCP) 2013 guidelines, a systematic review by Silvestri et al. incorporating 2,756 patients reported an overall median sensitivity of 89% (range 46–97%) and a median negative predictive value of 91%.[7] By way of comparison, the ACCP review data for cervical mediastinoscopy included 9,267 patients with a sensitivity of 78% for detecting N2/3 disease. The sensitivity for video-mediastinoscopy in 995 patients was 89%.

Yasufuku et al. reported the first prospective controlled trial to compare EBUS-TBNA with mediastinoscopy for mediastinal lymph node staging.[8] The sensitivity, negative predictive value, and diagnostic accuracy for EBUS-TBNA, which was performed under GA, were 81%, 91%, and 93% respectively. The corresponding results for mediastinoscopy were 79%, 90%, and 93%, respectively. There was no significant difference between EBUS-TBNA and mediastinoscopy for determination of nodal stage.

Taking a similar approach, Um et al. (2015) reported a prospective study whereby 138 patients underwent sequential EBUS-TBNA followed by cervical mediastinoscopy in order to determine the efficacy of these approaches for mediastinal staging.[9] Patients with no evidence of mediastinal disease underwent surgical resection with lymph node dissection. EBUS-TBNA was carried out using local anesthesia and sedation and mediastinoscopy was performed under GA. EBUS-TBNA was undertaken in all 138 patients and 127 had EBUS and mediastinoscopy. N2 or N3 disease was present in 59% of cases. The diagnostic sensitivity, negative predictive value, and accuracy of EBUS-TBNA were 88%, 85%, and 93%, respectively all of which were significantly higher than for mediastinoscopy where the corresponding values were 81%, 79% and 89%.

These publications showed that EBUS-TBNA is equivalent to surgical staging in terms of sensitivity and accuracy.

Adequacy of EBUS-TBNA aspirates for subtyping and genotyping lung cancer

In recent years, it has been shown that squamous and nonsquamous NSCLC are best treated with different chemotherapy regimens. Furthermore, the advent of agents designed to target tumors expressing specific mutations means that it is increasingly important for pathologists to have sufficient tumor material to allow for subtyping and genotyping. At the same time, the shift toward the use of techniques such as EBUS and endoscopic ultrasound (EUS), which provide smaller diagnostic samples, has provided a challenge for pathologists. Therefore, new tissue processing techniques such as liquid-based thin-layer cytology and cell blocks have been developed in order to make optimal use of limited sample material.

Navani et al.[10] investigated the utility of EBUS-TBNA samples in a large series involving 774 patients. They showed that accurate NSCLC subtyping of EBUS-TBNA samples was possible in 77% of cases and genotyping for epidermal growth factor (EGFR) mutations was possible in 90% of cases tested. Folch et al. in a series of 42 lung cancer patients, all diagnosed using EBUS-TBNA, demonstrated that overall success rate for mutation analysis was 95% for EGFR mutations, 90.5% for KRAS mutations, and 90.5% for anaplastic lymphoma kinase mutations.[11] These are similar values to those that can be obtained with histological biopsies.

Endoscopic ultrasound and combined EBUS/EUS

Linear EUS uses an esophageal approach to investigate lymph nodes in the inferior and posterior mediastinum – stations 2L, 4L, 7, 8, and 9. In addition, EUS can also provide access to the coeliac lymph nodes, the left lobe of the liver, and the left adrenal gland. As with EBUS, EUS is normally performed under local anesthesia with moderate sedation. When combined together in one procedure, EBUS and EUS can provide access to all mediastinal and hilar/interlobar lymph node stations with the exception of lymph nodes in the true aortopulmonary window (station 5) and prevascular position (station 6).

Combined EBUS and EUS

Using EBUS and EUS in combination takes advantage of the fact that EBUS provides excellent coverage of the anterior/superior mediastinum and EUS offers better access to the posterior/inferior mediastinal nodal stations.

Annema and colleagues undertook the first randomized controlled trial (the ASTER study) comparing EBUS/EUS with surgical staging.[12] Patients with (suspected) lung cancer were randomly allocated to either EBUS/EUS (under sedation and local anesthesia) or surgical staging (cervical mediastinoscopy, mediastinotomy or video-assisted thoracoscopy). In the endosonography arm, if there was no evidence of malignancy, surgical staging was performed prior to thoracotomy. The sensitivity for detection of malignancy in N2/N3 lymph nodes was 85% in the EBUS/EUS arm and 79% in the surgical arm – no significant difference. However, in patients who underwent surgical staging following a 'negative for malignancy' EBUS/EUS, the sensitivity for detection of malignancy increased to 94%. The 9% increase in sensitivity from 85% to 94% means that in order to identify one additional patient with mediastinal nodal disease, 11 additional surgical procedures are required.

More recently, the efficacy of combined EBUS/EUS versus surgical staging has been compared by Liberman et al (2014).[13] 166 patients with confirmed or suspected NSCLC requiring mediastinal staging underwent sequential EBUS, EUS and surgical mediastinal staging during a single procedure performed under general anesthesia. Each patient served as their own control. Patients with no evidence of nodal disease went on to resection with lymph node sampling. In this study the prevalence of mediastinal disease was 32%. The sensitivity, negative predictive value, and diagnostic accuracy of EBUS were 72%, 88%, and 91%, respectively. The equivalent results for EUS were 62%, 85%, and 88%. The results for combined EBUS/EUS were 91%, 96%, and 97%, respectively. It was calculated that the use of EBUS and EUS in combination prevented 14% of patients undergoing thoracotomy unnecessarily.

Combined EBUS and EUS using an EBUS bronchoscope

Although many centers undertake EBUS and EUS using separate EUS and EBUS scopes, EUS can be performed using an EBUS scope (termed EUS-B). In a prospective series of 150 patients with potentially operable (suspected) NSCLC who underwent EBUS, followed by EUS(B) the sensitivity, negative predictive value, and diagnostic accuracy of EBUS-TBNA for the detection of mediastinal disease were 84%, 93%, and 95% respectively.[14] With EUS(B) these outcomes increased to 91%, 96%, and 97% respectively. These results are similar to those that can be obtained by undertaking EBUS and EUS separately.

In practice, the choice of patients for EBUS or EUS or combined EBUS/EUS often depends upon the clinical situation. If the CT or PET-CT have shown extensive disease, biopsies from one or two lymph node stations should be sufficient to provide a histological diagnosis and confirm mediastinal disease. In this situation, EBUS or EUS can be selected depending on the position of the target nodes. However, if prebiopsy CT and/or PET-CT in conjunction with the clinical information indicates that treatment with potential curative intent is possible, then full systematic assessment of all mediastinal nodes using combined EBUS/EUS is recommended in order to fully stage the mediastinum.

Kang et al. (2014) explored the optimum order in which to perform EBUS and EUS(B).[15] They found that, whilst adding EUS-FNA to EBUS-TBNA did not significantly increase the accuracy or sensitivity of detecting mediastinal metastases, adding EBUS-TBNA to EUS-FNA increased the accuracy from 86.5% to 97.3%. This suggests that commencing mediastinal staging with EBUS-TBNA is probably the most efficacious approach.

RE-STAGING OF THE MEDIASTINUM FOLLOWING NEOADJUVANT CHEMOTHERAPY

When neo-adjuvant chemotherapy is employed, mediastinal re-staging is required prior to surgical resection. However, because of fibrotic change and adhesions induced by the initial mediastinoscopy and induction treatment, repeat mediastinoscopy is technically more difficult and the sensitivity for detection of residual malignant disease by re-mediastinoscopy has been reported to range from 29–74% in a series of studies by Mateu-Navarro et al. (2000), De Leyn et al. (2006), and Marra et al. (2008).[16-18]

At present there are few studies that have examined the role of EBUS for re-staging the mediastinum following induction chemotherapy. A retrospective review of 124 patients with stage IIIA N2 disease who had been treated with induction chemotherapy and undergone re-staging using EBUS-TBNA with subsequent surgical verification was was reported by Herth et al.[19] In this series the prevalence of persistent mediastinal disease was high at 94%. The sensitivity of EBUS for detecting residual malignancy in mediastinal nodes was 76% but the negative predictive value was low at 20%.

Szlubowski et al. (2014) used TEMLA as a re-staging tool in a prospective series of 106 patients who had already undergone combined EBUS/EUS following induction therapy for NSCLC. The prevalence of residual mediastinal nodal disease was 52%.[20] Overall, sensitivity, specificity and accuracy of EBUS/EUS for mediastinal metastases were 67%, 96% and 81% respectively and the negative predictive value was 73%.

Many groups now use EBUS and/or EUS for initial staging and re-staging. However, given the low negative predictive value of combined EBUS/EUS, it is recommended that negative findings be confirmed by surgical staging (mediastinoscopy), prior to resection.

INVESTIGATION OF ISOLATED MEDIASTINAL LYMPHADENOPATHY

EBUS is now regularly used as the first line investigation for isolated mediastinal lymphadenopathy. The most common final diagnoses in this situation are metastatic tumor from a known or unknown extra-thoracic primary, sarcoidosis or sarcoid, *M. tuberculosis,* and lymphoma. However, while EBUS can often provide a diagnosis, there may be some situations where a surgical biopsy is required for confirmation, and giving careful thought to the probability of the final diagnosis may help select the best initial test or combination of tests.

Diagnosis of metastatic extrathoracic malignancy

Several publications reporting the utility of EBUS-TBNA for diagnosing mediastinal lymphadenopathy in patients with known or suspected extrathoracic malignancy were the subject of a systematic review and meta-analysis performed by Yang et al. (2014).[21] Using pooled estimates from six studies comprising 533 patients, EBUS-TBNA had a sensitivity of 0.85 (95% CI 0.80–0.89) and a specificity of 0.99 (95% CI 0.95–1.00) for identifying malignancy in hilar or mediastinal lymph nodes. The overall diagnostic odds ratio was 179.77 (95% CI 66.29-487.50). The area under the receiver operating curve and the diagnostic accuracy were 0.92 and 0.86, respectively. Thus, evidence gathered from studies of moderate quality, as measured by the Quality Assessment of Diagnostic Accuracy Studies (QUADAS) tool, showed a high degree of diagnostic accuracy of EBUS-TBNA for diagnosing intra-thoracic lymph node metastases in patients with extra-thoracic malignancy.

Investigation of suspected sarcoidosis

Tissue verification of noncaseating granulomas in an appropriate clinical setting is recommended for the diagnosis of sarcoidosis. Historically, bronchoscopy with transbronchial lung biopsies has been the diagnostic standard. Since 2007, several groups have shown that biopsy of intrathoracic lymph nodes is a promising alternative for the investigation of suspected sarcoidosis. A systematic review and meta-analysis by Agarwal et al. identified 15 good quality, predominantly prospective, studies involving 553 patients.[22] This showed that the diagnostic yield of EBUS-TBNA ranged from 0.54–0.93 with a pooled diagnostic accuracy of 0.79 (95% CI 0.71–0.86). In the first randomized control trial comparing the diagnostic accuracy of EBUS-TBNA with transbronchial biopsy in patients with suspected sarcoidosis, von Bartheld et al. demonstrated that, amongst patients with suspected stage I or II pulmonary sarcoidosis, the diagnostic yield to detect granulomas using endosonography (80%) was significantly higher than using bronchoscopy with transbronchial biopsy (53%).[23] Gupta et al. (2014) showed that, compared to conventional transbronchial needle aspiration, EBUS-TBNA had the highest diagnostic yield, with values of 48% and 74.5%, respectively.[24] The addition of endobronchial and transbronchial lung biopsy to EBUS-TBNA increased the yield to 92%.

It should be noted that, on occasion, some cases of 'burnt out' sarcoidosis will require a surgical biopsy for confirmation, because the yield of diagnostic material showing non-caseating granulomas from fibrotic lymph nodes is very low on a fine needle aspirate.

Investigation of suspected *Mycobacterium tuberculosis*

The incidence of tuberculosis in industrialized countries has declined considerably, but thoracic tuberculous lymphadenopathy remains a common presentation in patients originating from countries with a high prevalence of tuberculosis. In cases of sputum 'smear negative' tuberculosis, sampling of thoracic lymphadenopathy is often required. Furthermore, given the emerging issue of drug-resistant tuberculosis, it is good practice to obtain samples for culture and sensitivities before commencing treatment.

Navani et al. (2011) examined the sensitivity of EBUS for diagnosing tuberculous intrathoracic-lymphadenopathy in 156 patients with a final clinical diagnosis of *M. tuberculosis.*[25] EBUS-TBNA provided the diagnosis of *M. tuberculosis* in 94% of cases. Pathology findings indicated *M. tuberculosis* in 86% of cases. In 47% of cases, a positive culture of *M. tuberculosis* was obtained. Geake et al. reported an Australian multicenter experience of 159 patients who underwent EBUS-TBNA with samples sent for mycobacterial culture.[26] In 39 cases (25%), *M. tuberculosis* was the final diagnosis. Sensitivity of EBUS-TBNA for microbiologically confirmed tuberculous mediastinal lymphadenitis was 62% and specificity was 100%. The negative predictive value and diagnostic accuracy for microbiological diagnosis was 89% (95% CI 82–93%) and 91% (CI 84–94%), respectively.

Overall, the literature suggests that, if the pre-test probability of *M. tuberculosis* is high, EBUS-TBNA appears to be a useful first-line investigation. The diagnostic yield obtained with EBUS is similar to that reported using other modalities, such as mediastinoscopy and EUS-guided biopsy.

Investigation of suspected lymphoma

EBUS-TBNA can be used to investigate suspected lymphoma. A number of retrospective studies show that the efficacy of EBUS-TBNA for diagnosis of lymphomas is quite variable with sensitivity ranging from 57% to 91%. Although the current British Thoracic Society guidelines do not recommend the use of EBUS for diagnosis of de novo cases of lymphoma recent reports suggest that EBUS may have an important role to play in this setting. Moonim et al. showed that by using rapid on-site pathology and taking multiple biopsies from lymph nodes with the most cellular aspirates, a diagnostic sensitivity of 89% was achievable in 100 patients with mediastinal lymphoma. However, in 28 cases, further surgical biopsy was required to fully characterize the lymphoma.[27]

Re-evaluation of current guidance through carefully designed prospective studies is needed. Until then, in cases of suspected lymphoma, close liaison between the lymphoma multidisciplinary team, chest physician, and thoracic surgeons is recommended to achieve the optimal approach to rapid diagnosis.

COST-EFFECTIVENESS OF EBUS AND EUS

Robust prospectively collected data on the cost-effectiveness of EBUS and/or EUS is limited to date. Indeed, the economic model for a number of diagnostic pathways in the 2011 National Institute for Health and Care Excellence guideline for lung cancer diagnosis and treatment was limited by the lack of published evidence and was largely based on expert opinion. Since then, two publications based on the ASTER trial have given further insight on resource use and cost-effectiveness. Sharples et al. reported on survival, quality of life (QoL), and resource use for patients from a UK perspective.[28] Cost-effectiveness using UK-based economic methods showed that the EBUS/EUS strategy was cheaper and patients had a better QoL during staging. Subsequently, Rintoul et al. undertook a country-specific cost-effectiveness analysis in the UK, the Netherlands, and Belgium, which showed that, in all three countries; the EBUS/EUS strategy had slightly higher quality-adjusted life-years over 6 months and was cheaper. Based on the clinical, QoL, and cost-effectiveness data, the authors concluded that mediastinal staging should begin with endosonography.[29]

Most recently, Navani et al. (2015) randomized patients to either initial EBUS-TBNA or to conventional approaches for lung cancer diagnosis and staging. Their cost analysis suggested that EBUS-TBNA, as an initial investigation after a CT scan, was not more expensive than conventional diagnostic staging. Furthermore, the patients in the EBUS group had a shorter time to treatment decision. The authors concluded that EBUS-TBNA was more cost-effective than conventional approaches.[30]

COMPLICATIONS OF EBUS-TBNA

Endobronchial ultrasound is regarded as a safe, minimally invasive technique in which major patient-related complications are rare. Most complications are minor and similar to those seen with flexible bronchoscopy: hypoxemia, cough, and post-procedure pyrexia. However, since the numbers of EBUS procedures being performed have begun to rise, case reports of more serious complications such as pneumothorax, lung abscess, mediastinitis, pericarditis, clinically significant airway injury, and hemopneumomediastinum have appeared. Two procedure-related deaths have been reported; one due to a postprocedure streptococcal septicemia likely caused at intubation as a result of nasopharyngeal carriage and one following cerebral infarction. In their meta-analysis, Gu et al.[5] reported only two complications in 1299 participants (0.15%). A systemic review by Von Bartheld et al.,[31] examined 190 studies including 16,181 cases. The serious adverse event rate and mortality rate for EBUS were 0.05% and 0%, respectively. However, a prospective registry study that evaluated 1317 EBUS-TBNA cases showed a complication rate of 1.44%.[32] A Japanese prospective survey of 7,345 cases reported a complication rate of 1.23% (95% CI 0.97–1.48%).[33] These latter studies suggest that there may be an underreporting bias in retrospective studies.

TRAINING AND SERVICE PROVISION

Training requirements for EBUS has received relatively little attention to date. Historically, bronchoscopy has been taught using an apprenticeship model, whereby trainees practice on patients under the supervision of an experienced practitioner. With the introduction of computer bronchoscopy simulators, trainees can now obtain basic bronchoscopy skills by practicing in a skills laboratory.

A study using cumulative sum analysis by Kemp et al., showed that there was considerable variability in length-of-time before competence was achieved among five experienced bronchoscopists.[34] Wahidi et al. conducted a multicenter cohort study to assess the learning experience of EBUS amongst trainees in respiratory medicine and suggested that these trainees needed an average of 13 procedures to achieve first independent successful performance of EBUS-TBNA following a training protocol that included a didactic curriculum and simulation-based practice.[35] As one might expect, Bellinger et al. showed that the diagnostic yield of both trainees and skilled bronchoscopists improved with increasing experience, with the latter group achieving a 90% yield after performing 50 procedures.[36] On the other hand, Stather et al. found that interventional respiratory medicine fellows were still demonstrating improvement in technical skill after 200 procedures and as many as one-third of participants did not achieve expert-level technical skill during their fellowship training.[37]

There are no specific guidelines on the training required to achieve competency at present. Rather than stipulating a specific number of procedures to be performed before an individual is deemed competent, the focus should be on monitoring an individual's performance and outcomes. The skill level of practice and expertise required for assessing and accurately staging the mediastinum, including biopsy of sub-centimeter nodes to achieve a high negative predictive rate, is considerably greater than the skill level required for taking a biopsy from a large station 4R or 7 lymph node for diagnostic purposes only.

REFERENCES

1. Krasnik M, Vilmann P, Larsen SS, Jacobsen GK. Preliminary experience with a new method of endoscopic transbronchial real time ultrasound guided biopsy for diagnosis of mediastinal and hilar lesions. Thorax 2003; 58:1083–1086.
2. Herth FJ, Eberhardt R, Vilmann P, et al. Real-time endobronchial ultrasound guided transbronchial needle aspiration for sampling mediastinal lymph nodes. Thorax 2006; 61:795–798.
3. Rintoul RC, Skwarski KM, Murchison JT, et al. Endobronchial and endoscopic ultrasound-guided real-time fine-needle aspiration for mediastinal staging. Eur Respir J 2005; 25:416–421.
4. Yasufuku K, Chiyo M, Sekine Y, et al. Real-time endobronchial ultrasound-guided transbronchial needle aspiration of mediastinal and hilar lymph nodes. Chest 2004; 126:122–128.

5. Gu P, Zhao YZ, Jiang LY, et al. Endobronchial ultrasound-guided transbronchial needle aspiration for staging of lung cancer: a systematic review and meta-analysis. Eur J Cancer 2009; 45:1389–1396.
6. Dong X, Qiu X, Liu Q, Jia J. Endobronchial ultrasound-guided transbronchial needle aspiration in the mediastinal staging of non-small cell lung cancer: a meta-analysis. Ann Thorac Surg 2013; 96:1502–1507.
7. Silvestri GA, Gonzales AV, Jantz MA, et al. Methods for staging non-small cell lung cancer: diagnosis and management of lung cancer, 3rd edn. American College of Chest Physicians evidence-based clinical practice guidelines. Chest 2013; 143:e211S–250S.
8. Yasufuku K, Pierre A, Darling G, et al. A prospective controlled trial of endobronchial ultrasound-guided transbronchial needle aspiration compared with mediastinoscopy for mediastinal lymph node staging of lung cancer. J Thorac Cardiovasc Surg 2011; 142:1393–1400.
9. Um SW, Kim HK, Jung SH, et al. Endobronchial ultrasound versus mediastinoscopy for mediastinal nodal staging of non-small-cell lung cancer. J Thorac Oncol 2015; 10:331–337.
10. Navani N, Brown JM, Nankivell M, et al. Suitability of endobronchial ultrasound-guided transbronchial needle aspiration specimens for subtyping and genotyping of non-small cell lung cancer: a multicenter study of 774 patients. Am J Respir Crit Care Med 2012; 185:1316–1322.
11. Folch E, Yamaguchi N, VanderLaan PA, et al. Adequacy of lymph node transbronchial needle aspirates using convex probe endobronchial ultrasound for multiple tumor genotyping techniques in non-small-cell lung cancer. J Thorac Oncol 2013; 8:1438–1444.
12. Annema JT, van Meerbeeck JP, Rintoul RC, et al. Mediastinoscopy vs endosonography for mediastinal nodal staging of lung cancer: a randomized trial. JAMA 2010; 304:2245–2252.
13. Liberman M, Sampalis J, Duranceau A, et al. Endosonographic mediastinal lymph node staging of lung cancer. Chest 2014; 146:389–397.
14. Hwangbo B, Lee GK, Lee HS, et al. Transbronchial and transesophageal fine-needle aspiration using an ultrasound bronchoscope in mediastinal staging of potentially operable lung cancer. Chest 2010; 138:795–802.
15. Kang HJ, Hwangbo B, Lee GK, et al. EBUS-centred versus EUS-centred mediastinal staging in lung cancer: a randomised controlled trial. Thorax 2014; 69:261–268.
16. De Leyn P, Stroobants S, De Wever W, et al. Prospective comparative study of integrated positron emission tomography-computed tomography scan compared with remediastinoscopy in the assessment of residual mediastinal lymph node disease after induction chemotherapy for mediastinoscopy-proven stage IIIA-N2 Non-small cell lung cancer: a Leuven Lung Cancer Group Study. J Clin Oncol 2006; 24:3333–3339.
17. Marra A, Hillejan L, Fechner S, Stamatis G. Remediastinoscopy in restaging of lung cancer after induction therapy. J Thorac Cardiovasc Surg 2008; 135:843–849.
18. Mateu-Navarro M, Rami-Porta R, Bastus-Piulats R, et al. Remediastinoscopy after induction chemotherapy in non-small cell lung cancer. Ann Thorac Surg 2000; 70:391–395.
19. Herth FJ, Annema JT, Eberhardt R, et al. Endobronchial ultrasound with transbronchial needle aspiration for restaging the mediastinum in lung cancer. J Clin Oncol 2008; 26:3346–3350.
20. Szlubowski A, Zielinski M, Soja J, et al. Accurate and safe mediastinal restaging by combined endobronchial and endoscopic ultrasound-guided needle aspiration performed by single ultrasound bronchoscope. Eur J Cardiothorac Surg 2014; 46:262–266.
21. Yang B, Li F, Shi W, et al. Endobronchial ultrasound-guided transbronchial needle biopsy for the diagnosis of intrathoracic lymph node metastases from extrathoracic malignancies: a meta-analysis and systematic review. Respirology 2014; 19:834–841.
22. Agarwal R, Srinivasan A, Aggarwal AN, Gupta D. Efficacy and safety of convex probe EBUS-TBNA in sarcoidosis: a systematic review and meta-analysis. Respir Med 2012; 106:883–892.
23. von Bartheld MB, Dekkers OM, Szlubowski A, et al. Endosonography vs conventional bronchoscopy for the diagnosis of sarcoidosis: the GRANULOMA randomized clinical trial. JAMA 2013; 309:2457–2464.
24. Gupta D, Dadhwal DS, Agarwal R, et al. Endobronchial ultrasound-guided transbronchial needle aspiration vs conventional transbronchial needle aspiration in the diagnosis of sarcoidosis. Chest 2014; 146:547–556.
25. Navani N, Molyneaux PL, Breen RA, et al. Utility of endobronchial ultrasound-guided transbronchial needle aspiration in patients with tuberculous intrathoracic lymphadenopathy: a multicentre study. Thorax 2011; 66:889–893.
26. Geake J, Hammerschlag G, Nguyen P, et al. Utility of EBUS-TBNA for diagnosis of mediastinal tuberculosis lymphadenitis: a multicentre Australian experience. J Thorac Dis 2015; 7:439–448.
27. Moonim MT, Breen R, Fields PA, Santis G. Diagnosis and subtyping of de novo and relapsed mediastinal lymphomas by endobronchial ultrasound needle aspiration. Am J Respir Crit Care Med 2013; 188:1216–1223.
28. Sharples LD, Jackson C, Wheaton E, et al. Clinical effectiveness and cost-effectiveness of endobronchial and endoscopic ultrasound relative to surgical staging in potentially resectable lung cancer: results from the ASTER randomised controlled trial. Health Technol Assess 2012; 16:1–75.
29. Rintoul RC, Glover MJ, Jackson C, et al. Cost effectiveness of endosonography versus surgical staging in potentially resectable lung cancer: a health economics analysis of the ASTER trial from a European perspective. Thorax 2014; 69:679–681.
30. Navani N, Nankivell M, Lawrence DR, et al. Lung cancer diagnosis and staging with endobronchial ultrasound-guided transbronchial needle aspiration compared with conventional approaches: an open-label, pragmatic, randomised controlled trial. Lancet Respir Med 2015; 3:282–289.
31. von Bartheld MB, van Breda A, Annema JT. Complication rate of endosonography (endobronchial and endoscopic ultrasound): a systematic review. Respiration 2014; 87:343–351.
32. Eapen GA, Shah AM, Lei X, et al. Complications, consequences, and practice patterns of endobronchial ultrasound-guided transbronchial needle aspiration: Results of the AQuIRE registry. Chest 2013; 143:1044–1053.
33. Asano F, Aoe M, Ohsaki Y, et al. Complications associated with endobronchial ultrasound-guided transbronchial needle aspiration: a nationwide survey by the Japan Society for Respiratory Endoscopy. Respir Res 2013; 14:50.
34. Kemp SV, El Batrawy SH, Harrison RN, et al. Learning curves for endobronchial ultrasound using cusum analysis. Thorax 2010; 65:534–538.
35. Wahidi MM, Hulett C, Pastis N, et al. Learning experience of linear endobronchial ultrasound among pulmonary trainees. Chest 2014; 145:574–578.
36. Bellinger CR, Chatterjee AB, Adair N, et al. Training in and experience with endobronchial ultrasound. Respiration 2014; 88:478–483.
37. Stather DR, Chee A, MacEachern P, et al. Endobronchial ultrasound learning curve in interventional pulmonary fellows. Respirology 2015; 20:333–339.

Chapter 29 Electromagnetic navigation bronchoscopy

Amit K Mahajan, Sandeep J Khandhar

INTRODUCTION

Peripheral pulmonary nodules represent a diagnostic challenge for physicians. The gold standard of care for patients with high-risk lung nodules is surgical resection. Yet, the most effective approach for patients with lung nodules considered intermediate risk for malignancy or those deemed poor surgical candidates for resection remains controversial. Flexible bronchoscopy is an excellent tool for accessing and biopsying bronchoscopically visible pulmonary lesions.[1] Unfortunately, more than two thirds of lung nodules are located in the peripheral lung zones not accessible to the bronchoscope due to the constantly narrowing branches of the bronchial tree.[2] As a result of this limitation, diagnostic yield for sampling peripheral lesions by conventional bronchoscopy is low.[3-6] Peripheral lesions in the outer third of the chest less than 2 cm in diameter have a diagnostic yield of only 14% using conventional flexible bronchoscopy.[7] Traditionally, nonsurgical modalities for sampling peripheral lesions have been limited to transthoracic needle aspiration (TTNA). While such an approach is effective, with yields of approximately 80%, the risk of pneumothorax associated with TTNA range anywhere from 5% to 64%.[8-14] Additionally, specimens obtained by CT guided needle biopsies may be inadequate for molecular marker analysis in non-small cell lung cancer.

Electromagnetic navigation bronchoscopy (ENB) is a minimally invasive procedure used to sample peripheral lung nodules. This image-guided localization procedure utilizes steerable catheters combined with highly specialized navigation software to create three-dimensional (3D) anatomical maps to reach targeted lesions. By directing the locatable guide (LG) along the created pathway to peripheral lesions, in a manner similar to that of global positioning software, a bronchoscopist can navigate to peripheral lesions and perform brushings, biopsies, and washings. Utilization of ENB in conjunction with use of an endobronchial ultrasound radial probe (EBUS-RP) results in a yield of approximately 88%.[15] Additionally, the safety of the procedure is excellent, with a pneumothorax rate anywhere from 0–10%.[16,17] The advent of ENB has provided a reliable and safe avenue for sampling peripheral pulmonary nodules unreachable by conventional bronchoscopy.

THE ELECTROMAGNETIC NAVIGATION BRONCHOSCOPY SYSTEM

The ENB system is comprised of virtual bronchoscopy planning software, an electromagnetic location board, a locatable guide, an extended working channel (EWC), and a steering catheter. Used in concert, the system can direct the LG to a peripheral lung nodule and allow sampling of the lesion under fluoroscopic guidance. While multiple ENB systems exist, each remains dependent on electromagnetic fields and LGs.

Planning

During the planning phase, a high-quality CT scan of the chest in Digital Imaging and Communications In Medicine (DICOM) format is loaded into navigation software via hard disk or through a network connection. The digital information is then used to reconstruct axial, coronal, and sagittal images of the subject's chest anatomy (**Figure 29.1**).

Additionally, 3D views of the tracheobronchial tree are created and provide a virtual airway map toward the targeted lesion. The detail and quality of the reconstruction is dependent on the slice thickness of the CT scan, with cuts of 1.5 mm or less and a 1.0-mm overlay being most effective.

The planning phase involves identifying and marking the desired lesion to be targeted in axial, coronal, and sagittal CT views using planning software. While earlier versions of ENB required a bronchoscopist to manually create the path to the lesion by leaving virtual markers from the lesion to the proximal trachea, latest versions merely require

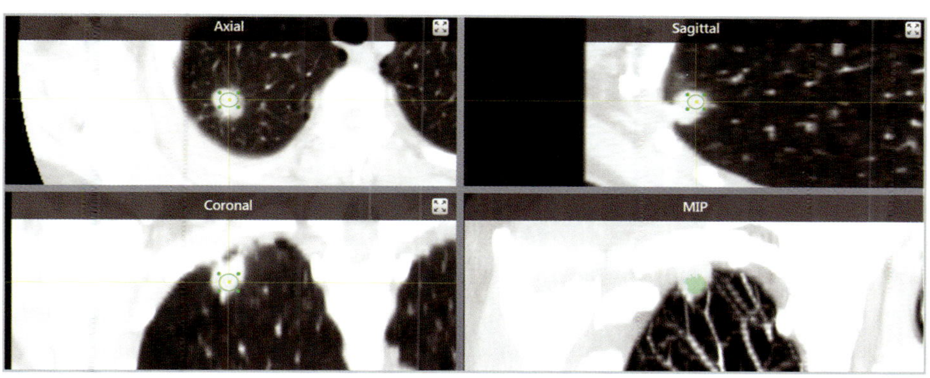

Figure 29.1 Reconstructed CT views of a right upper lobe lung nodule in the axial, coronal, and sagittal planes. The nodule can be marked in each plane to create an accurate path to the target.

identification of an airway entering the target, after which the software automatically suggests the most direct pathway (**Figure 29.2**).

The bronchoscopist is able to view the created pathway through the virtual map on a planning laptop prior to the actual procedure. The planning information is then exported to a memory stick and is uploaded into the ENB console.

Procedure set-up

The ENB procedure can be performed with general anesthesia or moderate sedation. Accurate navigation and effective sampling requires a patient to move minimally, thus establishing an airway and avoiding coughing is ideal. The patient is positioned supine on a designated stretcher that seats an electromagnetic board below the mattress (**Figure 29.3**).

This board creates a low frequency electromagnetic field around the patient extending approximately 50 cm above the patient. Metallic objects may interfere with the electromagnetic field and therefore care should be taken to avoid metal within 1 meter of the subject. Positioning of the patient, specifically the targeted lesion, within the electromagnetic field is essential for accurate navigation. Three adhesive location pads are placed upon the patient's chest in a triangular formation, which allows the system to follow the LG within the patient's airways as it is navigated to the targeted lesion.

Registration

Merging the CT images to the patient's actual bronchoscopic anatomy is known as the registration phase. Sensor probes located on the tip of the LG allow the ENB system to track the position and 3D orientation of the LG as it passes through the electromagnetic field. The bronchoscopist places the LG through the EWC via the biopsy channel of the bronchoscope and extends the LG approximately 10 mm from the distal end of the bronchoscope. The scope is then systematically advanced into each lobar bronchus, during which data collected by the software to merge the virtual map to the patient's actual anatomy. Confirmation of adequate registration is achieved when production of a 3D map is visualized on the ENB screen and movement of the LG through the patient's airways as visualized bronchoscopically matches that of the computerized reconstruction.

Navigation

The bronchoscope is wedged into the segmental airway leading to the target lesion at which time the steering catheter, telescoped through the EWC, is used to navigate the LG through peripheral airways to the target lesion. A colored line on the virtual reconstruction images represents the path needed to follow in order to reach the target lesion, which is represented by a green sphere.

When the bronchoscope can no longer advance due to the ever-narrowing diameter of the distal airways, the EWC and LG are advanced toward the lesion. Throughout the navigation procedure, the distance of the LG from the lesion is continuously being displayed and updated for the bronchoscopist. Multiple simultaneous views are displayed to track the LG advancing along the path to the target lesion (**Figure 29.4**).

Once the LG is directed in close proximity to the lesion, usually within 1 cm, the EWC is locked into place. The LG can be removed from within EWC and an EBUS-RP can be passed under fluoroscopic guidance to confirm position within the target lesion.

Tissue sampling

Following successful navigation to the target lesion, sampling can be performed. Brushes, needles, and forceps can be passed through the EWC to sample the lesion under fluoroscopic guidance. Sampling tools are pre-marked to the length of the EWC to prevent the operator from advancing tools past the lesion. Each operator will have his or her own preference for sampling tools, but typically two cytology brushings and ten transbronchial forcep biopsies are obtained. Finally, the operator performs a bronchoalveolar lavage by instilling sterile saline through the EWC. A number of adjunct modalities can be used in concert with

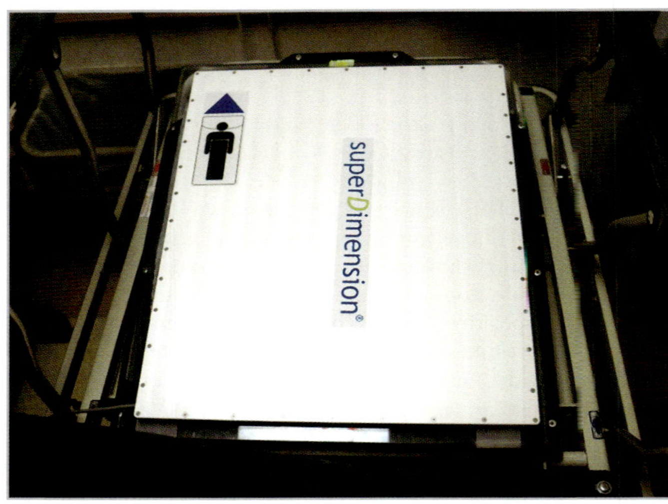

Figure 29.3 The navigation board used to create the electromagnetic field during the ENB procedure.

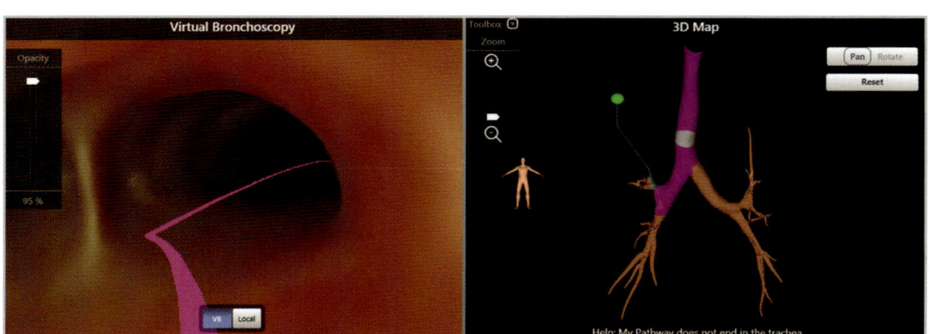

Figure 29.2 Computer generated 3-dimensional reconstruction of the patient's airways with a path leading to the right upper lobe nodule.

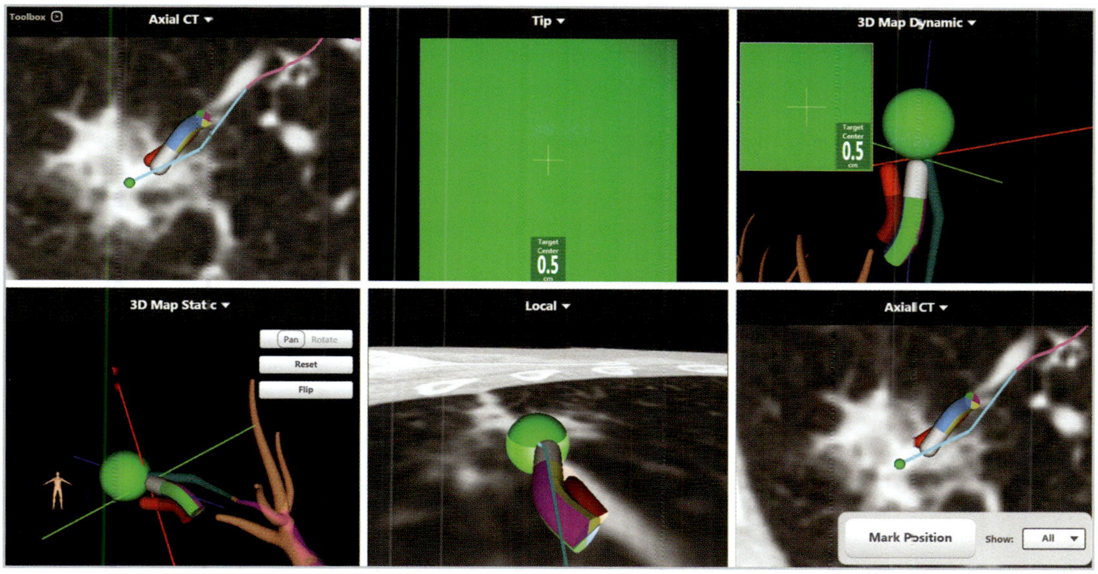

Figure 29.4 Multiple views of the LG approaching the target lesion, which is represented as the green ball.

ENB, including rapid on-site cytological evaluation (ROSE). While use of ROSE is operator dependent, it provides confirmation of target sampling at the time of the procedure.

EFFECTIVENESS OF ELECTROMAGNETIC NAVIGATION BRONCHOSCOPY

The diagnostic yield of ENB has been reported as high as 88%, with pneumothorax rates as low as 0–10%.[16-18] Reproducibility of these results is highly variable and is dependent on a number of factors including operator experience and presence or absence of an airway into the lesion, also known as a 'bronchus sign'. Unfortunately, the definitions of accurate navigation and successful diagnostic yield are also variable. While biopsies yielding malignancy or infection can be considered true-positives, biopsies deemed benign cannot be considered truly negative unless appropriate follow-up or further diagnostic testing is performed for confirmation. Additionally, the majority of the reports documenting diagnostic yields and complication rates are limited to case studies, with few randomized trials available.

A myriad of studies have been published regarding the uses of ENB since the initial animal trials performed in 2003.[19] The first human studies were performed in 2006, demonstrating the safety and effectiveness of the procedure.[3] Since these studies a number of reports describing diagnostic yields and safety of ENB have been published. One of the largest studies to date, produced by Wilson et al., featured 279 patients with a diagnostic yield of 65%, with a complication profile of 3% pneumothorax, 1% moderate bleeding, 0.3% hematoma formation, and 0.3% pneumonia.[20] Eberhardt et al., published a study documenting a diagnostic yield of 67% independent of lesion size, contradicting the assumption that of lesion size is essential to a successful biopsy.[21] The latest comprehensive meta-analysis that examines the effectiveness and safety of ENB was published by Gex et al., in 2014. This study included 15 trials reporting yields for peripheral lung lesions. A positive yield and definitive diagnosis was obtained after 64.9% of all ENB procedures (95% CI 59.2–70.3). Overall diagnostic accuracy was 73.9% (95% CI 68.0–79.2). Sensitivity to detect cancer was 71.1% (95% CI 64.6–76.8). with a negative predictive value of 52.1% (95% CI 43.5–60.6). Pneumothorax was seen 3.1% of patients, requiring chest tube drainage in 1.6% of the cases.[22] Higher yields can be seen with a combination of adjunct modalities including EBUS-RD. Eberhardt et al. randomized patients to ENB alone, EBUS-RP alone, or combined ENB and EBUS-RP to confirm position of the LG in the lesion with diagnostic yields of 59%, 69%, and 88%, respectively. A 'bronchus sign', has great impact on diagnostic yield in ENB. A direct pathway into the lesion allows for biopsy within the target with forceps and brushings. If the airway is located tangentially to the desired target, biopsies may collect material only from the associated airway, missing the lesion completely. One study investigating the importance of the bronchus sign featured 51 consecutive patients undergoing ENB. Analysis of the 34 patients yielding a diagnosis, 88% had a bronchus sign leading into the lesion.[23] In lesions lacking a bronchus sign, the position of the nodule in relation to the airway can be visualized with EBUS-RP. The EBUS-RP can be passed through the EWC to confirm navigation to the lesion with a 360°, real-time ultrasound image. Multivariate analysis evaluating the success of EBUS-RP guided transbronchial biopsies described that position of the lesion in relation to the EBUS-RP independently predicted yields, with the RP located within the lesion demonstrating the highest yield of 88%.[15]

A number of factors must be considered when investigating methods to increase diagnostic yields in ENB. While each operator may have specific techniques and tools utilized during the procedure, such as fluoroscopic guidance, ROSE, or EBUS-RP for improving diagnostic yields, further research must be performed to determine the ideal approach for performing ENB.

FURTHER CLINICAL APPLICATIONS OF ELECTROMAGNETIC NAVIGATION BRONCHOSCOPY

The utility of fiducial marker placement using ENB has provided improved treatment for patients undergoing stereotactic radiotherapy. Use of stereotactic radiotherapy allows for more precise focusing of radiation to malignancies in patients who are poor surgical candidates or defer surgery. Fiducial markers can be effectively placed around a malignant lesion by utilizing ENB, allowing precise targeting and dosing of radiation without exposing surrounding healthy tissue.

The placement of fiducial markers has proven safe with multiple studies demonstrating the ability of the coils to remain in position following deployment. Nabivizadeh et al. followed 31 patients with 34 nodules after the placement of a total of 105 fiducial markers. Following placement, 103 of the 105 fiducials were identified on simulation CT scans (98.1%) with a pneumothorax rate of only 6%.[24] The ability to effectively and safely use ENB for fiducial placement provides an alternative therapy for patients deemed non-surgical candidates for the treatment of malignant lesion using stereotactic radiotherapy.

The ability to dye mark sub-centimeter nodules with ENB allows surgeons to identify areas of resection during video-assisted thoracoscopic surgery. Dyes, such as indigo carmine, can be injected following navigation to small lesions in order to mark the nodule and pleura so that a target can be visualized for resection. Such a function of ENB highlights the potential for such a modality in advancing the diagnosis and treatment of cancer.

CONCLUSION

The advent of ENB has provided a novel modality for sampling peripheral lung nodules unreachable by conventional flexible bronchoscopy. As the use of lung cancer screening becomes more prevalent internationally, the need to safely and effectively biopsy lung nodules in intermediate-risk patients will be essential. While current ENB technology is limited to sampling nodules and placing fiducial markers, future development of nodule ablative technology is on the horizon. As the move toward minimally invasive diagnosis of lung cancer grows, the need to further study and utilize ENB will continue to intensify.

REFERENCES

1. Rivera MP, Mehta AC, Wahidi MM. Establishing the diagnosis of lung cancer: Diagnosis and management of lung cancer, 3rd edn: American College of Chest Physicians evidence-based clinical practice guidelines. Chest 2013; 143:e142S–165S.
2. Rivera MP, Detterbeck F, Mehta AC. Diagnosis of lung cancer: the guidelines. Chest 2003; 123:129S–136S.
3. Schwarz Y, Greif J, Becker HD, Ernst A, Mehta A. Real-time electromagnetic navigation bronchoscopy to peripheral lung lesions using overlaid CT images: the first human study. Chest 2006; 129:988–994.
4. Funakoshi Y, Sawabata N, Takeda S, Okumura Y, Hayakawa M, Maeda H. Bronchoscopically undiagnosed small peripheral lung tumors. Interact Cardiovasc Thorac Surg 2003; 2:517–520.
5. Stringfield JT, Markowitz DJ, Bentz RR, Welch MH, Weg JG. The effect of tumor size and location on diagnosis by fiberoptic bronchoscopy. Chest 1977; 72:474–476.
6. Cortese DA, McDougall JC. Biopsy and brushing of peripheral lung cancer with fluoroscopic guidance. Chest 1979; 75:141–145.
7. Baaklini WA, Reinoso MA, Gorin AB, Sharafkaneh A, Manian P. Diagnostic yield of fiberoptic bronchoscopy in evaluating solitary pulmonary nodules. Chest 2000; 117:1049–1054.
8. Cox JE, Chiles C, McManus CM, Aquino SL, Choplin RH. Transthoracic needle aspiration biopsy: variables that affect risk of pneumothorax. Radiology 1999; 212:165–168.
9. Li H, Boiselle PM, Shepard JO, Trotman-Dickenson B, McLoud TC. Diagnostic accuracy and safety of CT-guided percutaneous needle aspiration biopsy of the lung: comparison of small and large pulmonary nodules. AJR Am J Roentgenol 1996; 167:105–109.
10. Westcott JL. Percutaneous transthoracic needle biopsy. Radiology 1988; 169:593–601.
11. Khouri NF, Stitik FP, Erozan YS, et al. Transthoracic needle aspiration biopsy of benign and malignant lung lesions. Am J Roentgenol 1985; 144:281–288.
12. Kazerooni EA, Lim FT, Mikhail A, Martinez FJ. Risk of pneumothorax in CT-guided transthoracic needle aspiration biopsy of the lung. Radiology 1996; 198:371–375.
13. Laurent F, Michel P, Latrabe V, et al. Pneumothoraces and chest tube placement after CT-guided transthoracic lung biopsy using a coaxial technique: incidence and risk factors. Am J Roentgenol 1999; 172:1049–1053.
14. Klein JS, Salomon G, Stewart EA. Transthoracic needle biopsy with a coaxially placed 20-gauge automated cutting needle: results in 122 patients. Radiology 1996; 198:715–720.
15. Eberhardt R, Anantham D, Ernst A, Feller-Kopman D, Herth F. Multimodality bronchoscopic diagnosis of peripheral lung lesions: a randomized controlled trial. Am J Respir Crit Care Med 2007; 176:36–41.
16. Lamprecht B, Porsch P, Pirich C, Studnicka M. Electromagnetic navigation bronchoscopy in combination with PET-CT and rapid on-site cytopathologic examination for diagnosis of peripheral lung lesions. Lung 2009; 187:55–59.
17. Mahajan AK, Patel S, Hogarth DK, Wightman R. Electromagnetic navigational bronchoscopy: an effective and safe approach to diagnose peripheral lung lesions unreachable by conventional bronchoscopy in high-risk patients. J Bronchology Interv Pulmonol 2011: 18:133–137.
18. Bertoletti L, Robert A, Cottier M, Chambonniere ML, Vergnon JM. Accuracy and feasibility of electromagnetic navigated bronchoscopy under nitrous oxide sedation for pulmonary peripheral opacities: an outpatient study. Respiration 2009; 78:293–300.
19. Schwarz Y, Mehta AC, Ernst A, et al. Electromagnetic navigation during flexible bronchoscopy. Respiration 2003; 70:516–522.
20. Wilson D, Bartlett R. Improved Diagnostic yield of bronchsoccpy in a community practice: combination of electromagnetic navigation system and rapid on-site evaluation. J Bronchology Interv Pulmonol 2007; 14:227–232.
21. Eberhardt R, Anantham D, Herth F, Feller-Kopman D, Ernst A. Electromagnetic navigation diagnostic bronchoscopy in peripheral lung lesions. Chest 2007; 131:1800–1805.
22. Gex G, Pralong JA, Combescure C, et al. Diagnostic yield and safety of electromagnetic navigation bronchoscopy for lung nodules: a systematic review and meta-analysis. Respiration 2014; 87:165–176.
23. Seijo LM, de Torres JP, Lozano MD, et al. Diagnostic yield of electromagnetic navigation bronchoscopy is highly dependent on the presence of a Bronchus sign on CT imaging: results from a prospective study. Chest 2010; 138:1316–1321.
24. Nabavizadeh N, Zhang J, Elliott DA, et al. Electromagnetic navigational bronchoscopy-guided fiducial markers for lung stereotactic body radiation therapy: analysis of safety, feasibility, and interfraction stability. J Bronchology Interv Pulmonol 2014; 21:123–130.

Chapter 30 Air leak and chest drain management

Cecilia Pompili

INTRODUCTION

Management of chest tubes remains a critical aspect in the postoperative course of patients following lung resection.

It is traditionally influenced by two factors: presence of air leak and daily pleural fluid output. The combination of these two factors has characterized protocols of chest tube removal.

PROLONGED AIR LEAK

Figures from the European Society of Thoracic Surgeons Database Annual report showed that the incidence of an air leak lasting longer than 5 days is about 8.9% after lobectomy, 6.4% after segmentectomy and 3.4% after wedge resection.

These data confirm that prolonged air leak (PAL) remains a frustrating complication. Several authors have shown that PAL is a major determinant of postoperative hospital stay and costs.[1,2] Varela et al. have shown that only 10% of patients with PAL are likely to be discharged by the 7th postoperative day, whereas 90% of those without PAL can be sent home by this time.[2] They found that the excess cost attributable to PAL (driven mainly by the increased length of stay) was about 39,000 euro in 21 patients with this complication; an average of 1,860 euro per patient.[2]

Although many patients can be safely sent home with a one-way valve or portable chest drainage system, this practice is not always well accepted by patients and not feasible in all settings, and is not possible for those patients with medium- to high-grade air leaks.

Prolonged air leak is not only a financial issue but has also been shown to increase the risk of other medical complications, particularly empyema.[3]

For this reason, several authors have attempted to predict the occurrence of this complication in an effort to identify high-risk patients in whom to apply preventative measures.

The most consistently reported risk factors are reduced pulmonary function indicative of a damaged and fragile lung parenchyma, use of steroids, performance of an upper lobectomy, low body mass index (BMI) and presence of pleural adhesions.[4] Brunelli et al. have recently developed an aggregate risk model stratifying the risk of PAL in four risk classes according to the presence of four weighted factors: age > 65 years, 1 point; presence of adhesions, 1 point; FEV_1 < 80%, 1.5 points; BMI< 25.5, 2 points. The sum of the individual points in each patient yields a cumulative score, which may range from 0 to 5.5. For instance, a 75-year-old patient with a FEV_1 of 70%, BMI of 24 and with pleural adhesions would have the maximum score of 5.5 points. According to the score, 4 risk classes were derived with an incremental risk of PAL. In the validation set, the risk of PAL was nil in class A (no risk factors present, score 0), 6.7% in class B (score 1), 10.9% in class C (score 1.5–3), and 25.7% in class D (> 3.5).

The best way to avoid the occurrence of prolonged air leak is to prevent this complication during surgery, by applying meticulous technique. However, once this complication is evident in the postoperative period, several measures have been tested in order to reduce the duration of air leak (chest tube management, autologous blood patching, reoperation, etc.).

Certainly one of the most studied methods used in the postoperative phase is the application of different protocols of chest tube management.

Several randomized clinical trials have been published comparing suction versus 'water seal/no suction'.

There are relative pros and cons in using suction versus no suction. Theoretically, suction promotes pleura-pleural apposition favoring the sealing of air leak and drainage of large air leaks. However, suction has also been shown to increase the flow through the chest tube proportional to the level of suction applied, and it is assumed that this increased airflow increases the duration of drainage. Also, the use of suction has historically been associated with reduced patient mobilization, particularly if wall suction is used. On the other hand, the so called 'water seal' or 'no suction' approach has been shown to be effective in some circumstances to reduce the duration of air leak, presumably by decreasing the air flow, while also favoring mobilization (since the patient is not attached to the wall suction). Nonetheless, the absence of suction makes this approach ineffective in the case of medium to large air leaks (particularly in the presence of a large pneumothorax) and is associated with an increased risk of further complications (particularly pneumonia and arrhythmia).

Table 30.1 summarizes the findings of randomized trials published on suction versus no suction in lung resection patients.

The table shows that these trials yielded mixed results. Some authors found a benefit by using 'water seal', others did not find any difference between the two modalities.

There are a number of problems with these studies. The most important is the lack of objective data for more sensitive measurements of air leak severity. This limitation has prevented the standardization of studies, and test and control groups within studies, resulting in a lack of accurate quantification and reproducibility. Further, a conceptual problem inherent to all these studies was the definition of 'water seal' and suction.

STANDARDIZATION OF TERMINOLOGY

A recent collaborative proposal from European Society of Thoracic Surgeons (ESTS), American Association for Thoracic Surgery (AATS), Society of Thoracic Surgeons (STS), and General Thoracic Surgery Club (GTSC) on standardization of nomenclature has helped clarify some controversial definitions based on physical and physiological principles.[6]

Among others the following terms were discussed and proposed:

- **Passive drainage** is when intrapleural pressure rises above atmospheric pressure
- **Active drainage** occurs when a subatmospheric pressure is applied to the pleural space either by an external suction device or by creating a column of liquid within the chest tube that extends below the level of the pleural space (siphoning effect). In this regard, the

Table 30.1 Summary of the randomized trials comparing suction versus no suction

Author	Algorithm	No. of patients	Suction	Benefit
Cerfolio[22]	no suction on POD2	33	no	larger air leak seal by POD3
Marshall[23]	no suction on ward arrival	68	no	shorter air leak duration
Brunelli[24]	no suction on POD1	145	yes	no difference in air leak duration, increased trend of complications
Brunelli[25]	Alternate suction	94	Alternate suction	shorter tube duration, length of stay, less PAL versus full time no suction
Alphonso[26]	Immediate no suction	234	yes	no difference

Abbreviations: PAL, prolonged air leak; POD, postoperative day

old term 'water seal' does not always correspond to 'no suction'. It may at times represent a form of uncontrolled, active drainage. Recent findings have shown large variations of values of pleural pressure measured during the last hour before chest tube removal in a series of uncomplicated pulmonary lobectomies, while the chest tube was maintained on water seal without external suction.[7] Pressure can vary from values above atmospheric pressure, exposing patients to the risk of tension pneumothorax to values as negative as –40 cmH_20 in the same patients during a relatively short period of time.

To simplify terminology and understanding active drainage, the situation where a subatmospheric pressure is created by an external suction device has been defined as 'external suction applied'. In all other cases (previously referred to as 'water-seal') the definition of 'no external suction applied' has been proposed.

Another important definition is the distinction between regulated (variable) suction and unregulated (fixed) suction. Regulated suction is a form of active drainage obtained through the application of an external source of suction capable of modifying its level of suction (negative pressure) in response to the feedback coming from the pleural space. In other words, the suction source applied to the chest drainage system is capable of varying its activity to maintain a preset value of pressure. As a consequence, these systems can be best described as suction when needed by the patient and non-suction when not. Non-regulated or fixed suction is a form of active drainage provided by an external source of suction not capable to vary its level based on the intrapleural pressure level (i.e. wall suction).

ELECTRONIC DRAINAGE SYSTEMS

Recent chest drainage systems feature built in electronic components able to measure the air flow and pleural pressure.

There are several reports already published that detail the clinical characteristics and benefits of these novel devices.

In summary the main features of the commercially available digitalized chest drainage systems are as follows:

- Objective measurement of air leak, which improve reproducibility and interobserver agreement
- Graphic display of trends of air flow, which assists in chest tube management
- Recording of data for later export, retrospective analysis and medico legal purposes
- Compact, light and portable design
- Built-in pump, no need to attach to chest wall for suction
- Provide regulated, variable suction to generate a stable intrapleural negative pressure
- Intelligent systems, which work only when needed to maintain preset negative levels in the presence of air leak (suction when needed, non-suction when not)
- They are unaffected by gravity and the position of the system relative to the patient

One of the most important studies about digital systems is the one published from the Salamanca group.[8] They found a high interobserver variability among staff surgeons in deciding when to remove a chest tube when using a traditional device. On the other hand, the interobserver agreement was almost perfect when a digital system was used to assess air leak. The main reason explaining the difference is the availability of objective data about air leak upon which to base the decision on whether to remove the chest tube.

The objective unequivocal quantification of the air leak is likely to be the most important factor explaining the clinical benefits found in two randomized clinical trials comparing digital versus traditional devices.[9,10]

Cerfolio et al. found that patients connected to a digital system had a shorter duration of chest tube (0.8 days less) and hospital stay (0.7 days less) compared to those connected to a traditional device. One interesting aspect of this study was the cross-over of patients with an air leak on both devices, which made correlation of the readings from both systems possible.[9]

The authors were able to find a certain linear correlation between the median air flow measured by the digital device and the intensity of the bubbling.

Brunelli et al. randomized 160 patients submitted to lobectomy into two groups.[10] The group connected to a digital system had a significantly shorter duration of chest tube placement which resulted in a reduced hospital stay of about 1 day, and translated into a cost saving of approximately 500 euro per patient. Additionally, 51% of patients with the digital drainage device had their chest tube removed by the second postoperative day compared to only 12% of those with the analog device. One of the most important aspects of this study was the use of a standardized fast track chest tube removal protocol taking advantage of the objective information about air leak recorded in the system. The protocol does not rely on instantaneous assessment of air leak anymore but rather on average values of air leak, expressed in mL/min, recorded during the last 3–6 hours.

Both these randomized trials were conducted using a system, called Digivent, no longer available in the market.

PLEURAL PRESSURE

Some new electronic chest drainage systems are not only able to measure the air flow but also the pleural pressure. Little is known about the influence of the pleural pressure on the duration of air leak and even less on the importance of it to the recovery of the lung after surgery.

A recent paper combining patients from Ancona and Mayo Clinic has shown that the differential pressure (difference between minimum pressure and maximum pressure) calculated from measurements taken during the 6th postoperative hours following lobectomy was associated with the duration of air leak and the risk of a prolonged air leak.[11]

Patients with an air flow greater than 50 mL/min and a differential pressure greater than 10 cmH_2O have a risk of PAL > 72 hours as high as 52%.

This work may have clinical implications by modifying the differential pressure (narrowing the 'swing' between maximum and minimum pressure) there may be the possibility to influence the duration of air leak.

These findings were derived from data recorded by using the Digivent system, which is no longer available in the market. That system featured separate flow and pressure sensors located at the canister level, which allowed for influence by external factors such as siphoning effects and positioning of the patient.

New systems, like the Thopaz (Medela Healthcare, Switzerland), provide more sophisticated data and clinical results. They feature a pressure sensor that measure the intrapleural pressure at the chest and contain an intelligent algorithm that controls the pump, meaning they are capable of reacting to the feedback coming from the sensor. The air flow is accurately measured (with less than 1% error rate) by the activity of the pump to maintain a preset level of pressure. In a sealed environment and in the case of no air leak, the pump function ceases to work once the preset negative pressure is reached, turning these systems into no suction devices. In the absence of air leak, Thopaz will simply observe and record the pressure driven by the patient.

One of the greatest potential advantages of regulated suction devices (i.e. Thopaz) is the capability to maintain stable the pressure even in case of air leak with a minimal variability in the range of 0.1 cmH_2O (**Figure 30.1**). Furthermore, when the preset pressure is at or below −8 cmH_2O and there is no air leak the device works passively, as a one-way valve, only monitoring and recording the pleural pressure driven by the patient themselves (**Figure 30.2**).

What you set in the device is what you get inside the pleural space. In contrast to a traditional chest drainage system, the oscillations around the preset value are minimal, a fact that can contribute to reduce the duration of air leak, according to the above mentioned paper.[11]

The introduction of these types of novel electronic chest drainage systems in the clinical practice has been shown to be effective and safe. In a previous investigation, Pompili et al. used propensity score case-matched analysis to compare the first consecutive 51 lobectomy patients managed with Thopaz with 51 counterparts managed with a traditional device.[12]

Patients managed with Thopaz had approximately a 2-day shorter chest tube duration and 1.5 days' shorter hospital stay, with a consequent saving of approximately 750 euro per patient.

From the start, compared to patients managed with a traditional system, those connected to the Thopaz had a consistently shorter chest tube duration. The 'learning curve' sloped down for the first 40 patients before reaching a plateau, when the maximum benefit of the electronic device was evident.

Modern chest drain devices, which are able to apply regulated suction to maintain the preset intrapleural pressure, represent the ideal instruments to reliably assess the effect of different levels of negative pressures on the duration of air leak. They may overcome the main limitation of previous trials using traditional devices by continuously monitoring the real intra-pleural pressure and relative air flows.

A recent trial compared the effect of different levels of pleural pressure on the duration of air leak under controlled conditions by using a regulated chest drainage system (Thopaz).[13]

One hundred patients submitted to pulmonary lobectomy were randomized to receive two different types of chest drainage management: Group 1, regulated individualized suction mode, with different pressure levels depending on the type of lobectomy and ranging from −11 cmH_2O to −20 cmH_2O based on a previous investigation,[7] group 2, regulated seal mode (−2 cmH_2O). At this low level of suction,

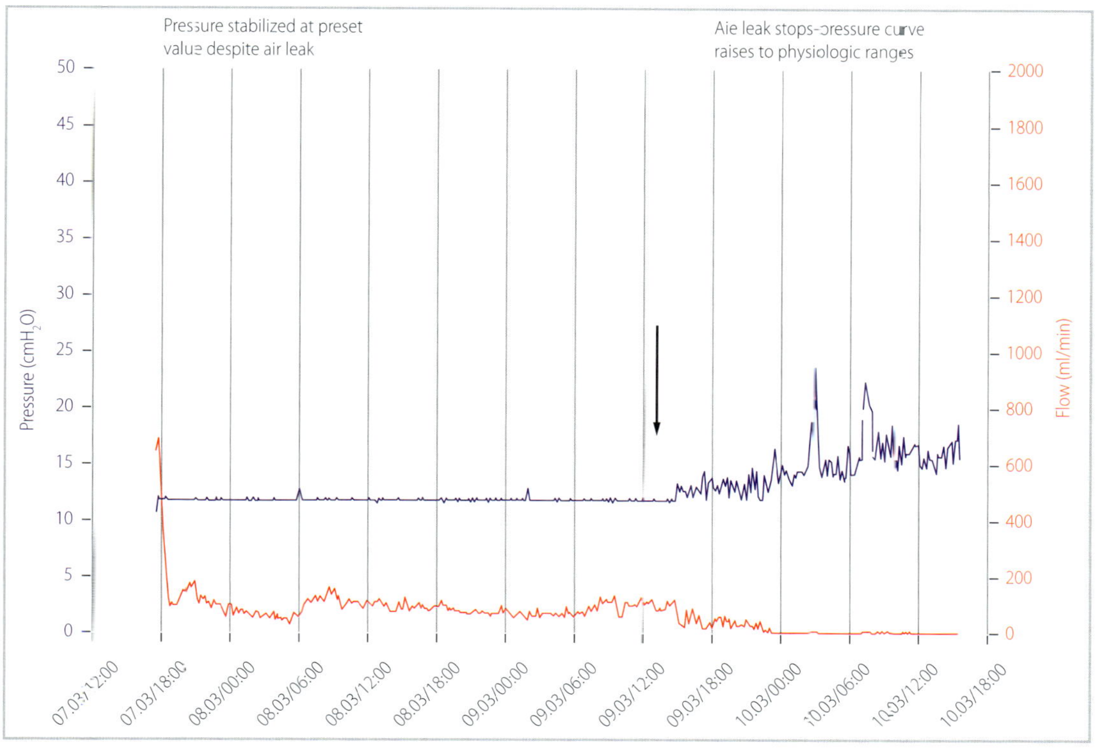

Figure 30.1 Air-flow-pleural pressure graph downloaded from a regulated-pressure chest drainage system in a patient submitted to pulmonary lobectomy. The red line represents airflow and the blue line the pleural pressure recorded at the chest. In this patient there was a period of air leak lasting approximately 48 hours. The device worked to maintain the pleural pressure stable at the preset value (−12 cmH_2O) without oscillations in spite of the airflow. Once the airflow stopped, the patient stabilized his own pleural pressure within physiological values. The device simply observed without exerting any suction.

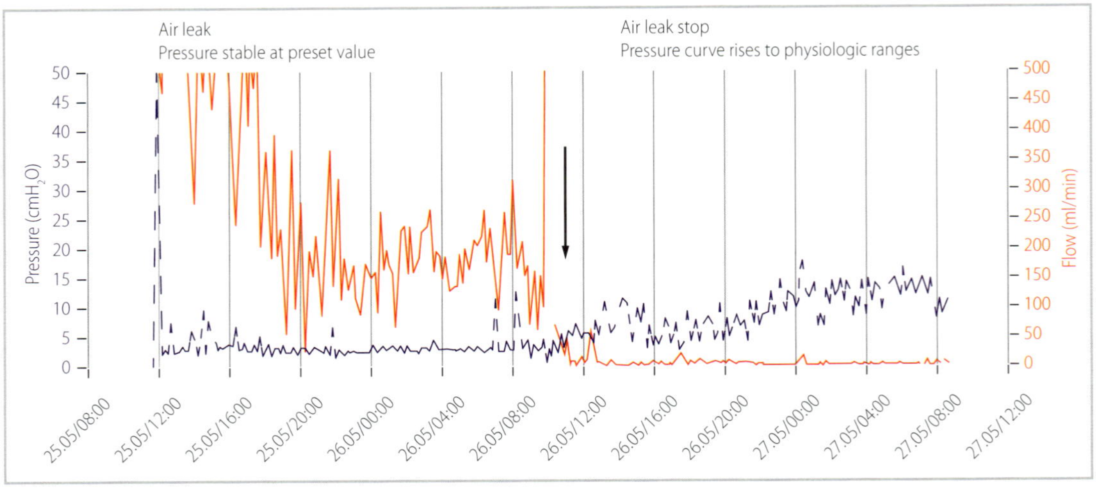

Figure 30.2 Air-flow-pleural pressure graph downloaded from a regulated-pressure chest drainage system (Thopaz) in a patient submitted to pulmonary lobectomy. The red line represents airflow and the blue line the pleural pressure recorded at the chest. There was an initial period of few hours with some air leak and in which the pleural pressure was maintained stable at -2 cmH_2O (which was the preset value in this case). Once the airflow stopped, the patient stabilized his own pleural pressure within physiological values. The device simply observed without exerting any suction.

the system works only to compensate the occurrence of values more positive than -2 cmH_2O in case of air leak. Otherwise, it works passively as a regulated, no suction device. We found that the average air leak duration and the number of patients with prolonged air leak were similar between the groups, showing that regulated seal is as effective and safe as regulated suction in managing chest tubes following lobectomy. Although this experience can be refined by the application of different levels of suction or different endpoints, it will contribute to set the basis for future investigation on active pleural management based on regulated pleural pressure.

The objective new advantages achieved with the use of an electronic device, have been linked to more subjective endpoints by an international randomized trial comparing digital versus traditional drainage devices in terms of chest tube removal and patient satisfaction.[14] The authors demonstrated that patients managed with digital devices had a 1-day shorter duration of chest tube placement and hospital stay compared with those managed with a traditional device. Furthermore, despite cultural differences (patients from Europe, USA and Asia were included in the trial), they found that patients managed with the electronic device had a more positive perception of the chest drainage system, in particular related to its comfort, portability, and convenience for personnel and patients compared with those managed with the traditional device. These results, have confirmed previous small trials which were assessing the subjective preferences by patients of the electronic devices favoring early mobilization.[15]

CONCLUSION

Several papers have tried to address the issue of the best chest tube management after thoracic surgery. There is no absolute answer to this problem. The first step to help surgeons has been in standardizing the current terminology with the efforts of the ESTS, AATS, STS and GTSC. The other support came from industry, with the development of new devices capable to transform measurement of air leak from a subjective interpretation to an objective and recordable observation. These devices will enable new trials and studies to help define proper guidelines for the management of chest tubes following thoracic surgery.

REFERENCES

1. Irshad K, Feldman LS, Chu VF, et al. Causes of increased length of hospitalization on a general thoracic surgery service: a prospective observational study. Can J Surg 2002; 45:264–268.
2. Varela G, Jiménez MF, Novoa N, Aranda JL. Estimating hospital costs attributable to prolonged air leak in pulmonary lobectomy. Eur J Cardiothorac Surg 2005; 27:329–333.
3. Brunelli A, Xiume F, Al Refai M, et al. Air leaks after lobectomy increase the risk of empyema but not of cardiopulmonary complications: a case-matched analysis. Chest 2006; 130:1150–1156.
4. Brunelli A, Cassivi SD, Halgren L. Risk factors for prolonged air leak after pulmonary resection. Thorac Surg Clin 2010; 20:359–364.
5. Brunelli A, Varela G, Refai M, et al. A scoring system to predict the risk of prolonged air leak after lobectomy. Ann Thorac Surg 2010; 90:204–209.
6. Brunelli A, Beretta E, Cassivi SD, et al. Consensus definitions to promote an evidence-based approach to management of the pleural space. A collaborative proposal by ESTS, AATS, STS, and GTSC. Eur J Cardiothorac Surg 2011; 40:291–297.
7. Refai M, Brunelli A, Varela G. The values of intrapleural pressure before the removal of chest tube in non-complicated pulmonary lobectomies. Eur J Cardiothorac Surg 2012; 41:831–833.
8. Varela G, Jiménez MF, Novoa NM, Aranda JL. Postoperative chest tube management: measuring air leak using an electronic device decreases variability in the clinical practice. Eur J Cardiothorac Surg 2009; 35:28–31.
9. Cerfolio RJ, Bryant AS. The benefits of continuous and digital air leak assessment after elective pulmonary resection: a prospective study. Ann Thorac Surg 2008; 86:396–401.
10. Brunelli A, Salati M, Refai M, et al. Evaluation of a new chest tube removal protocol using digital air leak monitoring after lobectomy: a prospective randomised trial. Eur J Cardiothorac Surg 2010; 37:56–60.
11. Brunelli A, Cassivi SD, Salati M, et al. Digital measurements of air leak flow and intrapleural pressures in the immediate postoperative period predict risk of prolonged air leak after pulmonary lobectomy. Eur J Cardiothorac Surg 2011; 39:584–588.
12. Pompili C, Brunelli A, Salati M, Refai M, Sabbatini A. Impact of the learning curve in the use of a novel electronic chest drainage system after pulmonary lobectomy: a case-matched analysis on the duration of chest tube usage. Interact Cardiovasc Thorac Surg 2011; 13:490–493
13. Brunelli A, Salati M, Pompili C, Refai M, Sabbatini A. Regulated tailored suction vs regulated seal: a prospective randomized trial on air leak duration. Eur J Cardiothorac Surg 2013; 43:899–904.
14. Pompili C, Detterbeck F, Papagiannopoulos K, et al. Multicenter international randomized comparison of objective and subjective outcomes between electronic and traditional chest drainage systems. Ann Thorac Surg 2014; 98:490–496.
15. Rathinam S, Bradley A, Cantlin T, Rajesh PB. Thopaz Portable suction systems in thoracic surgery: an end user assessment and feedback in a tertiary unit. J Cardiothorac Surg 2011; 6:59.

Chapter 31 Pleuroscopy

Sumit Chatterji, Pasupathy Sivasothy

INTRODUCTION

Pleuroscopy (also called thoracoscopy) is a procedure whereby an endoscope, either rigid or semirigid, is inserted through an incision in an intercostal space into a pneumothorax created in the pleural cavity. It enables direct inspection of the pleura and lungs, and biopsies or therapeutic interventions can be performed. The procedure can be performed under conscious sedation and local anesthetic, or general anesthesia.

BACKGROUND

In the early 20th century, Hans-Christian Jacobaeus, a Swedish internist and widely considered the founder of thoracoscopy, introduced the technique together with laparoscopy.[1] He used the procedure for the diagnosis of tuberculous pleural effusions and defined three requirements that remain fundamental: (1) The introduction of a trocar safely into the pleural cavity without damaging internal organs or causing too much pain, (2) Introduction of air into the pleural space to create a pneumothorax and (3) an endoscope of dimensions small enough to be introduced through the trocar. By 1913, he had used the technique for therapeutic purposes in patients with pulmonary tuberculosis who had developed adhesions between visceral and parietal pleura that prevented the artificial pneumothorax lung collapse therapy used in the pre-antibiotic era. By using endoscopic cauterization these adhesions could be lysed and the lung collapsed. With the advent of antibiotic therapy for tuberculosis in the 1950s, the therapeutic use of thoracoscopy in this setting subsided, but, with the development of better endoscopic illumination techniques, optics and video-processing technologies, the procedure has become increasingly popular for the diagnosis and treatment of a variety of pleural and pulmonary disorders. Medical thoracoscopy (MT) is typically performed by interventional pulmonologists or respiratory physicians and video-assisted thoracoscopic surgery (VATS) by thoracic surgeons, with a wider range of treatment options. MT is now typically offered in North American interventional pulmonology training programs and is incorporated in various guidelines for the investigation of unilateral exudative pleural effusions and for the management of malignant pleural effusions.[2]

MEDICAL VERSUS SURGICAL THORACOSCOPY

The two techniques differ in methodology, equipment used and are performed by different practitioners. In general, surgical thoracoscopy is performed under general anesthesia and MT under sedation with local anesthesia. However, some practitioners prefer performing MT under general anesthesia and VATS has been described with sedation and local anesthesia.[3] For MT, either a single-port or dual port technique can be used – one port for the examination scope and the other for accessory instruments. In VATS, typically three ports are used, though this can vary. An overview of indications for MT versus VATS is provided in **Table 31.1**.

Table 31.1 General indications for medical thoracoscopy (MT) versus video-assisted thoracoscopic surgery (VATS)

Medical thoracoscopy	Video-assisted thoracoscopic surgery
Pleural effusions of unknown etiology	Pneumonectomy/lobectomy
Draining pleural effusions	Lung biopsy
Diagnosis of pleural disease (diffuse or localized)	Decortication
Talc pleurodesis	Pleurectomy/bullectomy (pneumothorax)
Drainage of empyema (stage 1/2)	Drainage/decortication of empyema (stage 3)
Drainage of early hemothorax	Lung volume reduction
	Resection of masses, cysts
	Esophagectomy
	Fundoplication
	Sympathectomy
	Thoracic duct ligation
	Pericardial window

EQUIPMENT AND PERSONNEL

An example of equipment needed for MT is given in **Figure 31.1**. The usual diameter of the rigid thoracoscope is 4–9 mm, and that of the semirigid pleuroscope 7 mm. Rigid thoracoscopes with 0°, 30°, 45° and 50° fields of view are available (**Figure 31.2**). The wider views are used for initial inspection of the thoracic cavity, with the 0° scope used for closer inspection and in combination with instruments for biopsies (**Figure 31.3**). The trocar, comprising a blunt conical, or sharp-tipped obturator and cannula can vary in size from 5–10 mm. Trocars with diameter greater than 10 mm are generally more painful for the patient and can be harder to manipulate between the ribs. The cannula allows air to enter and leave the pleural space freely but typically a detachable rubber stopper and often a closable side port allow conversion to an airtight seal. For electrocautery, trocars with insulated tips and interiors should be used.

A semi-rigid pleuroscope (**Figure 31.4**; LTF 260 pleuroscope, Olympus Medical Systems, Tokyo, Japan) is available as an alternative and often appeals to respiratory physicians, due to similarity in appearance and technique with bronchoscopes. Other advantages include autoclavability and compatibility with existing processors and light sources used for bronchoscopy by the same manufacturer, thereby saving equipment costs. Typically, the flexible distal end can angulate 160° up and 130° down and has a 2.8-mm working channel to permit access for biopsy forceps, needles and other accessories.

The set of equipment is completed with an oxygen supply, continuous monitoring devices (pulse oximetry, heart rate, blood pressure), large sterile drapes to cover the area of intervention, local anesthetic

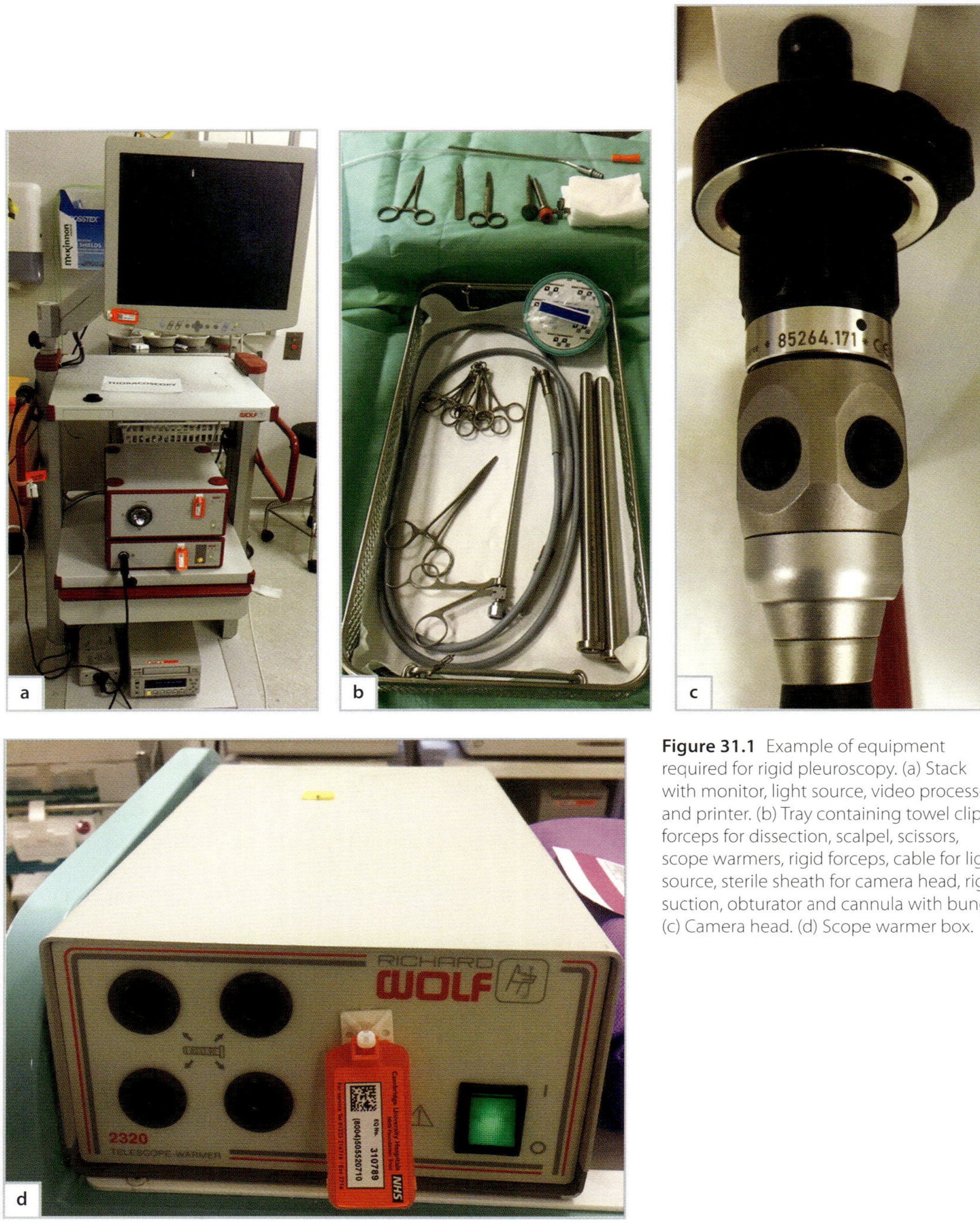

Figure 31.1 Example of equipment required for rigid pleuroscopy. (a) Stack with monitor, light source, video processor and printer. (b) Tray containing towel clips, forceps for dissection, scalpel, scissors, scope warmers, rigid forceps, cable for light source, sterile sheath for camera head, rigid suction, obturator and cannula with bung. (c) Camera head. (d) Scope warmer box.

(often with adrenaline to reduce bleeding), sutures, a talc insufflation kit, chest drains (minimum 20F size), underwater drainage sets to accommodate potentially large volumes of pleural fluid and for evacuation of the pneumothorax post-procedure.

The location for the procedure should allow the operator to perform under strict sterile conditions, with sufficient room for the patient trolley, video equipment, light source, monitoring devices and other equipment trolleys. A resuscitation kit and cardiac defibrillator should be available in case needed.

Personnel typically required for the safe performance of MT include the primary operator and a scrubbed assistant, nursing staff to monitor the patient's vital signs, comfort and sedation and to open or provide equipment. It is also useful to have another assistant, usually called a runner, to be on hand to obtain things out of the immediate environment if needed.

All procedures need to be recorded accurately and samples sent for a variety of tests, so information technology systems including radiology viewing need to be in the immediate vicinity.

PERFORMING THE PROCEDURE

Preprocedure evaluation

All patients being considered for MT should have a thorough history and clinical examination to determine important comorbidities, performance status, ventilatory status, ability to lie flat and contra-

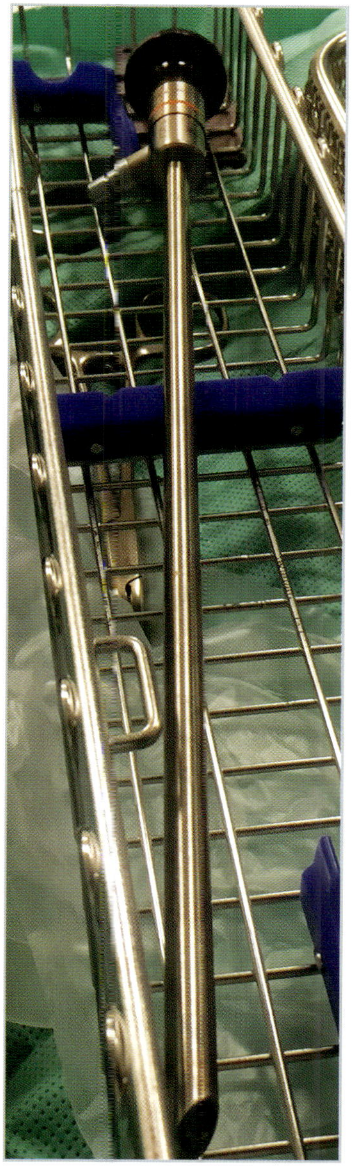

Figure 31.2 Rigid 7 mm 50°oblique viewing scope. Once attached to the camera head it can be used for the initial inspection of the pleural cavity.

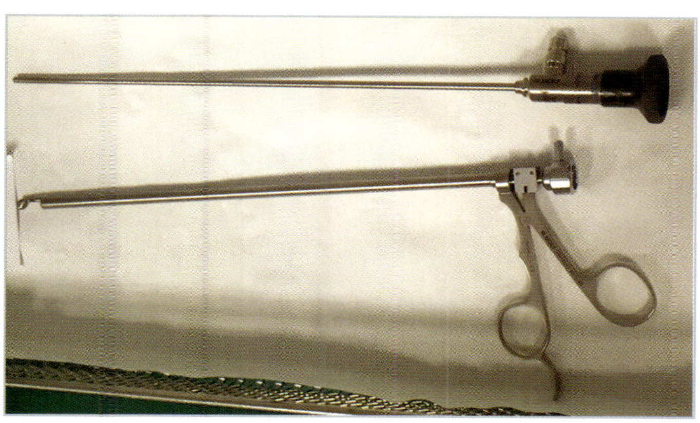

Figure 31.3 Rigid biopsy forceps and 4 mm 0° rigid scope. The scope is inserted into the rigid forceps and secured with a locking mechanism at the proximal end.

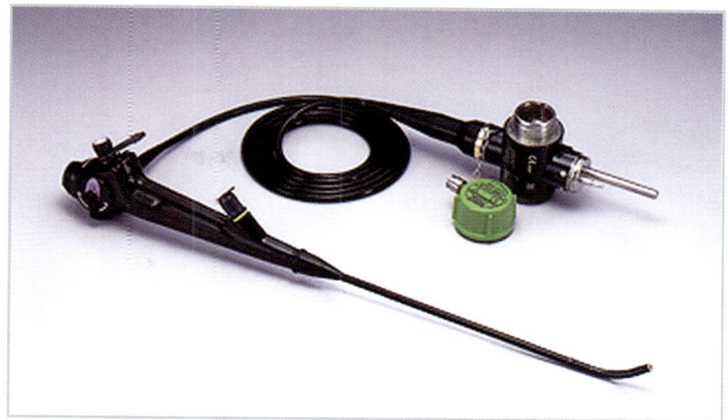

Figure 31.4 LTF 260 pleuroscope, Olympus Medical Systems, Tokyo, Japan. Semi-rigid pleuroscope with a working channel to permit instrumentation.

indications or considerations for the procedure. Pleural and pulmonary pathology will be visualized with chest radiography and often computed tomography (CT) as part of the workup. The authors also perform a pre-procedure thoracic ultrasound assessment of the patient in the thoracoscopy position to ensure adequate pleural fluid volume, measure skin-pleura depth, presence of adhesions or septations and assess patient comfort.

Standard blood screening includes a full blood count and coagulation screen. Depending on comorbidities, additional testing including serum electrolytes, glucose, electrocardiogram, blood gas analysis, or spirometry may be required.

All patients should provide informed written consent on the day of the procedure. Antibiotic prophylaxis is not indicated as the risk of bacteremia is considered low, unless the pleural space is known or thought to be infected, in which case antibiotic therapy is appropriate, especially in individuals at risk of endocarditis.[4]

Anesthesia

Medical thoracoscopy can be performed under local, regional or general anesthesia. Typically, rapid-acting sedatives administered intravenously (e.g. midazolam or propofol) are combined with analgesics (e.g., morphine, fentanyl) and local anaesthesia (e.g. lidocaine 0.5–2% with or without adrenaline) to skin and subcutaneous tissues to achieve patient comfort. Particularly painful steps in the MT procedure include infiltration of local anesthesia and breaching the parietal pleura, levering the cannula on the ribs during endoscope examination, removal of adhesions by coagulation, biopsies of the parietal pleura and the minutes after talc insufflation. Younger patients and those with macroscopically normal pleura tend to be more sensitive to pain and the analgesic medications need to be titrated according to patient response during the procedure.

One must be aware of the potentiating effects of benzodiazepine and opiate combinations, increasing the likelihood of respiratory depression, hypoxemia and cardiac arrest in elderly patients and those with chronic cardiac, hepatic or renal failure. Doses should be adjusted accordingly and specific antagonists of opioids (e.g. naloxone) and benzodiazepines (e.g. flumazenil) should be available if needed.

Patient positioning

The thoracoscopist typically faces the patient during the procedure. The procedure is performed with the patient in the lateral decubitus position with the healthy side down. The patient can be asked to place palm-to-palm with their arms raised up and a pillow can be positioned under the chest – both procedures to increase separation of the ribs to permit easier access to the pleural space. Alternatively, the uppermost arm can be raised above the head and placed in a sling. The couch height should be adjusted for operator comfort and the assistants positioned in their respective positions around the patient. The monitor and stack face the operator from the other side of the patient. Following this, the point of entry is determined by imaging, the presence of pleuropulmonary adhesions and location of fluid on thoracic ultrasound. The chest is then prepared and draped as for thoracotomy.

Creating a pneumothorax

A requirement for MT is the induction of a pneumothorax to allow introduction of the trocar without risk to underlying lung. In the case of a large pneumothorax or pleural effusion, after confirmation of air/fluid with the anesthetic needle, a tract can be dissected between the ribs and the trocar inserted with a gentle twisting and pushing motion till a sudden lack of resistance indicates entry to the pleural space. The obturator is then removed and atmospheric air allowed to freely enter the pleural space via the cannula. Suctioning of pleural effusion is performed to remove fluid, whilst allowing this volume to be replaced with air, thereby preventing rapid lung re-expansion.

With smaller pleural effusions, thoracic ultrasound can either allow insertion under direct guidance of a cannula into the pleural space allowing insufflation of air, or specific needles such as a Boutin needle can be used for the same purpose. If the volume of fluid is too small even for these techniques, or if adhesions prevent induction of pneumothorax, careful blunt dissection to the pleural space with a finger sweep to break adhesions can achieve the same result.

Some operators prefer to induce a pneumothorax with a cannula in the pleural space prior to the procedure. This has the advantage of allowing radiological evaluation using either standard posteroanterior chest radiography or lateral decubitus imaging, to confirm an adequate pneumothorax and exclude adhesions which may hamper pleural entry.

Access to the pleural space

An anterolateral approach via the 5th or 6th intercostal space in the mid-axillary line is commonly chosen as it permits good inspection of all lobes of the lung. If MT is being performed for pneumothorax, a higher point of entry in the 3rd or 4rth intercostal space may be chosen to allow better inspection of the lung apex. Conversely, if a metastatic pleural effusion is suspected, the point of entry is typically basal where most pleural metastases tend to be found.[5] Ultrasound immediately preceding pleural access is invaluable in locating a safe point of entry.

For a single-port technique, the cannula serves as the entry point for suction and optical biopsy forceps which typically suffices in simple effusions with diagnostic pleural sampling. In cases where adhesiolysis, coagulation or extended pleural/lung sampling are required, a dual-port technique is preferred. Here, two incisions are made in separate intercostal spaces allowing the insertion of cannulas for separate scope and instrument access. The operator then coordinates the movement of scope and instrument together to achieve fully visualized interventions.

Inspection

A methodical approach is required when inspecting the thoracic cavity so that landmarks can be identified and the location and extent of pathology determined, typically with a view to a subsequent sampling procedure. With rigid scopes, a variety of oblique viewing systems are available, allowing the scope to be inserted and rotated like a periscope to achieve good overall views. With semi-rigid thoracoscopy, the tip can be flexed with a thumb lever to achieve a range of viewing angles.

Typically, the endoscope is advanced toward the posterior thorax and then directed toward the costophrenic recess and diaphragm first. Using a rotational and sweeping movement, the parietal pleura, diaphragm, lung surface and mediastinal structures are visualized in turn. The scope can be advanced toward the lung apex for extended inspection. On the left, the oblique fissure can be used for orientation and on the right, the intersection of oblique and horizontal fissures denotes the position where all three lobes meet. The diaphragm can be recognized typically by its movement with respiration, the heart by its transmitted pulsations, great vessels by side (aorta and subclavian vessels on the left; vena cava, innominate vein and subclavian artery on the right) and ribs, intercostal vessels and fat by typical appearances. The normal lung surface has a pink sheen with reticulations, often with some anthracotic pigmentation. Atelectactic changes are purplish-red with well demarcated edges. Bullae/blebs are easily recognized and protrude from the lung surface. Nodules on the pleural surfaces or from the substance of the lung are obvious and imply pathology – typically malignancy. Pleural changes, including diffuse thickening, erythema and an amorphous appearance can represent benign or malignant pleural processes and require multiple sampling sites.

Pleural sampling

The appearance of the pleural surface at thoracoscopy can vary enormously from normal appearances on one hand to gross nodularity on the other. The preceding imaging investigations can indicate the likely findings, with ultrasound typically more sensitive than CT for detecting parietal and hemidiaphragm pleural nodularity and pleural space septations. The most common malignancies that metastasize to the pleura are lung and breast, accounting for two-thirds of malignant pleural effusions.[6] Malignant mesothelioma is increasingly common, with a peak incidence expected within the next 5 years in the United Kingdom (Cancer Research UK, 2016). Thoracoscopic appearances do not differentiate between the various primary tumors, but share common macroscopic appearances which should make the operator suspicious of malignancy. These include pleural nodules or masses (37%), pleural thickening (26%), a combination of both (21%). Lymphangitis and non-specific erythema is also commonly observed. Areas of abnormality can be biopsied directly with rigid biopsy forceps, or with flexible forceps introduced through the working channel of a semi-rigid scope. Typically 2 to 6 biopsies of a suspicious lesion will establish a diagnosis (**Figure 31.5**). Sufficient material should be obtained if hormone receptor studies or genetic mutational analysis is anticipated. In malignant mesothelioma, which can be a patchy process with areas of normal appearing mucosa infiltrated with tumor and other areas of erythematous, thickened pleura with non-specific inflammatory or fibrotic infiltrate, 10 to 12 biopsies of multiple areas are required to achieve reasonable diagnostic sensitivity.

In tuberculosis, where diagnostic sensitivity approaches 100% with pleural biopsies, samples should be sent in saline for acid fast bacilli staining and culture.

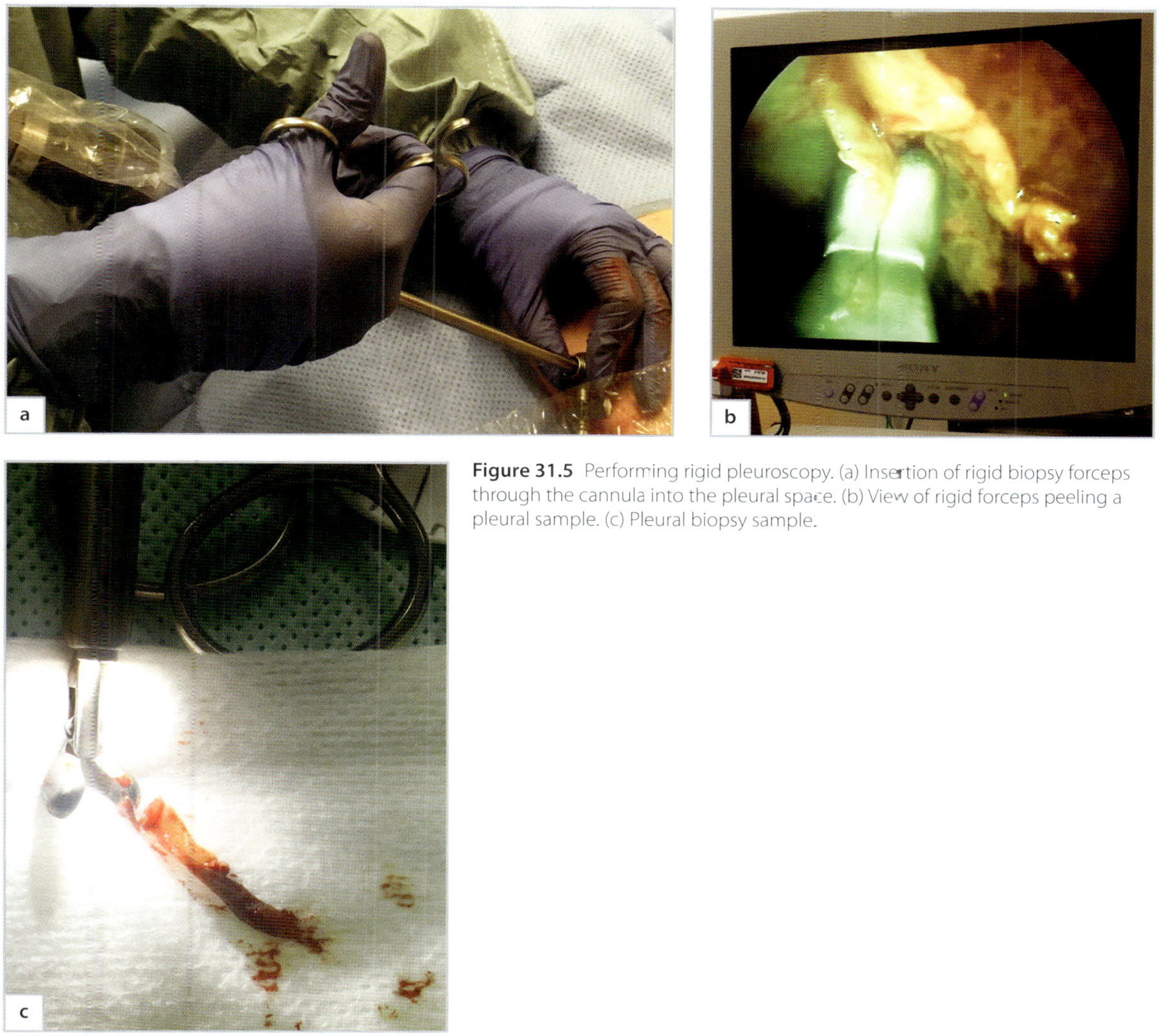

Figure 31.5 Performing rigid pleuroscopy. (a) Insertion of rigid biopsy forceps through the cannula into the pleural space. (b) View of rigid forceps peeling a pleural sample. (c) Pleural biopsy sample.

Talc insufflation

Talc insufflation at MT is an effective way of achieving pleural symphysis[7] and a current prospective randomized trial is evaluating its efficacy compared to talc slurry administered via intercostal drain for malignant pleural effusions (TAPPS trial, 2014).[8] Typically 4–8 g sterile, graded talc is insufflated after complete pleural fluid drainage, with the catheter directed at all surfaces to ensure a widespread coating. To encourage pleural apposition, pleural suction is often administered via the intercostal drain after the procedure at 10–20 cmH_20, till the daily fluid output is less than 200 mL and radiologically the lung is fully inflated with no residual fluid.

Chest tube

At the end of every procedure an intercostal drain is inserted to drain the residual pneumothorax and to ensure there is no persisting air leak or bleeding. After talc instillation, the drain allows the talc and fluid to drain as the pleural surfaces unite. Some centers performing day-case MT remove the chest drain a few hours after the procedure after radiological confirmation of lung re-expansion, thus allowing the patient home later in the day. Drain sizes used in MT typically range from 20–36F with larger drains preferred for hemothorax or significant air leak.

Documentation

A systematic and detailed written or electronic record of the procedure is essential as it forms part of the patient's permanent medical history and is a tool to communicate findings to other specialists involved in their care. Documentation should include details about the pre-procedural radiological findings, procedural steps including macroscopic appearance, fluid volume drained, location and number of biopsies taken and the tests requested. Administration of medications and talc should also be recorded, along with any complications and the postprocedure care should be listed. Video recordings, or static images should be saved if possible and ultrasound examinations (where indicated) should be uploaded to local image archiving systems.

POTENTIAL COMPLICATIONS

Medical thoracoscopy is a safe and effective method for the diagnosis and treatment of a variety of pleuropulmonary diseases with an overall complication rate reported in one meta-analysis of 10.2% in 2566 cases.[9] Mortality is extremely rare with a reported incidence of 0.01%. A list of possible complications is detailed in **Table 31.2**.

In general, complications can be avoided or mitigated by adherence to standard operating protocols which include: careful selection of patients, well-trained staff working with familiar equipment in a suitable environment, patient preparation for the procedure, bedside imaging to determine a safe trocar insertion site, continuous patient monitoring and adequate oxygenation, safe operative technique, then good post-operative care including analgesia, pleural suction and chest drain management protocols. All practicing MT units should have a bleed management protocol and regular staff training to deal with the issues that may be encountered perioperatively.

Table 31.2 Potential complications of medical thoracoscopy (MT) before, during and after the procedure

Preprocedure	During the procedure	Postprocedure
Hypersensitivity to local anesthetic or other medication Over-sedation with hypnotic and/or opiates	Pain Hypoxemia Over-sedation and hypoventilation Hypotension Hemorrhage Injury to diaphragm, intrathoracic or sub-diaphragmatic organs Cardiac arrhythmias	Pain Postoperative fever Empyema Wound infection Re-expansion pulmonary edema Subcutaneous emphysema Prolonged air leak Persisting pneumothorax Drain displacement Talc-related side effects including pain and respiratory distress syndrome Seeding of tract and chest wall with tumor cells

CONCLUSION

The principles of MT have not changed in over a century, but technical advances and improvements in operative monitoring, sedation and postoperative care mean this technique is simple, safe and effective for diagnosing and managing a range of benign and malignant pleuropulmonary diseases. Attractive features include the ability to perform the procedure under local anesthesia and 'conscious sedation' often meaning patients can be discharged home the same day, with high diagnostic sensitivity and low complication rates. For this reason, as well as its incorporation in diagnostic algorithms for the investigation and/or management of undiagnosed and malignant pleural effusions, its use is increasingly prevalent and likely to increase into the 21st century.

REFERENCES

1. Jacobeus HC, Uber die Moglichkeit, die Zystoskopie bet Untersuchung seriöser Höhlungen anzuwenden [About the possibility of using the cystoscope for examining hollow cavities]. Munch Med Wschr 1910; 57:2090–2092.
2. Hooper C, Lee GYC, Maskell N, et al. Investigation of unilateral pleural effusions in adult patients: British Thoracic Society pleural disease guidelines. Thorax 2010; 65:ii4–17.
3. Pompeo E. Nonintubated video-assisted thoracic surgery under epidural anesthesia—Encouraging early results encourage randomized trials. Chinese Journal of Cancer Research 2014; 26:364–367.
4. Bratzler DW, Houck PM. Antimicrobial prophylaxis for surgery: an advisory statement from the National Surgical Infection Prevention Project. Am J Surg 2005; 189:395–404.
5. Sureka B, Thukral BB, Mittal MK, et al. Radiological review of pleural tumors. The Indian J Radiol Imaging 2013; 23:313–320.
6. Laisaar T, Palmiste V, Vooder T, et al. Life expectancy of patients with malignant pleural effusion treated with video-assisted thoracoscopic talc pleurodesis. Interact Cardiovasc Thorac Surg 2006; 5:307–310.
7. Kolschmann S, Ballin A, Gillissen A. Clinical efficacy and safety of thoracoscopic talc pleurodesis in malignant pleural effusions. Chest 2005; 128:1431–1435.
8. Bhatnager R, Laskawiec-Szkonter M, Piotrowska H, et al. Evaluating the efficacy of thoracoscopy and talc poudrage versus pleurodesis using talc slurry (TAPPS trial): protocol of an open-label randomised controlled trial. BMJ Open 2014; 4:e007045.
9. Villanueva AG, Beamis JF. Medical thoracoscopy. Diagnosis of pleural pulmonary disorders. In: Beamis J F, Mathur PN, Mehta AC, (Eds). Interventional Pulmonary Medicine. Lung Biology in Health and Disease. New York, Marcel Dekker 2004:431–449.

Index

Note: Page numbers in **bold** or *italic* refer to tables or figures respectively.